Spreading Germs

Spreading Germs discusses how modern ideas on the bacterial causes of communicable diseases were constructed and spread within the British medical profession in the last third of the nineteenth century. Michael Worboys revises many existing interpretations of this pivotal moment in modern medicine. He shows that there were many germ theories of disease, and that these were developed and used in different ways across veterinary medicine, surgery, public health and general medicine. A central theme is the importance of the metaphor of 'seed and soil' in medical discussions of germs and their effects, and in the management of infections in individuals or populations. Professor Worboys shows that British doctors gave the same attention to the receptivity of the human body or 'soil' as to the nature of the germs or 'seeds' of disease. Thus, the growth of bacteriology is considered in relation to the evolution of medical practice, rather than as a separate science of germs. Professor Worboys also demonstrates that, while they incorporated many ideas and practices from the stronger institutions of medical science in France and Germany, British germ theorists and their medical followers had their own research programmes, germ 'discoveries' and innovations. The best known of these technical changes, Joseph Lister's antiseptic surgery, is shown to be just one of many germ-related preventive, diagnostic and therapeutic methods that were used to transform many features of medical practice.

T0297755

Cambridge History of Medicine

Edited by

CHARLES ROSENBERG, Professor of History and Sociology of Science, University of Pennsylvania and COLIN JONES, University of Warwick

Other titles in the series:

Continued on page following the index

Spreading Germs

Disease Theories and Medical Practice in Britain,
1865–1900

MICHAEL WORBOYS

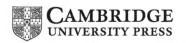 CAMBRIDGE
UNIVERSITY PRESS

CAMBRIDGE UNIVERSITY PRESS
Cambridge, New York, Melbourne, Madrid, Cape Town, Singapore, São Paulo

Cambridge University Press
The Edinburgh Building, Cambridge CB2 2RU, UK

Published in the United States of America by Cambridge University Press, New York

www.cambridge.org
Information on this title: www.cambridge.org/9780521773027

First published 2000
This digitally printed first paperback version 2006

A catalogue record for this publication is available from the British Library

Library of Congress Cataloguing in Publication data

Worboys, Michael, 1948–
     Spreading germs: diseases, theories, and medical practice in Britain,
1865–1900 / Michael Worboys.
          p.   cm. – (Cambridge studies in the history of medicine)
     Includes bibliographical references and index.
     ISBN 0-521-77302-4 hardback
     1. Public health – Great Britain – History – 19th century.   2. Social
medicine – Great Britain – History – 19th century.   3. Diseases –
Causes and theories of causation – Great Britain – History –
19th century.   4. Medicine – Great Britain – History – 19th century.
I. Title.   II. Series.

RA427. W68 2000
610´.941´09034 – dc21   00–023501

ISBN-13 978-0-521-77302-7 hardback
ISBN-10 0-521-77302-4 hardback

ISBN-13 978-0-521-03447-0 paperback
ISBN-10 0-521-03447-7 paperback

To my late parents
Ben Worboys
and
Joy Worboys (née Loveday)

CONTENTS

ILLUSTRATIONS

ABBREVIATIONS

AAMR	Association for the Advancement of Medical Research
BAAS	British Association for the Advancement of Science
BIPM	British Institute of Preventive Medicine
BMJ	*British Medical Journal*
CRA	Clinical Research Association
LGB	Local Government Board
MAB	Metropolitan Asylums Board
MOH	Medical Officer of Health
MOsH	Medical Officers of Health
NAPC	National Association for the Prevention of Consumption
NVE	National Vaccine Establishment
RCVS	Royal College of Veterinary Surgeons
RAMC	Royal Army Medical Corps
RASE	Royal Agricultural Society
RVC	Royal Veterinary College
UCL	University College London

PREFACE

I have had it in mind to write a book on germ theories of disease for more than twenty years. I first had the idea when I tried to place my early work on tropical medicine and parasitology in the wider context of the development of microbiology and new theories of disease, and found the literature on such an important topic to be very scant. Little had changed over a decade later when I began work on the project. I was awarded a Research Leave Grant by the Wellcome Trust for 1988–89 that enabled me to spend a very fruitful year at the Wellcome Unit of the History of Medicine at the University of Manchester. My intention then was to write a history of laboratory medicine and bacteriology in the late Victorian period, but I soon ran up against the problem that there were in fact very few bacteriological laboratories, as such, and that bacteriology as an institution was a relatively late developer in Britain. My task was made more difficult still by the dearth of substantial primary sources for the main institutions and leading figures, apart from Joseph Lister. My reading of published and unpublished sources on the topic soon convinced me that the most important issues in British medicine after 1865 were the debates and development of theories of disease and new disease management practices. Laboratories were not unimportant, though far more significant were the negotiations about the meanings and standing of germ theories of disease in the fields of clinical and preventive medicine.

Also, much 'laboratory' work took place in the field, in operating theatres, clinics and when managing infectious diseases. I have worked mainly from published sources. This was both from choice and circumstances. Given that I am mainly interested in the negotiations over the constructions, meanings and uses of germ theories and practices, professional discourses of knowledge in-the-making were a necessary focus, especially for such a wide-ranging topic. As mentioned above, primary material for the leading germ theorists was scarce, and in the papers of doctors not centrally involved in the topic, mentions of germs were scattered. This is a significant finding on its own account, but it is not one that will support a monograph. That said, I have used primary material as appropriate, but mostly I have read as widely as possible in the provincial and specialist literature, as well as the different editions of texts and the many shades of opinion expressed on topics in the national journals. As the volume shows, there was no shortage of work on germs, their nature, their transmission, their effects and the body's reactions to them.

In the protracted process of researching and writing this book I have received help and support from many people and organisations. First I would like to thank the Wellcome Trust for its financial support and for sustaining such an excellent infrastructure for the history of medicine, especially the Wellcome Institute Library and its staff. I would like to thank the archivists at the Wellcome Institute Library, the Royal College of Physicians; University College, London; the Royal College of Surgeons; John Rylands University Library, Manchester; and the Royal Veterinary College for their help. Michele Minto, Wellcome Photographic Library; and John Woodhouse, Pat Cummings and Dr. Dorothy Clayton, John Rylands University Library, Manchester, provided the illustrations. An earlier version of Chapter 2 was published in *Medical History,* 1991, 35: 308–327, and the material is reproduced by permission of The Trustee, The Wellcome Trust. I have received excellent support and guidance from Alex Holzman of the New York Office of Cambridge University Press and my copy editor Elise Oranges improved my manuscript in many ways. Many colleagues and friends also helped in various ways, including Sanjoy Bhattacharya, David Cantor, Roger Cooter, Jon Harwood, Elsbeth Heaman, Chris Lawrence, Sharon Mathews, Malcolm Nicolson, Paolo Palladino, Steve Sturdy, John Woodward and others too many to mention. Many of the ideas have been aired and discussed at seminars and conferences, so I would like to thank all those who have commented. My two referees provided constructive advice that led me to rethink a number of lines of argument. I must acknowledge separately four people who have provided particularly valuable and timely advice on the whole project: the Series Editor, Charles Rosenberg, Bill Bynum, Mark Harrison, and especially John Pickstone, who has been a constant sounding board for ideas throughout the project. Needless to say, I alone am responsible for the views expressed in the volume. Finally, I would like to thank Carole, Liam and Julia for their help in so many ways, their patience and in the last few months their constructive impatience with this project.

Michael Worboys

Introduction

The pivotal role of the germ theory of disease in modern medicine is widely acknowledged in medical history and beyond. Typical comments are that it was 'probably the most important single concept for the history of modern medicine'[1] and that in the late nineteenth century it helped 'transform every aspect of medicine'.[2] Historians have also argued that it was central to the 'scientific revolution in medicine' of the last quarter of the nineteenth century, which was forged around the growing role and authority of the laboratory in medical investigation and practice.[3] There are perhaps more celebratory histories of 'the microbe revolution' than of any other episode in medical history.[4] The names of Louis Pasteur (1822–95), Robert Koch (1843–1910) and Joseph Lister (1827–1912) – the key 'discoverers' and 'innovators' – are well known. Their lives and work have been the subject of many academic studies, as well as popular biographies and radio and television programmes.[5] There are a number of histories of medical bacteriology and many journal articles on the changing understanding of specific diseases. However, there is no recent study of the development and spread of the germ theory in medicine.[6] In this volume I begin to make good this deficiency by explor-

1 R. E. McGrew, *Encyclopaedia of Medical History*, London, Macmillan, 1985, 25.
2 C. E. Rosenberg, *The Care of Strangers*, Baltimore, MD, Johns Hopkins University Press, 1987, 141.
3 A. Youngson, *The Scientific Revolution in Victorian Medicine*, London, Croom Helm, 1979; J. V. Pickstone, 'Ways of Knowing: Towards a Historical Sociology of Science', *BJHS*, 1993, 26: 433–58.
4 The genre began with P. de Kruif, *The Microbe Hunters*, London, Jonathan Cape, 1926. Cf. A. L. Baron, *Man Against Germs*, London, Robert Hale, 1958; R. Reid, *Microbes and Men*, London, BBC, 1974; P. E. Baldry, *The Battle Against Bacteria*, Cambridge, Cambridge University Press, 1965; H. Koprowski and M. B. A. Oldstone, eds., *Microbe Hunters: Then and Now*, New York, Medi-Ed Press, 1996.
5 On the three heroes see: R. Dubos, *Pasteur and Modern Science*, Madison, WI, SciTech, 1960, rep. 1988; G. L. Geison, 'Louis Pasteur', in C. C. Gillispie, ed., *The Dictionary of Scientific Biography*, New York, Charles Scribner, 1974, 350–416; idem., *The Private Science of Louis Pasteur*, Princeton, NJ, Princeton University Press, 1995; P. Debré, *Louis Pasteur*, Baltimore, MD, Johns Hopkins University Press, 1998; T. D. Brock, *Robert Koch: A Life in Medicine and Bacteriology*, Madison, WI, Science Tech, 1988; F. F. Cartwright, *Joseph Lister*, London, Longmans, 1963; R. B. Fisher, *Joseph Lister, 1827–1912*, New York: Stein and Day, 1977.
6 W. Bulloch, *The History of Bacteriology*, London, Oxford University Press, 1938; W. D. Foster, *A History of Medical Bacteriology and Immunology*, London, Heinemann Medical, 1970. On disease his-

ing how, why and to what extent germ ideas and practices were used, and with what effect, by the medical profession in Britain in the period 1865–1900. I do so around four propositions: (i) Rather than discussing a single germ theory, we need to explore the many *germ theories of disease* (and germ theories of other phenomena) current after 1865; (ii) we should give equal place to germ *practices*; (iii) we must always consider ideas on how the *body reacts to germs* and not leave this question until the emergence of formal immunological models from the mid-1880s; and (iv) we examine the *new meanings of science in medicine* that were linked with the new knowledge of germs.[7]

The first and most important theme to acknowledge is the range of *germ theories of disease* current between 1865 and 1900.[8] In the 1860s and 1870s, there were many views on what disease-germs were, for example, chemical poisons, ferments, degraded cells, fungi, 'bacteria' or a class of parasites. Indeed, it was likely that there was a spectrum of disease agents, from simple chemical poisons through to worms. The plurality of germ theories was acknowledged by some contemporary doctors and scientists; for example, John Drysdale (1817–92), in his *Germ Theories of Infectious Disease* in 1878, identified at least ten types of 'infectious miasms': 'chemical ferments', 'organised ferments', morphologically specific parasites, physiologically specific parasites, saprophytes, animal graft-germs, vegetable graft-germs and chemical septic products (liquid or gaseous).[9] However, the key issues in the mid-1860s were

tories see, for example, R. and J. Dubos, *The White Plague: Tuberculosis, Man and Society*, Boston, Little Brown and Co., 1952; A. M. Brandt, *No Magic Bullet: A Social History of Venereal Disease in the United States since 1880*, 2nd edition, New York, Oxford University Press, 1987; N. Rogers, *Dirt and Disease: Polio Before FDR*, New Brunswick, NJ, Rutgers University Press, 1992. Further studies can be expected following the impact of C. E. Rosenberg and J. Golden, *Framing Disease: Studies in Cultural History*, New Brunswick, NJ, Rutgers University Press, 1992.

7 S. E. D. Shortt, 'Physicians, Science and Status: Issues in the Professionalisation of Anglo-American Medicine in the Nineteenth Century', *MH*, 1983, 27: 51–68.

8 The notion that there were many germ theories was the basis of the work of Richard Shryock and Phyllis A. Richmond, though the implication of their work was that after 1870 the 'true' germ-theory was finally accepted. R. H. Shryock, 'Germ Theories in Medicine Prior to 1870: Further Comments on Continuity in Science', *Clio Medica*, 1972, 7: 81–109; P. A. Richmond, 'The Germ Theory of Disease', in A. M. Lilienfield, ed., *Times, Places and Persons: Aspects of the History of Epidemiology*, Baltimore, MD, Johns Hopkins Univeristy Press, 1980, 84–93. Margaret Pelling and Christopher Hamlin have been the strongest advocates of *theories* rather than *the theory*. M. Pelling, *Cholera, Fever and English Medicine, 1835–65*, Oxford, Oxford University Press, 1978; idem., 'Contagion/Germ Theory/Specificity', in W. F. Bynum and R. Porter, eds., *Companion Encyclopaedia of the History of Medicine*, London, Routledge, 1993, 309–34; C. Hamlin, 'Politics and Germ Theories in Victorian Britain: The Metropolitan Water Commissions of 1867–9 and 1892–3', in R. MacLeod, ed., *Expertise and Government: Specialists, Administrators and Professionals, 1860–1919*, Cambridge, Cambridge University Press, 1988, 111–23.

9 J. J. Drysdale, *The Germ Theories of Infectious Diseases*, London, Baillière, Tindall and Cox, 1878. John James Drysdale was a Liverpool doctor who published homeopathy, scientific materialism, theories of life and 'pyrogens' – fever-producing chemicals in the blood. In the early 1870s, he published a number of articles on microorganisms with W. H. Dallinger (1842–1909). R. G. H., 'Obituary: Rev. W. H. Dallinger', *JRMS*, 1909, 29: 699–702.

around the boundary of complex chemicals and life-forms: Were disease-agents living or not, could they arise *de novo* or were they always 'ancestral'? There was also great uncertainty over whether germs were cause, consequence or mere concomitants of disease, not to mention which diseases were associated with germs. One problem for my emphasis on germ theories of disease is that contemporaries usually wrote of a single theory.[10] I shall return to this question in the Conclusion, but it is worth noting that part of the reason was political. Proponents of all of the theories of disease advanced their ideas as firm principles, because to admit that there were many theories would have weakened their position. Conversely, critics were only too happy to highlight the number of theories to show the uncertainties amongst germ-theorists.

After 1880, there was a growing consensus in medicine that most disease-germs were 'bacteria', and more agreement on their properties and how they were transmitted. However, there was never closure on even a single bacterial model for germs or their actions in any branch of the profession. In medicine, although not in the wider culture, the word 'germ' began to be used less and less over the period, as 'bacteria' and 'microorganisms' became the *lingua franca* of modern medicine.[11] In 1881, the germ theory of disease was defined in a medical lexicon as 'the idea that the origin of many diseases lay in the pathogenic actions of certain micro-organisms when introduced into the body'.[12] This definition indicates that the 'reality' of germs was no longer disputed. However, questions about how different 'bacteria', in different diseases, produced their 'pathogenic actions' and how they were 'introduced into the body' remained open. There was also, of course, the major issue of the body's reactions to the 'pathogenic actions' of 'introduced' bacteria. The change from germs to 'bacteria', as we will see, was not without its problems. Many 'bacteria' remained beyond the capture of microscopy and the new laboratory techniques. Equally, it proved difficult to determine their physical, chemical and biological effects in the body, and to construct accounts of the relations between their often localised presence and the systemic effects seen in clinical syndromes. Thus, I have to explain why, despite these uncertainties and against quite concerted opposition, bacterial theories of disease continued to gain supporters and spread.

In Britain, as elsewhere, there was a group of germ-theorists, mostly

---

10 One of the first histories wrote as though there was a single theory. E. M. Crookshank, 'The History and Present Position of the Germ Theory of Disease', *PH*, 1888–89, 1: 16–9, 53–6.

11 For a model study of the public reception and uses of germs in the United States, see: N. Tomes, *The Gospel of Germs: Men, Women and the Microbe in American Life*, Cambridge, MA, Harvard University Press, 1998.

12 This definition is derived from the *Oxford English Dictionary* is based on the one given in H. Power and L. W. Sedgwick, *New Sydenham Society's Lexicon of Medicine and the Sciences*, London, New Sydenham Society, 1881. J. K. Crellin, 'The Dawn of Germ Theory: Particles, Infection and Biology', in F. N. L. Poynter, ed., *Medicine and Science in the 1860s*, London, WIHM, 1966, 57–76.

doctors and scientists, who developed and championed the new ideas and practices. However, the differences between germ-theorists were often as great as those between them and their opponents. I pay particular attention to the latter and to alternative explanations of disease, avoiding the common presumption that there were no theories of disease before germs, or that alternatives were undeveloped and 'unscientific'.[13] Indeed, histories of germ theories of disease have tended to give too much emphasis to germs and ignored the medically much more important story of 'theories of disease'. This is somewhat surprising, as germ theories, and then bacteriology, have been seen as important factors in a major shift in the dominant conception of disease in Western medicine.[14] This change has been described in many ways, but at its simplest it can be seen as moving from defining diseases by their symptoms and results to defining them in terms of processes and causes. The changing constructions can be illustrated by reference to tuberculosis.[15] In the early nineteenth century, the disease was known as consumption, or *phthisis*, from the Greek word for 'wasting'. This characterisation was based on a holistic view of the symptoms and results; patients wasted away as their body literally consumed itself. In the first half of the nineteenth century, the term 'tuberculosis' came to be used, referring to the localised pathological process of tubercle (nodule) formation in the lungs.[16] Thus, the disease was defined by a process and its results, but these were now described at the tissue and cellular levels. However, the identification and acceptance of the *Tubercle bacillus* in the 1880s as the essential cause, over an extended period it must be said, led to the creation of an aetiological definition of the disease. Indeed, the disease eventually took on the name of its cause – TB, short for *Tubercle bacillus*, the entity that entered the body and started the process of tubercle formation, which impaired respiration and circulation, to produce wasting.

13 P. A. Richmond, 'Some Variant Theories in Opposition to the Germ Theory of Disease', *JHM*, 1954, 9: 290–303. But note the comments on Richmond's approach in N. Tomes, "American Attitudes toward the Germ Theory of Disease: Phyllis Allen Richmond Revisited', *JHM*, 1997, 52: 17–50.

14 O. Temkin, 'Health and Disease', O. Temkin, in *The Double Face of Janus and Other Essays in the History of Medicine*, Baltimore, MD, Johns Hopkins University Press, 1977, 436–8; K. Codell Carter, 'The Development of Pasteur's Concept of Disease Causation and the Emergence of Specific Causes in Nineteenth Century Medicine, *BHM*, 1991, 65: 528–48.

15 Andrew Cunningham's interesting argument that there is no continuity between pre- and post-bacteriological constructions of disease is addressed implicitly throughout the volume. I think he is wrong for three main reasons: first, he overestimates the degree of difference between pre- and postgerm models of disease; second, he neglects the coexistence of different models amongst different groups of practitioners; and third, many contemporary doctors found no problem recognising continuities, despite epistemological differences. A. Cunningham, 'Transforming Plague: The Laboratory and the Identity of Infectious Disease', in A. Cunningham and P. Williams, eds., *The Laboratory Revolution in Medicine*, Cambridge, Cambridge University Press, 1992, 209–44.

16 Tubercles were small rounded projections or nodules of a particular grey-yellow consistency that became the defining postmortem sign of consumption. Its root is the same as the botanical term 'tuber'.

Historians have often preferred to characterise the overall change as one in the dominant ideal-type model of disease, with the physiological conceptions of disease being replaced by the so-called ontological ones. The physiological view fashioned diseases as disturbances in normal functioning or structure that resulted from the patient's predisposition interacting with a configuration of personal and environmental influences, including injuries and poisonings. Diseases were inseparable from the sick person; indeed, they were often seen positively as the body's way of healing itself. Ontological models made diseases 'things' or entities that were separate from the patient. On this view, diseases developed when pathogenic entities arose in the body (e.g. cancer cells) or entered the body (e.g. bacteria) and spread their effects locally or systemically. Ontological conceptions were associated more directly with causal definitions of disease and were seen by many doctors to open up new approaches to diagnosis, prevention and treatment by recognising and removing causes. While accepting that there was an overall transition from physiological to ontological models as ideal types, I suggest that this change was complex and uneven.[17] For example, in 1900, the terms 'phthisis', 'consumption', 'tuberculosis' and 'TB' were all used concurrently and often as alternatives, despite their distinct origins and meanings. The dominant medical view was that the development of the disease required both the *Tubercle bacillus* and a vulnerable human constitution, and there was a growing awareness that bacilli only produced disease in a minority of those infected.

My second proposition is that *germ practices* – seeing, killing, culturing, altering and representing germs – deserve as much attention as germ theories.[18] However, I do not want to concentrate on laboratory practices because those developed in the field were just as important, as were relations between the two areas of practice. Many existing medical and sanitary procedures, such as disinfection, isolation, antisepsis, anti-inflammatory remedies and vaccination, were redefined as germ practices after 1865. The style of laboratory work was carried into the field, as in antiseptic surgery, and field experience set the parameters for laboratory investigations of aetiology and pathogenesis.

The neglect of practice in extant histories of germs is exemplified by the emphasis given to Koch's postulates – the steps necessary to prove disease causation by germs – compared to attention given to his technical innovations in microscopy, culturing and experimental pathology, not to mention his work in clinical and preventive medicine and his technically innovative publications.[19] The extent to which the development of bacteriology as a technical specialism contributed to the eclipse of 'germs' in the 1880s is debat-

17 J. M. Bruce, 'The Dominance of Etiology in Modern Medicine, *BMJ*, 1910, ii: 246–7.
18 A. S. Evans, 'Causation and Disease: The Effects of Technology on Postulates of Causation', *Yale Journal of Biological and Medicine*, 1994, 64, 513–28.
19 K. Codell Carter, 'Koch's Postulates in Relation to the Work of Jacob Henle and Edwin Klebs', *MH*, 1985, 29: 353–74. An exception is Brock's biography of Robert Koch.

able. The terms of debate certainly changed, as speculation and principles were replaced by facts, practical demonstrations and precise models. Certainly, 'bacteria' were made available for doctors to see and attempts were made to spread knowledge of the techniques. However, in other ways things became less certain. The adoption of new methods of investigation produced more aetiological claims from more sources, so it became harder to keep up and assess the proliferation of ideas. Many suspected 'bacteria' continued to elude the new practices, or their properties could not be fixed; hence the notion of 'germs' remained useful, not least for the possibility that many diseases were due to the germs of bacteria, in the sense of their ultramicroscopical, uncul-turable and hence uninoculable 'spores' – the 'seeds' of the seeds of disease. I include some discussion of 'failed' aetiological claims, although not as many as I expected. I suspect that there would be more in a study of Germany or France, but in Britain the volume of laboratory investigations of germs and bacteria was smaller, and not always targeted towards constructing aetiologi-cal claims and achieving recognition.

I am also interested in the interactions between theory and practice, although I do not assume that the two are necessarily or simply linked. Indeed, with antiseptic surgery, one of the great icons of the germ era, I suggest that for long periods theory and practice were deliberately decou-pled. In public health, practice was often said to be ahead of theory. This issue requires careful handling, as germ theorists and then bacteriologists were always keen to claim that their ideas and laboratory work led to practical benefits. In other words, they promoted a linear module of innovation: pure science leading to applied science, to technologies and then social consequences.

My third theme is that disease-germs cannot be considered in isolation from ideas about *the body's reactions to them*. Contemporaries were only too aware that most people recovered from infections, and hence germ theories of disease necessarily implied theories of health. One powerful and persistent argument against any germ-theory was that germs did not invariably produce disease. The need to look at explanations of the body's defences has been recognised by historians for the period after 1885, but then only in terms of the development of immunological theories. There has been little consider-ation of the less specific immunological thinking developed earlier, around notions of the body's refractoriness, predisposition, openness, diathesis or constitutional strength, which continued to be used well into the twentieth century.[20] I will argue that in Britain the dominant metaphor in germ the-ories of disease and health was the botanical one of 'seed and soil'. In many cases this was literally true. Bacteria were classified as plants, as were other likely pathogenic organisms, for example, fungi and fern spores. Only in the

---

20 P. H. Mazumdar, 'Immunity in 1890', *JHM*, 1972, 27: 312–24; S. MacKenzie, 'The Powers of Natural Resistance, or the Personal Factor in Disease of Microbe Origin', *TMSL*, 1902, 25: 302–18.

1890s was the now more popular military analogy of invading germs in conflict with the body's defences used extensively.

Fourth, I will suggest that germ theories and practices were not just theoretical and practical innovations; they were also carriers of *new meanings for
science in medicine.*[21] The place of scientific knowledge and methods in medicine was debated vigorously from the mid-nineteenth century, being central
to the transition of medicine from a status to an expert profession, in which
science became the basis for identity and work. The notion of there having
been a 'scientific revolution in Victorian medicine' once hinged on the
assumed impact of germ theories. There has been a move in medical history
to downplay the clinical and social benefits of germ and other medical laboratory sciences, and to play up their ideological value in modernising the
profession.[22] I take issue with those historians who have suggested that laboratory medicine was promoted on its promise rather than its actual results.
Instead, I argue that laboratory-derived ideas and practices were important
resources in the reshaping of prevention, diagnosis, treatment and patient
management, although they make no assessment of specific outcomes.

I want to emphasise at the outset that this volume is a *medical history of
germs.* It explores how different groups of practitioners within medicine
understood and used the new germ science and technology. I have not
written a history of bacteriology,[23] microbiology,[24] immunology[25] or even laboratory medicine.[26] I discuss themes such as spontaneous generation,[27] pleomorphism,[28] classification and evolution,[29] but only when they were relevant
to the making and spread of germs ideas and practices in medicine.[30] My
approach is to consider in turn different areas of practice, looking at how

21 J. H. Warner, 'Science in Medicine', *Osiris*, 1983, 1: 37–85; idem., 'Ideals of Science and Their
  Discontents in Late Nineteenth Century American Medicine', *Isis*, 1991, 82: 454–78;
22 Youngson, *Scientific Revolution, passim.*
23 The standard works that focus on medical bacteriology are: Bulloch, *History of Bacteriology*, and
  Foster, *Medical Bacteriology*. On other aspects of the subject, see: K. Vernon, 'Pus, Sewage, Beer and
  Milk: Microbiology in Britain, 1870–1940', *History of Science*, 1990, 28: 289–325.
24 Microbiology was very much a French term. See: C. Salomen-Bayet, 'The First Bio-medical
  Revolution: Slow Shaping of Microbiology, France', in Y. Kawaita et al., eds., *History of Therapy:
  Proceedings of the Tenth International Symposium of Comparative Medicine: East and West,* Tokyo, Ishiyaku
  EuroAmerica Inc., 1990, 173–92, and C. Salomen-Bayet and B. Lécuyer, *Pasteur et la Revolution
  pastorienne,* Paris, Payot, 1986. Also see: H. A. Lechevalier and M. Solotorovsky, *Three Centuries of
  Microbiology,* New York, McGraw Hill, 1965; P. Collard, *The Development of Microbiology,* Cambridge,
  Cambridge University Press, 1976.
25 A. M. Silverstein, *A History of Immunology,* San Diego, CA, Academic Press, 1989; D. J. Bibel, ed.,
  Milestones in Immunology: A Historical Exploration, Madison, Science Tech, 1988.
26 Cunningham, *Laboratory Revolution, passim.*
27 J. E. Strick, *The British Spontaneous Generation Debates of 1860–1880: Medicine, Evolution and
  Laboratory Science in the Victorian Context,* Unpublished PhD Thesis, Princeton University, 1997.
28 M. Wainwright, 'Extreme Pleomorphism and the Bacterial Life Cycle: A Forgotten Controversy',
  Perspectives in Biology and Medicine, 1997, 40: 407–14.
29 W. F. Bynum, 'Darwin and the Doctors: Evolution, Diathesis and Germs in Nineteenth Century
  Britain', *Gesnerus,* 1983, 40: 43–53.
30 The volume that is closest to mine is Foster, *Medical Bacteriology.*

different professional groupings attempted to understand diseases and to prevent, diagnose, control, manage and treat diverse afflictions. The distinct interests and resources of different groups enabled them to produce distinct theories and meanings, and to fashion diverse germ practices. The different discourses on germs that I explore were not developed in isolation from one another; hence, I consider the interactions between different groups within Britain and internationally. One advantage of this method is that it offers the opportunities for comparative history and to test just how 'local' medical cultures were in the late nineteenth century. My comparisons with the construction and use of germ theories in other countries are not as extensive as I would have liked.[31] Needless to say, Bruno Latour's *The Pasteurisation of France* was a major influence on my work, less for its philosophical propositions than for its ambitious attempt to account for the ways in which germ ideas and practices were spread and used.[32] Relations between British germ theorists and those in France and Germany, especially the powerful schools of Pasteur and Koch, are important parts of the story. However, I suggest that we need to revise any notion of British backwardness or inferiority. For most of the period I discuss, Lister was as important an international figure as Pasteur or Koch. There were many British germ workers, and there was no shortage of publications and debate. British investigators were more than willing to challenge their continental colleagues; for example, Charlton Bastian (1837–1915) (see Figure 3) took on Pasteur over spontaneous generation in the late 1870s and Edward Klein (1844–1925) (see Figure 2) disputed Koch's work on cholera through the late 1880s and early 1890s.

Germ theories had no essential meaning, nor did germ practices dictate specific preventive or therapeutic strategies. As Tomes and Warner have recently argued, the historical task is not to study 'the acceptance of the germ-theory of disease but to fix its meaning', although I think that 'meanings' better captures their intent.[33] This is, of course, a potentially huge venture, especially if germ theories did 'transform every aspect of medicine'. Thus, I have been necessarily selective in the local cultures that I have studied, concentrating on veterinarians, surgeons, public health doctors and general practitioners and physicians through the lens of tuberculosis. Given time and space, I would like to have included an analysis of nurses' germs,[34] patholo-

31 The value of such work is evident in Mendelsohn's outstanding study of France and Germany. J. A. Mendelsohn, *Cultures of Bacteriology: Foundation and Transformation of a Science in France and Germany, 1870–1914*, Unpublished PhD thesis, Princeton University, 1996.

32 B. Latour, *The Pasteurization of France*, Cambridge, MA, Harvard University Press, 1988. But see: S. Sturdy, 'The Germs of a New Enlightenment', *Studies in the History and Philosophy of Science*, 1991, 22: 163–73, and S. Schaffer, 'The Eighteenth Brumaire of Bruno Latour', Ibid., 174–92.

33 N. J. Tomes and J. H. Warner, 'Introduction to Special Issue on Rethinking the Reception of Germ Theory of Disease: Comparative Perspectives', *JHM*, 1997, 52: 16.

34 On nurses' germs see: A. Bashford, *Purity and Pollution: Gender, Embodiment and Victorian Medicine*, Houndmills, Hants., Macmillan, 1998.

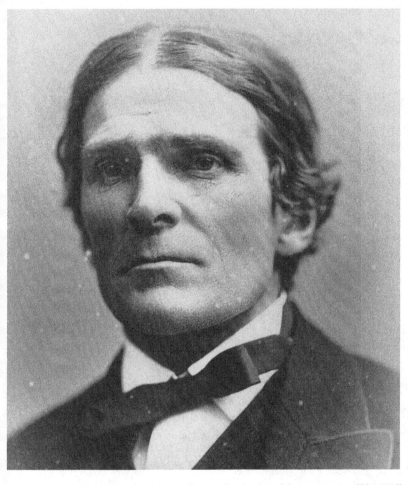

Figure 1. John Burdon Sanderson (Reproduced by courtesy of the Wellcome Institute Library, London)

gists' germs, obstetricians' germs,[35] colonial doctors' germs[36] and, of course, bacteriologists' germs. I have not ignored the latter, but there are a number of good histories of medical bacteriology, and until the twentieth century this was a small group. Until then, most germ workers were part-time bacteriologists with interests and loyalties in other professional domains. The groups and topics that I consider are those where germ theories and practices were most developed, debated and used. However, I have not been rigid

35 I. S. L. Loudon, *Childbed Fever: A Documentary History*, London, Garland, 1996.
36 M. Worboys, 'From Miasmas to Germs: Malaria, 1860–1880', *Parassitologia*, 1994, 36: 61–8.

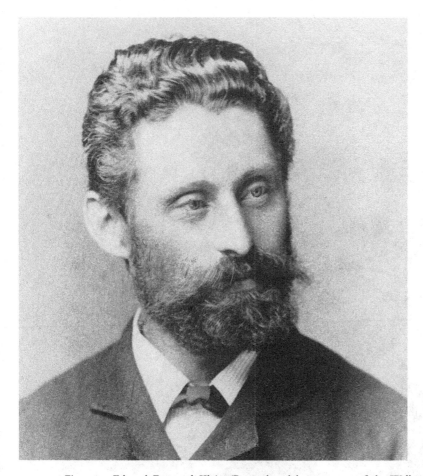

Figure 2. Edward Emanuel Klein (Reproduced by courtesy of the Wellcome Institute Library, London)

about boundaries and do consider interactions and translations between these and other medical subcultures, as well as nonmedical groups. After 1880, germs were mainly associated with communicable and septic diseases, but they were also linked with many other conditions, from arthritis to scurvy, and from cancer to constipation. Restrictions of space and time mean that I have not been able to look at the full range of diseases in which germs were implicated, so I have concentrated on the major debates and changes as experienced by practitioners.

My approach, through practitioners and their interests, means that I do not privilege the 'discovery' of specific germs and the establishment of disease aetiologies. Germs may have been 'discovered', in the sense of being first

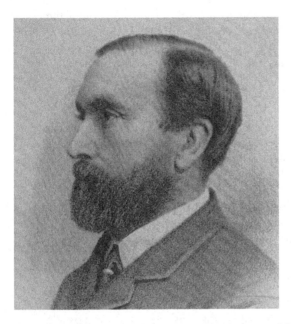

Figure 3. Charlton Bastian (Reproduced by courtesy of the Wellcome Institute Library, London)

revealed as physical 'objects', but the leaps to how these 'objects' produced disease were inventions of the human mind. Theories are, of course, imposed on nature by investigators not taken from it. I have little discussion of 'Eureka!' moments of discovery; instead I discuss the processes by which germ accounts of disease were developed, and how knowledge claims were spread and adopted, or not adopted, by groups of practitioners. I assume that this was not simply because they were 'true' or 'false'. Rather, I seek to explain the various reasons why individuals and groups were persuaded, or not persuaded, of the value of holding germ beliefs and adopting or adapting germ practices. I always try to do this in relation to the full spectrum of existing and alternative disease theories and medical practices. Thus, I avoid the temptation to write about the 'impact' of germ theories on medicine. Germ theories of disease were, of course, largely constituted *within* medicine; they did not arrive from elsewhere, discrete and ready-formed. I show that the role of germs in disease was debated and various positions taken long before there was any agreement on their character. Also, even when plausible models of their form and function were developed, these were continually reinterpreted and changed. For the small number of ideas and practices that did arrive, as it were, 'out of the blue' from marginal practitioners or serendipitous practice, there remain problems with the notion of 'impacts'. Too often the term is used in a mechanistic, billiard ball, concept of causation – something 'hits' something and produces a reaction. While physical objects coming together react in this way, social institutions, human behaviour and ideas do not. They are rarely discrete entities, and they interact rather than react. More-over, there are numerous possible resolutions to the interactions of social forces, individuals and beliefs. In the debates on germs, in some instances all parties were converted to germ accounts of a disease, and in others none. In most cases one sees uneven and combined patterns of belief and action, depending on the disease, circumstances and interests.

If my prime focus is not the 'discovery' of germs, or the 'impact' of germ theories and practices, what is it? My preference is to say that I am inter-ested in the 'construction' and 'use' of germ theories and practices by local medical cultures.[37] One advantage of these terms is that they bring *agency* to the fore, that is, I have to say who was making and employing new ideas and practices, and when, where, how and why they were spread and used. This is a valuable counter to histories that are content to talk about ideas being 'in the air' or see 'unit ideas' influencing one another or combining in largely disembodied ways. Historians are now rightly wary of speaking of the diffu-sion of ideas because of associations with passive processes and the possible neglect of human agency, hence my preference for thinking about the 'use' and 'spread' of germ theories and practices.

The metaphor of 'construction' is valuable because it suggests a process, taking place over a time, in particular settings. It raises questions about the materials from which new knowledge was produced and about its various builders. Was construction a cooperative or competitive venture? Were there competing plans and even rival structures? Were new ideas and practices forged by first demolishing the old ones, by building on the old foundations or by modifying existing forms? In what stages were knowl-edge claims put together, and how was it known when they were complete or usable? How did the new structures appear from the perspective of different groups? There are dangers in the metaphor, not least the possible tendency to think of knowledge as like a physical structure, concrete and rigid, although in these days of computer graphics and virtual realities it is perhaps easier than it was to maintain notions of fluidity, malleability and contingency.

I have chosen to use 'construction' rather than the currently more popular terms of *social construction* and *framing*.[38] The 'social' in social constructivism is largely redundant and sometimes carries with it the connotation that knowl-

37 J. Golinski, *Making Natural Knowledge: Constructivism and the History of Science*, Cambridge, Cambridge University Press, 1998.
38 R. A. Aronowitz, *Making Sense of Illness: Science, Society and Illness*, Cambridge, Cambridge University Press, 1998, 1–23.

edge is the product of social relations alone. I see knowledge and practice being produced from social and material interactions.[39] Thus, I agree with those who argue that historians of medicine cannot ignore 'biology' and the ways this shapes ideas and actions.[40] I think this is best expressed by extending an analogy that E. P. Thompson suggested for historical study. He wrote of concepts being like carpenters' tools, while historical evidence was the wood to be worked on. He argued that it is generally easier to work with the grain of the wood than against it, and that different types of wood are better suited to certain purposes than others. Different tools are suited to different types of wood, and different purposes. Nonetheless, powerful tools (and imaginations) allow surprising things to be made from wood, even though this often requires immense effort and investment and produces outcomes that are difficult to sustain. It seems to me that much science is like this; while nature underdetermines our knowledge, there is still a degree of determination by nature that involves both impetuses and constraints.

The currently favoured notion of 'framing', with its explicit use of the analogy of the viewing of 'pictures', can tend to realism. Framing can appear to be nothing more that the context or setting in which nature is viewed, rather than a process where it is actively shaped. That said, some historians have used a dynamic notion of framing, where, as in constructivism, intellectual, manual and social work has to be undertaken on nature to produce 'pictures' in a specific context. Thus it would be argued that the anthrax bacillus was not just framed by Koch's microscope lens; he had previously isolated the organism from its natural habitat, nurtured it in special conditions, treating it as a unicellular plant and parasite, made artificial inoculations of tissues and so on.[41] He produced data that were constituted in ways that were acceptable to certain, but by no means all, audiences. In this sense Koch was doing more than just *framing* nature, he was both materially and metaphorically *reconstructing* nature, or, as Clarke and Fujimura might have it – making the 'right germs for the job'.[42]

My approach is contextual. I analyse changes in theories of disease in relation to shifts in the social organisation and culture of medicine, exploring how ideas were used politically as well as practically. There are three major shifts in medical culture in which germ theories and practices were mobilised. The first shift was the slow, uneven and ongoing movement of medicine to an expert, science-based profession. Various meanings and uses of science had

39 L. Jordanova, 'The Social Construction of Medical Knowledge', *SHM*, 1995, 3: 364–82; M. Bury, 'Social Construction and the Development of Medical Sociology', *Sociology of Health and Illness*, 1986, 8: 131–69.
40 C. E. Rosenberg, 'Framing Disease: Illness, Society and History', in Rosenberg *Framing Disease*, xv–xvi.
41 For details see: Brock, *Robert Koch*, 27–53.
42 A. E. Clarke and J. H. Fujimura, eds., *The Right Tools for the Job: At Work in Twentieth Century Life Sciences*, Princeton, NJ, Princeton University Press, 1992.

been enlisted in the medical reform movement from the 1830s, but after 1860 laboratory science came to play a larger role. Initially, physiology was the model medical science, although from the mid-1870s pathology became much more important, especially when linked with bacteriology in the 1880s. The rapidity of this change highlights the likely importance of generational differences in the Victorian profession. Second, the institutionalisation of the study of germs and bacteria offers insights into the processes of specialisation in medicine, including the emergence of new research agencies, as well as changes within existing institutions such as hospitals, medical schools and government departments. Third, I also look at individual alliances and rivalries. The number of doctors involved in the construction and dissemination of germ theories and practices remained quite small, and many of the controversies and collaborations were personal as well as intellectual and intraprofessional.

A book on germ theories and modern medicine that has Britain as its principal focus, if the existing histories are any guide, should be a rather slim volume. British scientists and medical practitioners have been portrayed as spectators in an unfolding drama, where all of the action takes place in France or Germany. And when the location moved, as it did to the British Empire with cholera in the 1880s and the plague in the 1890s, it was French and German scientists who continued to take the star roles. The list of credits for germ discoveries and innovations is full of German and French scientists. Only Joseph Lister is routinely given a major part in histories of germ theory for his pioneering of antiseptic surgery, although Edward Jenner (1749–1823) sometimes appears incongruously for his work on vaccinia almost a century earlier. The only other British figures who sometimes make the Hall of Fame are Alexander Ogston (1844–1929), for the discovery of the role of staphylococci in septic infection;[43] Ronald Ross (1857–1932), when the story is widened to include parasitology;[44] and Almroth Wright (1861–1947), who appears as both hero (anti-typhoid vaccine) and villain (vaccine therapy) in histories of immunology.[45] Different professional priorities and better news management by the British medical elite might have seen credit given to Edward Klein for the discovery of the scarlet fever germ,[46] William Greenfield (1846–1919) for pioneering anthrax vaccines[47] and Herbert Durham (b. 1866) and Albert Grunbaum, later Leyton (1869–1921) for the

43 I. A. Porter, 'Sir Alexander Ogston (1844–1929)', in G. P. Milne, ed., *A Bicentennial History, 1789–1989*, Aberdeen, Aberdeen Medico-Chirurgical Society, 1989, 179–89.

44 R. Ross, *Memoirs: With A Full Account of the Great Malaria Problem and Its Solution*, London, John Murray, 1923.

45 H. J. Parish, *Victory with Vaccines*, Edinburgh, E. & S. Livingstone, 1965; idem., *A History of Immunization*, Edinburgh, E. & S. Livingstone, 1965; H. W. Dowling, *Fighting Infection: Conquests of the Twentieth Century*, Cambridge, MA, Harvard University Press, 1977.

46 L. G. Wilson, 'The historical riddle of milk-borne scarlet fever', *BHM*, 1986, 60: 321–42.

47 W. D. Tigertt, 'Anthrax: William Smith Greenfield, MD, FRCP, Professor Superintendent, The Brown Animal Sanatory Institute', *Journal of Hygiene*, 1980, 85: 415.

invention of serum diagnosis for typhoid fever.[48] In the 1880s, when parasitic worms counted as germs, Patrick Manson (1844–1922) was often in the list of discoveries for his work with Filarial worms.[49] Better luck and more cooperative germs might have allowed John Burdon Sanderson (see Figure 1) (1825–1905) to claim the smallpox germ in 1869–70 and Klein the typhoid germ in 1874.[50] And what if Lister had decided to do experimental work on pus and septic tissues rather than turnip infusions and milk? Putting aside such counterfactual speculation, there were many British workers who undertook important investigations and interpretative projects. The work and influence of the following deserve to be better known and understood: Charlton Bastian and Lionel Beale (1828–1906), William Watson Cheyne (1852–1932), (see Figure 4), Edgar Crookshank (1858–1928), Charles B. Lockwood (1856–1914), John M'Fadyean (1853–1941), William Roberts (1830–99) and the physicist John Tyndall (1820–93). That said, the quantity and quality of germ work in continental Europe was much higher than in Britain, so an important element in my story is the international movements of people, ideas and practices, especially their adaptations to different professional and cultural conditions. I am interested in determining whether there were any 'peculiarities of the British' concerning germs, for example, over the distinction between germ theories of putrefaction and germ theories of fermentation, the influence of the seed and soil metaphor, and the extent to which clinical interests shaped the cognitive, practical and institutional development of the subject.

Each chapter in what follows is thematic and explores a particular area of medical practice or group of practitioners. The periodisation of many chapters runs in parallel, although there is a broad chronological shift from the 1860s towards 1900 through the volume. I analyse how germ theories of disease were constructed, spread and used, as well as how, if at all, professional, practical and cognitive trajectories were affected by the new culture of germs. Later chapters consider the elaboration and maturation of germ theories and practices in the institutionalisation of the new germ-based medical specialism of bacteriology.

In Chapter 1, I set the scene by discussing the character of the medical profession and theories of disease in the mid-1860s. I introduce the three main areas of practice to be discussed – medicine, surgery and public health – and set out the main medical ideas on the nature of disease, introducing key ideas about the zymotic theory of disease and its use in surgery and public health. Chapter 2 focuses on the relatively unfamiliar terrain of vet-

48 Bulloch, *History of Bacteriology*, 266–7.
49 A. Smart, 'A Chronological History of the Discovery of Germs, *BMJ*, 1884, ii: 565; J. Farley, 'Parasites and the Germ Theory of Disease', in Rosenberg, *Framing Disease*, 33–49.
50 See Chapters 4 and 7. Also see: T. Romano, *Making Medicine Scientific: John Burdon Sanderson: Medical Science in Victorian Britain*, Unpublished PhD Thesis, Yale University, 1993.

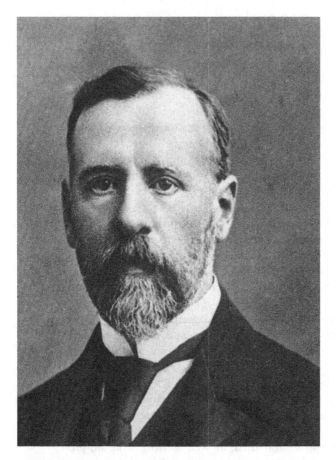

Figure 4. William Watson Cheyne (Reproduced by courtesy of the Wellcome Institute Library, London)

erinary medicine and shows just how contingent the elaborations and deployments of germ theories were over the period 1865–90. In terms of chronology, this chapter jumps ahead of those that immediately follow, which is justified because discussions of germs in veterinary medicine were relatively autonomous between the late 1860s and the late 1880s. A key moment in the modern history of germs in Britain was the cattle plague of 1866. Indeed, John Simon argued that it was 'the start of everything' in Britain regarding germs, communicable diseases and laboratory research.[51] My main contention is that veterinarians at all levels found germ theories a valuable resource for

51 *Report of the Medical Officer of the Privy Council and Local Government Board*, New Series, No. 3, Report on Scientific Investigations, 1874, BPP. 1875, [C.1068], xxxi, 5.

political reasons, principally because they used them to reinforce their commitment to contagion, quarantines and veterinary policing, and to support a professional identity that looked to the state rather than science for authority. I also suggest that, while veterinarians embraced germ theories, they eschewed germ practices. The elite believed that vaccination and other methods threatened their preferred administrative methods of controlling epizootics.

The best-known feature of the germ landscape in Britain was and is antiseptic surgery, which is considered in Chapters 3 and 5. Although Lister is a central figure in the story, I have attempted to set his ideas and work in the wider technical and ideological development of surgery. The central threads in these chapters are the developing innovations and ideas on wound management. In Chapter 3, which deals with the period 1865–76, these are considered mainly in the context of debates on hospital hygiene and the role of theory in surgery. I suggest that Listerian antiseptic practice made little headway in British surgery before the mid-1870s, and that his advocacy of Pasteurian germ-theory hindered rather than helped his cause. Events between 1877 and 1900 are discussed in Chapter 5, and follow the ways surgeons increasingly used bacterial germ theories to support both Listerian and non-Listerian practices. Brieger's suggestion that surgeons were important pioneers of bacteriology is borne out in Britain, although I show that this role was short-lived.[52] The growth of surgical practice and limited support for laboratory work in Britain drew key figures back to clinical work. Also, surgeons' interest in germs was largely around how to avoid them and how to destroy them, not to nurture and study them. Finally, I consider the development of aseptic surgery and argue, against much recent work, that its practical and ideological roots were in Listerism and not in the alternative project of surgical 'cleanliness'.

In the 1860s and 1870s, 'germ-theory', as it was then written, was associated almost exclusively with septic diseases arising in damaged or dead tissues; only in the late 1870s and early 1880s were the *contagium viva* of epidemic diseases routinely seen as germs and linked to a 'germ theory of infectious diseases'. Thus, the chapter on public health that splits the two on surgery discusses this important broadening of the scope of 'germ-theory', focusing on laboratory scientists and medical officers of health (MOsH). I discuss debates on germs within sanitary science and state medicine between the cholera epidemic of 1866 and the threats of the same disease in the early 1880s. To illustrate changes in the understanding and preventive management of fevers I focus on three important public health diseases – cholera, smallpox and typhoid fever. My central argument is that germ theories were incorporated unevenly into public health medicine, but that they were used

52 G. H. Brieger, 'American surgery and the germ theory of disease', *BHM*, 1966, 40: 135–45.

extensively before the 'bacteriological era' after 1880. The key issue in the use
of germ theories in public health before 1880 was their use in the conflict
between supporters of 'inclusive' and 'exclusive' preventive measures, usually
presented as hostilities between anticontagionists and old-style sanitarians on
the one hand, and contagionists and the new model army of MOsH on the
other. Most MOsH assumed that there was a spectrum of diseases between
the highly contagious and the noncontagious, with most occupying the
middle ground, being contingently and variably contagious. Germ theories
were used on all sides, although a key issue was the extent to which epidemics could arise *de novo* or whether they always had so-called *ancestral*
origins, that is, where every disease had a specific origin in another person
and was transmitted from person-to-person.

In Chapter 6, I explore the changing understanding and management of
consumption as the means to analyse the emerging uses of germ theories by
physicians and clinicians. I also chart the purported change from 'germ
theory' to 'germ fact' with the establishment of bacteriology – the science of
germs – in the early 1880s. Tuberculosis was the major killer disease of the
nineteenth century and the one whose aetiology is said to have been most
radically transformed by its new germ aetiology, changing from a hereditary
to an infectious disease. I dispute this view, suggesting instead that physicians
accommodated the *Tubercle bacillus* with hereditarian views through the seed
(bacillus) and soil (human constitution) metaphor. Only a minority of public
health doctors sought to remake consumption as a contagious, preventable,
zymotic disease. Thus, there was no direct or simple shift from physiological
to ontological conceptions of the disease. That said, I maintain that Koch's
Tubercle bacillus, and especially the techniques that he developed to see, grow
and manipulate it, were the key resources in the creation of bacteriology.
Finally, while accepting that the announcement of the *Tubercle bacillus* and all
that went with it was a turning point for the standing of germ theories and
practices in medicine, I show that there were major continuities in physicians' understanding and management of the disease, and that attacking the
germ was a relatively minor factor in the preventive campaigns of the 1890s.

Chapter 7 considers preventive medicine in the 1880s and 1890s. I consider the problems that bacteriology posed for supporters of smallpox
vaccination, not least the failure of laboratory scientists to be able to show
the smallpox germ by microscopy or culturing. With cholera, I look at the
neglected cholera threats of the 1880s and 1890s, focusing on the anti-Koch
line that was adopted by leading British bacteriologists between 1884 and
1894. The most important public health disease of the period was diphtheria, which in many ways became the definitive bacterial disease. It was an
infectious disease whose pathophysiology was well understood and where the
long-promised therapeutic benefits of laboratory medicine were first experienced. Socially, diphtheria was a child killer for which medical researchers

produced a miracle cure in 1894 – the diphtheria antitoxin. I consider changes in diphtheria control strategies before and after antitoxins, and show how the technologies of diagnosis and treatment developed for the disease became the basis upon which bacteriological laboratory work was routinised in hospitals, universities and local health authorities. Lastly, I look at the ways in which bacteriological ideas and practices were used in the prevention and control of disease c. 1900, highlighting the contrast between typhoid fever, for which bacteriologists had produced a preventive vaccine or diagnostic test, but as yet no therapy, and scarlet fever, the germ of which remained elusive and which continued to be managed by notification, isolation and disinfection.

1

Medical Practice and Disease Theories, c. 1865

To set the scene for the construction, use and spread of germ theories of disease after 1865, in this chapter I consider the mid-Victorian medical profession and the prevailing ideas on the nature of disease. My discussion of the profession concentrates on the areas in which major developments in germ theories and practices originated or gained the greatest currency, that is, in surgery and with the new groupings in state medicine and laboratory medicine. In considering disease theories, I start with the transition from hospital to laboratory medicine, and midcentury developments in physiology and cellular pathology. To reveal the relations between theory and practice, I focus on the ideas that informed both disease management with individual patients and disease prevention in populations. I also discuss the changing beliefs about septic and zymotic diseases, the ailments first remade as germ afflictions after 1865. I show that not only was the rise of germ theories of disease not anticipated, but that in the decades before the 1860s the tide had actually turned against explanations of disease as entities and as due to external, exciting causes.[1]

MEDICAL PRACTICE

The Medical Act of 1858 formally unified the medical profession in Britain, but there were few immediate signs of uniformity with practitioners remaining an extremely varied group.[2] The separate qualifications in medicine and surgery persisted, and only after 1886 did dual qualifications become mandatory. The great majority of the profession, who were almost exclusively men until the 1880s, were general practitioners (GPs), who plied their trade in both branches, mostly amongst the middling and lower classes. The commonest qualifications amongst older GPs were from the Royal College of Surgeons and the Society of Apothecaries, the latter's Licentiate having

1 M. Pelling, *Cholera, Fever and English Medicine, 1825–65*, Oxford, Oxford University Press, 1978.
2 J. M. Peterson, *The Medical Profession in Mid-Victorian London*, Berkeley, University of California Press, 1978.

become a general medical qualification rather than one merely for dispensing drugs. Younger doctors, in line with the requirements of the 1858 Act, were increasingly trained in medicine, surgery and midwifery at medical schools or hospitals linked to universities. However, the change was not just in formal certification; older doctors had trained in a variety of routes including apprenticeship – the new regime was more formal, standardised, science-linked and expensive, signalling and supporting the rise in social position of the profession overall. As the name suggests, general practitioners did a bit of everything: medicine, surgery, midwifery, dispensing drugs, and many held part-time appointments with the Poor Law, local authorities, voluntary agencies and private employers.[3] Patterns of work varied regionally, between rural and urban areas, and amongst different social classes and occupational groups. So too did the degree of economic success and security that practitioners gained from their small businesses in an overcrowded market.[4] The majority of GPs were professionally isolated; their social networks and identities were predominantly those of the middling classes in general rather than a technical cadre. Nonetheless, doctors were interested in new practices and therapies, not least when their adoption promised to improve their market position. As well as improving patient care and their own personal standing as a sympathetic family doctor, such developments were important in the wider ideology of improvement that was central to the professional middle class in mid-Victorian Britain.[5] Some GPs maintained professional links through membership in local medical associations, subscriptions to journals such as the *British Medical Journal* and *Lancet* and personal contacts. Some doctors had the inclination and time to follow developments in knowledge and even communicate their own ideas to fellow practitioners, but very few had the opportunities to make their own investigations.

An elite of group of physicians, who only dealt with 'internal' diseases, remained at the tip of the professional pyramid. Many enjoyed honorary posts as consultants in voluntary hospitals, which brought social connections along with wide experience and association with advanced practice. They worked part-time in hospitals with working-class patients, while the rest of their time was devoted to rich and middle-class private patients who they treated at home. There were differences between London, provincial and Scottish physicians. Metropolitan physicians played a major role in the Royal Colleges, while those in Scotland had close links with universities and developments in the natural sciences. In the English provinces and Wales situations varied greatly, and only in the largest towns and cities was it possible to practice as a pure physician. The aspirations and self-image of

3 I. Loudon, *Medical Care and the General Practitioner, 1750–1850*, Oxford, Clarendon Press, 1986.
4 A. Digby, *Making a Medical Living: Doctors and Patients in the English Market for Medicine, 1720–1911*, Cambridge, Cambridge University Press, 1994, 105–96.
5 H. Perkin, *The Rise of the Professional Society: England Since 1880*, London, Routledge, 1989.

physicians, if not of general practitioners, was to be a gentleman first and doctor second.[6] Professional success depended as much on social skills, general learning and experience as on technical expertise or medical knowledge. Clinicians sought to cut a figure that was resourceful, wise and insightful. Many practitioners seemed to be able to diagnose on sight from a patient's posture, demeanour, character or other features. The confidence that such powers inspired in patients was said to be important in maintaining the morale necessary for successful treatment. In part, this was because changes in ideas in the first half of the century had led physicians to treat less often and with less vigour than previously. They abandoned many so-called heroic therapies, such as bleeding and drugging, trusting more to the healing powers of nature and specific remedies, whose outcomes they monitored closely.[7]

Medicine per se, that is, the work of physicians and the nonsurgical activities of general practitioners, was the area in which modern germ theories of diseases were adopted last. In one sense this is not surprising, as 'internal' diseases were generally held to have internal origins and many conditions, such as functional diseases of the circulation and nerves, were never candidates for germ status. That said, doctors did not always regard 'disease-germs' as external contaminants or invaders; indeed, in the 1860s the most popular theories supposed that they arose within the body. Also, all doctors saw the external environment as an important factor in the origin and development of all manner of internal diseases, acting directly on tissues, as with the effects of colds and chills, or indirectly, as when predisposing the body to particular conditions, as with dampness leading to rheumatism. In the 1860s, the notion of 'germs of disease' was also used in a nonspecific sense to refer to the origins or cause of an illness. Yet, by the 1870s, the term was firmly linked to the modern concept of the 'germ theory of disease' – the aetiological construction of disease in which external agents entered the body to produce septic, infectious and other diseases.

Extensive debates about external, disease-causing germs took place first in surgery, with regard to septic infection, and then in public health, with zymotic diseases. Surgeons were also an elite group who had been below physicians in the pecking order because their work was manual, but who were rapidly gaining status and influence.[8] The nature of surgery in the 1860s needs careful delineation. To begin with, only in London and large towns,

6 C. Lawrence, *Medicine and the Making of Modern Britain, 1700–1920*, London, Macmillan, 1994, 57; C. Lawrence, '"Incommunicable Knowledge": Science, Technology and the Clinical "Art" in Britain, 1850–1910', *Journal of Contemporary History*, 1985, 20: 503–20.
7 W. F. Bynum, *Science and the Practice of Medicine in the Nineteenth Century*, Cambridge, Cambridge University Press, 1994, 226.
8 J. V. Pickstone, *Medicine in an Industrial Society: A History of Hospital Development in Manchester and its Region, 1752–1946*, Manchester, Manchester University Press, 1985, 191–3; R. Cooter, *Surgery and Society in Peace and War: Orthopaedics and the Organisation of Modern Medicine, 1880–1948*, Basingstoke, Macmillan, 1993.

especially the university towns of Scotland, was there a significant body of men who made a living solely from surgical practice. Most surgeons had dual qualifications, and had mixed businesses where they made their living from consultations and operations in 'surgeries' in their homes or, more usually, in their patients' homes.[9] Senior local surgeons often had part-time appointments in voluntary hospitals, where they offered their services gratis in return for the opportunity to hone skills and build up experience with the large number and variety of patients. Hospital appointments also provided opportunities to meet and attract private patients from amongst the wealthy and influential who served on boards of governors or were major subscribers. In the middle decades of the nineteenth century, surgeons' work changed, moving progressively from the 'exterior' to the 'interior' of the body, which was associated with hospital medicine and the development of localised pathology.[10] Yet, despite the availability of anaesthesia, surgeons performed relatively few elective operations and much of their work remained that of caring for external lesions and injuries.[11] Surgical practice was not an unmitigated round of blood, pus and sepsis. A typical pattern of work was that reported by William Lyons at the Glasgow Royal Infirmary over a six-month period in 1865. Half of his caseload comprised externally managed problems: bruises and lacerations (16%), fractures (14%), skin ulcers (13%) and scalds and burns (7%).[12] However, he chose to emphasise his operative work, which involved compound fractures, the excision of joints, the removal of malignant disease, amputations and hernias. Only with amputations and certain new operations, like ovariotomies, would his scalpel have penetrated deep into the body. Surgery in the 1860s may have had a nascent, heroic ideology, but practice tended to be limited and reactive.

Discussions on the future of surgery after midcentury offered a variety of prospects. Some surgeons looked to the refinement and extension of operations, while others welcomed the trend of surgery becoming more 'conservative' and even 'medical'. The elite Scottish surgeons James Miller (1812–64) and William Fergusson (1808–77) spoke of the 'head' having become more important than the 'hand', and the pen being substituted for the knife.[13] For

9 D. Hamilton and M. Lamb, 'Surgeons and Surgery', in O. Checkland and M. Lamb, eds., *Health Care as Social History*, Aberdeen, Aberdeen University Press, 74–80; C. Lawrence, ed., *Medical Theory, Surgical Practice*, London, Routledge, 1992.

10 O. Temkin, 'The Role of Surgery in the Rise of Medical Thought', *BHM*, 1951, 25: 248–59; R. C. Maulitz, *Morbid Appearances: The Anatomy of Pathology in the Early Nineteenth Century*, Cambridge, Cambridge University Press, 1987, 227–9.

11 Hamilton and Lamb, 'Surgeons', 77–80. On the complex impact of anaesthesia in the United States, see: M. J. Pernick, *A Calculus of Suffering: Pain, Professionalism and Anaesthesia in Nineteenth Century America*, New York, Columbia University Press, 1985.

12 *GMJ*, 1865–66, 13: 139–44.

13 J. Miller, *BMJ*, 1853, 342; W. Fergusson, *Lancet*, 1865, ii: 59. Fergusson, who had trained in Edinburgh, was Professor at King's College, London, 1840–1870. He was said to have invented the term 'conservative surgery'. See obituary notice in *EMJ*, 1876–77, 22: 856–61; G. Gordon Taylor, 'Sir William Fergusson, FRCS, FRS', *MH*, 1961, 5: 1–14.

example, in the treatment of syphilis, the cauterisation or excision of primary
lesions on the skin was regarded as ineffectual and surgeons relied on the
constitutional effects of mercury.[14] Key notions were that surgery now
required and displayed greater 'technique', 'precision' and 'exactness'.[15] Conservative methods, so-called because they avoided open operations, were routinely singled out for special praise, as too was the importance of after-care.[16]
Thus, the ideal surgeon was no longer a figure like Robert Liston, famed for
his boldness and speed, but the careful operator who used exact methods and
cared for the whole person before, during and after the operation.[17]

In the 1860s, the improving status of surgery was threatened when hospitals began to be criticised by sanitarian campaigners for their unhygienic conditions and consequent epidemics of septic diseases.[18] The determinants of a
purported 'crisis' were said to be the location of hospitals, their size and overcrowding, which together produced the great evils of smell, dirt and poor
ventilation. The principal manifestation of the problem was the prevalence of
so-called hospital diseases, which, because their origins lay in environmental
conditions, ought to be preventable. While the main targets of sanitarians were
hospital managers and patrons, surgeons were made complicit, not least when
comparisons were made between the higher mortality rates of hospital operations over those in private practice. The critics, with Florence Nightingale
amongst their leaders, were more generally critical of medical and surgical
practice for being reactive, waiting to undertake the usually hopeless task of
treating already developed diseases rather than proactively trying to prevent
illness arising in the first place.[19] Such comments usually missed their target,
partly because surgeons did not share sanitarians' views on the environmental origin of the hospital disease, and partly because surgeons, along with most
other doctors, were in fact very interested in disease prevention. Much advice
on regimen was preventive, treatments aimed to prevent the progress of
disease within the body and the convalescence advice aimed to halt the recur-
rence of disease.

Disease prevention applied to communities rather than individuals had

14 J. E. Erichsen, *The Science and Art of Surgery*, London, J. Walton, 1869, 8.
15 J. Miller, *Principles of Surgery*, Edinburgh, Adam and Charles Black, 1853.
16 See review of Erichsen's 1853 edition *BMJ*, 1853, 1065, where it is argued that the different mortality rates between surgeons is not due to their skill but their constitutional treatments.
17 G.Y. Heath, *BMJ*, ii, 1870, 163. F. F. Cartwright, *The Development of Modern Surgery*, London, Arthur
 Barker, 1967.
18 J. Farr, 'Miss Nightingale's "Notes on Hospitals"', *MTG*, 1864, i: 186–8, 491–2, and J. S. Bristowe
 and T. Holmes, 'The Hospitals of England', *Sixth Report of the Medical Officer of the Privy Council
 on the State of Public Health for 1863*, BPP 1864 [3416] xxviii, 1; A. J. Youngson, *The Scientific Revolution in Victorian Medicine*, London, Croom Helm, 1979, 164–71; J. H. Woodward, *'To Do the Sick
 no Harm': A Study of the British Voluntary Hospital System until 1875*, London, Routledge Kegan
 Paul, 1974.
19 On Florence Nightingale and sanitarianism, see: C. E. Rosenberg, 'Florence Nightingale on Contagion: The Hospital as Moral Universe', in C. E. Rosenberg, ed., *Healing and History: Essays for
 George Rosen*, New York, SHP, 1979, 116–36.

become the responsibility of a new group within medicine in the 1850s – the Medical Officers of Health (MOsH). They had emerged from the wider sanitary reform movement with the specific brief of reducing 'preventable deaths' from contagious and infectious diseases, and assisting with the administrative work of local boards of health. Various names were given to the medical side of this public health work – sanitary science, state medicine, hygiene and, latterly, preventive medicine. I use the term 'public health medicine' to emphasise that I am concentrating on the medical aspect of a much broader enterprise that included chemistry, meteorology, civil engineering, the law and other disciplines.[20] The preferred term within the profession in the 1860s was 'state medicine', which had been coined by Henry Rumsey (1809–76) in 1846 but only gained currency after the appointment of John Simon to lead the Medical Department of the Privy Council in the mid-1850s.[21] The operation of Simon's department was seen to define the term in Britain and also exemplify its difficulties. The department inherited from Chadwick's Board of Health the task of fulfilling the state's responsibility to ameliorate the health problems of urbanisation and industrialisation, by protecting the public from preventable diseases.[22] Established as a central agency, the department had to operate through legislation that local authorities were supposed to implement. However, the permissive character of many of the acts, and the limited powers of the department to enforce compliance, showed where the balance between state intervention and *laissez faire* had been struck in mid-Victorian Britain.

At the end of the 1860s, local authorities in England and Wales had appointed only fifty MOsH.[23] Many posts were part-time and tenure precarious, while low pay and poor conditions ensured that the position was not a prestigious one. For many newly qualified doctors, the post of MOH was the first step on the career ladder, while older practitioners either found the extra income useful or welcomed the opportunity to promote local 'improvements'.[24] In many ways MOsH occupied administrative rather than medical posts. They had to contend with a strong lay interest and involvement, plus the fact that engineers and other functionaries controlled many sanitary services. Through the British Medical Association (BMA) and local groupings,

20 D. E. Watkins, *The English Revolution in Social Medicine, 1889–1911*, Unpublished PhD Thesis, University of London, 1984. The preferred term within the profession in the 1860s was 'state medicine', and this continued to be used well into the 1880s, before being replaced by 'preventive medicine' and 'hygiene'.

21 R. MacLeod, 'The Anatomy of State Medicine', in F. N. L. Poynter, ed., *Medicine and Science in the 1860s*, London, Wellcome Institute for the History of Medicine, 1968, 199–227.

22 On Edwin Chadwick (1800–1890) see: C. Hamlin, *Public Health and Social Justice in the Age of Chadwick: Britain, 1800–54*, Cambridge, Cambridge University Press, 1998.

23 J. L. Brand, *Doctors and the State: The British Medical Profession and Government Action in Public Health, 1870–1912*, Baltimore, MD, Johns Hopkins University Press, 1965, 108–15.

24 C. Lawrence, 'Sanitary Reformers and the Medical Profession in Victorian England', T. Ogawa, ed., *Public Health: Proceedings of the Fifth International Symposium on Comparative History of Medicine: East and West*, Toyko, Saikon, 1980, 145–68.

such as the Metropolitan Society of MOsH from 1856, public health doctors became organised and, according to Porter, developed an identity distinct from that of the profession as a whole.[25] The day-to-day work of MOsH involved both sanitary regulation and disease control. They supervised teams of sanitary inspectors who were responsible for the collection of statistics and for monitoring housing, drains, the water supply, nuisances (which included human wastes as well as fly-tips, abattoirs and industrial hazards) and food adulteration. Local MOsH had a strategic role in recording, coordinating and publishing much of this information, adjudicating in disputes and negotiating with the local council and other vested interests. More directly medical and technical duties were also involved: the diagnosis of epidemic diseases, the disinfection of homes and people, the management of any smallpox or isolation hospital and, though it was formally the responsibility of the Poor Law Guardians, often the oversight of vaccinations. These duties were normally routine and mundane, but during local and national epidemics their work could be demanding and very high profile. However, MOsH felt that their work was circumscribed and that they had neither the professional power nor the administrative autonomy to protect public health effectively.

Simon developed the role of his central department as one of providing information and advice to local boards of health and then MOsH. The policy was evident in the mass of inquiries and reports made by the department's peripatetic inspectors.[26] Simon trusted in the first instance to the power of statistics and critical reports to shame local authorities into action, except on vaccinations and medical registrations where compulsion was used. The Sanitary Act, 1866, introduced compulsion into sanitary affairs in a limited way, a departure that was thought in no small measure to be the precedents established during the cattle plague crisis of 1865–66. However, the new legislation brought so many administrative complications and conflicts that within two years a Royal Commission was appointed to sort out the mess and rationalise measures.[27] Despite all of the problems, public health medicine had a high national profile, due to the continuing work of sanitary reformers, national and local sanitary associations and the social impact of epidemics.

Simon, through his own work and that funded by the Medical Department, was also a pioneer of medical science in Britain. Before moving to state medicine he practised as a surgeon, and was also well known as a

25 D. Porter, 'Stratification and its Discontents: Professionalisation and Conflict in the British Public Health Service, 1848–1944', in E. Fee and R. Acheson, eds., *A History of Education in Public Health: Health that Mocks the Doctors' Rules*, Oxford, Oxford Medical Publications, 1991, 83–113.

26 R. Lambert, *Sir John Simon 1816–1904 and English Social Administration*, London, MacGibbon and Kee, 1963.

27 A. P. Stewart and E. Jenkins, *The Medical and Legal Aspects of Sanitary Reform*, 1866, (Reprinted, with an introduction by M. W. Flinn), Leicester, Leicester University Press, 1969, xvii–xxiv. The importance of the cattle plague to public health has recently been reassessed by historians. See: A. Hardy, *The Epidemic Streets: Infectious Disease and the Rise of Preventive Medicine, 1856–1900*, Oxford, Clarendon Press, 1993, 6.

pathologist, being elected a Fellow of the Royal Society. Scientific investigations had been important in public health since the 1830s, first in statistical studies and then in chemical analyses of air, water, wastes and other matter. Simon's department was given authority for 'Laboratory Investigations' in 1865 and employed, on a part-time basis, several doctors who became leading medical scientists of the last quarter of the century, most notably John Burdon Sanderson and Edward Klein. Although the number of workers was small, their investigations limited and their results often inconclusive, the influence of their investigations was cumulatively significant. Simon's position and skill ensured that the findings received maximum publicity, which was facilitated by the fact that they were often on topics of medical and social importance, such as cholera, smallpox and tuberculosis. The investigations also represented state endorsement of the scientific laboratory as a source of medical knowledge, which in the 1860s was not uncontroversial within the profession or in the wider society due to the strength of antivivisection sentiments.

The teaching of the physical and biological sciences had long been an important part of medical education, as knowledge of physics, chemistry and botany was the basis for many medical ideas and practices. As these sciences became more specialised and technical, medical schools could no longer rely on part-time lecturers drawn from the ranks of the profession or from outside. There was no shortage of potential recruits to new teaching posts as many of the leading scientists of the day, for example, T. H. Huxley (1825–95) and Michael Foster (1836–1907), had first trained in medicine, this being the only route to higher learning in the biological sciences. However, the attempts to make science a profession led reformers to argue that full-time positions ought to be established in medical schools, backed up by appropriate facilities. Those responsible for the basic sciences in the medical curriculum also argued that the proper training of doctors required experience of experimental methods to illustrate scientific principles and methods. Such claims were advanced strongly by advocates of the reborn discipline of physiology, which claimed to be the leading biological science and the essential basis of medical knowledge and practice.[28]

As important as the generation of new knowledge were the methods of physiological science, principally (animal) experimentation, plus physical measurements, chemical analysis and microscopy. These symbolised the shift to new scientific styles, though reformers tried to moderate this by stressing continuities with apprenticeship, learning by doing and broader educational

28 S. E. D. Shortt, 'Physicians, Science and Status: Issues in the Professionalisation of Anglo-American Medicine in the Nineteenth Century', *MH*, 1983, 27: 51–68; J. V. Pickstone, 'Physiology and experimental medicine', in R. Olby et al., eds., *Encyclopaedia of the History of Science*, London, Routledge, 1989, 728–42; S. V. F. Butler, *Science and the Education of Doctors in the Nineteenth Century: a Study of British Medical Schools with Particular Reference to the Uses and Development of Physiology*, Unpublished PhD thesis, University of Manchester Institute of Science and Technology, 1982.

values. Physiological work was said to teach student doctors logical thought and analytical reasoning, to make them better observers and to inculcate a research orientation. Enthusiasts for physiology and established clinicians agreed about the virtues of science for the profession and its ideology, however, they were often talking about different features and meanings of science.[29]

DISEASE THEORIES, C. 1865

There are two main difficulties in characterising disease theories in the mid-1860s. The first is that medicine was very diverse, with many types of practices, interests and conflicting as well as common ideas. The second is that one of the few things that doctors did agree on was to avoid 'theory' and to try to be empiricists who did not have overarching principles. Antipathy to theory was central to the identity of the modern profession as it celebrated the abandonment of the 'systems', 'rationalism' and speculation that had characterised eighteenth-century medicine. Medicine was portrayed by its mid-Victorian propagandists as based on experience, with doctors working inductively, building up their knowledge and practice from careful observation.

The key conceptual revolution of the first half of the nineteenth century – localised pathology – was said by the profession's leaders to be the great result of this empirical and positivist turn.[30] This new construction of disease had been produced by the opportunities that hospital work had given doctors to see many more sick people, to compare and contrast cases, and to correlate symptoms and signs in life with tissue changes observed post mortem. Physicians and surgeons produced new classifications of diseases (nosologies) based on precise symptoms and anatomical changes. The critical change was that disease was increasingly seen, literally in dissections, to be contained in lesions within particular tissues or organs, and not to be a property of the whole body. Other changes were associated with localised pathology. Doctors defined specific diseases largely in terms of their morbid anatomy, introducing conceptions of disease as altered structures. This notion, sometimes referred to as solidism, contrasted with the earlier humoralism that was characterised by fluidism. The rise of the localist views of disease and anatomical constructions of the body owed much to the growing influence of surgeons relative to holist-oriented physicians. The *structural–anatomical* construction of the body provided new possibilities for surgical intervention, for example, in repairing or removing damaged parts.[31] Sigerist made this point

---

29 Lawrence, 'Incommunicable Knowledge', 505–12; J. H. Warner, 'Ideals of Science and Their Discontents in Late Nineteenth Century American Medicine', *Isis*, 1991, 82: 454–78.
30 N. D. Jewson, 'The Disappearance of the Sickman from Medical Cosmology, 1770–1870', *Sociology*, 1978, 10: 225–44.
31 R. C. Maulitz, 'The Pathological Tradition', in W. F. Bynum and R. Porter, eds., *Companion Encyclopaedia of the History of Medicine*, London, Routledge, 1993, 169–91.

when he observed that 'Surgery became great, not because anaesthesia and antisepsis were introduced, but anaesthesia and antisepsis were found because surgery was to become great; because surgery was the anatomical method of therapy.'[32]

Hospital patients were often treated by doctors as mere bodies, in part because they lost certain rights on entry to state or voluntary institutions and in part because they were often of the lowest social caste. Enjoying considerable power over patients, doctors became less inhibited about physical examinations. Many new kinds of 'hands-on' examinations were developed in the first half of the nineteenth century, and new investigative technologies were invented, such as the stethoscope, laryngoscope, speculum and clinical thermometer. Doctors were also under less pressure than in private practice to show that they were having an effect, so they were able to wait and see, which allowed them to observe the natural history of disease. Such opportunities made hospitals and their patients valuable resources for research and teaching; they literally became 'museums' of disease, at least for medical students and medical investigators. The large numbers of patients enabled statistics to be collected about the fate of various diseases and the success of treatments. Such studies revealed that many common remedies had little or no influence on the outcome of diseases, and these were a key force behind the 'therapeutic scepticism' and trust in the healing powers of nature that came into vogue in the mid-Victorian period. Doctors were able to describe and diagnose diseases more finely but bemoaned that this was not matched by their ability to treat effectively.

By the 1860s, the frontier of medical understanding was shifting from morbid anatomy and the style of natural history to physiology and experimental biology.[33] Accounts of diseases were being recast in terms of disordered functions as well as altered structures. The social basis of this change was that the hospital was being displaced by the laboratory as the source and arbiter of medical knowledge.[34] In the hands of Claude Bernard (1813–78) in France, physiology was made an overarching medical science, with the ambition of exploring normal and abnormal functions.[35] Physiological institutes in Germany developed similar methods, although with a programme to explain physiological processes by reducing them to physics and chemistry. The general aim of physiologists was to be able to manipulate and control bodily systems, to reveal the causes of deviations from normal function and perhaps to show where interventions in these processes could prevent or cure

32 C. Lawrence, 'Democratic, Divine and Heroic', in Lawrence, *Medical Theory*, 24.
33 J. V. Pickstone, 'Ways of Knowing: Towards a Historical Sociology of Science', *BJHS*, 1993, 26: 449–52.
34 E. Ackerknecht, *Medicine at the Paris Hospital, 1794–1848*, Baltimore, MD, Johns Hopkins University Press, 1967.
35 Bynum, *Science and the Practice*, 94–109.

diseases.[36] In Britain, only a few investigators pursued the trajectory of developing an applied medical science; most physiologists studied general principles in plants and lower animals, not abnormal function in humans or other mammals. There were many reasons for this, particularly the dominance of university departments over those in medical schools; the role of physiology in medical schools as a basic, preclinical science; the influence of antivivisection sentiment and the continuing power of the natural history tradition in British biology as exemplified by the publication of Darwin's *On the Origin of Species* in 1859.[37]

From the perspective of hospital and laboratory medicine, many doctors advanced the claim that diseases were specific, that is, disease states could be precisely defined, like plant or animal species, and were universal – being very similar entities in every body, place and time.[38] Within this framework, they proposed that treatments could and should also become specific, even standardised.[39] In the eyes of older doctors, the notion of disease specificity went hand-in-hand with ontological conceptions of disease and was an anathema. And it was not just older doctors who felt this. The new ideas of disease as an altered structure or abnormal function seemed quite congruent with physiological conceptions of disease. So constituted, 'diseases' were the manifestation of alterations and abnormalities, perhaps positive bodily responses to be encouraged as much as combated. Henry Letheby explained the point as follows in 1869:

We recognise that disease, as Sir John Forbes expressed it, 'is not a new thing superadded to the living body, and constituting a special entity in *revum naturâ* but is merely the result or an expression of an effect of nature to get rid of the poison which has been introduced from without, or developed within the body by a process of modified or abnormal nutrition'.[40]

This statement is all the more significant because Letheby went on to give his firm backing to the idea that the contagia of smallpox, syphilis, cholera and probably most zymotic disease were due to 'the operation of specific molecular living things' or 'living germs' when they meet with 'a congenial nidus'.

36 W. Coleman and F. L. Homes, eds., *The Investigative Enterprise: Experimental Physiology in Nineteenth Century Medicine*, Berkeley, University of California Press, 1988; J. H. Warner, 'Physiological Theory and Therapeutic Explanation in the 1860s: The British Debate on the Medical Uses of Alcohol', *BHM*, 1980, 54: 253–57.
37 G. L. Geison, *Michael Foster and the Cambridge School of Physiology*, Princeton, NJ: Princeton University Press, 1978.
38 M. Pelling, 'Contagion/Germ Theory/Specificity', in Bynum, *Companion Encyclopaedia*, 321–30.
39 J. H. Warner, 'From Specificity to Universalism in Medical Therapeutics: Transformation in the Nineteenth Century United States, in Y. Kawaita et al., eds., *History of Therapy: Proceedings of the Tenth International Symposium of Comparative Medicine: East and West*, Tokyo, Ishiyaku EuroAmerica Inc., 1990, 193–223.
40 H. Letheby, 'Introductory Lecture at the London Hospital, *BMJ*, 1869, ii: 297. Letheby was MOH for the City of London. Sir John Forbes (1787–1861) was a physician and founder of the *British and Foreign Medical Review*.

The notion of disease specificity was also interpreted in terms of uniqueness rather than universalism. Older physicians linked the idea to the position that disease-states were peculiar to individual bodies, and to time and place. This allowed them to fashion diseases as the unique result of an interaction between an individual's physical constitution, their lifestyle and behaviour, all acting in the context of their social and physical environments.[41] The singularity of diseases meant that each illness required custom-made therapy, as explained in a *Lancet* editorial in 1869:

Physicians who have learned their lesson at the bedside, and who know that the object of the healing art is not to cure a disease, but to treat a patient, will not waste their labour in the vain search after specific methods. In every case they will find scope for a wise eclecticism, and for the judicious administration of well-chosen remedies.[42]

In practice, doctors did not have to choose between the different meanings of specificity, as the individual case could be pictured as a variation, perhaps a subspecies, of a universal type of disease. For example, in the 1860s doctors still diagnosed English and Asiatic cholera, and saw cases where the former transmuted into the latter more serious condition. In their therapies, doctors would use standard drugs, such as quinine, in combination with prescriptions they thought appropriate to the particular case. Therapies were still used in holistic ways, aiming to 'lower' the system in cases of fever or inflammatory diseases, or to 'raise' the system in cases of degenerative or debilitating illnesses. However, therapies were increasingly given physiological rationales, such as improving tissue nutrition, aiding circulation and vitality, lowering nervous activity or increasing excretion.

Underlying the differences in professional ideologies and conceptions of disease was a commitment to rooting medicine in the natural sciences, and to naturalistic explanations of health and sickness. Rosenberg sums up this change by saying that, after midcentury, 'whether one emphasised anatomical change [solidism] or physiological function [humoralism or fluidism], symptoms were the consequence of specific material mechanisms'.[43] Doctors saw diseases as the visible manifestation of underlying biological changes, where each illness had a 'beginning' (pathogenesis), a 'middle' (pathophysiology) and an 'end' (morbid anatomy). Interestingly, the development of medicine in the nineteenth century worked backwards through this sequence. Morbid anatomy and pathology were the most developed and dominant subjects in 1850. Their position was displaced by physiology and pathophysiology by 1875, with bacteriology and experimental pathology, with their

41 C. E. Rosenberg, *Explaining Epidemics and Other Studies in the History of Medicine*, Cambridge, Cambridge University Press, 1992, 9–31.
42 *Lancet*, 1869, i: 164. J. E. Pollock observed that specific treatment in consumption should be aimed at correcting the diathesis not attacking the tubercular deposits. J. E. Pollock, *The Elements of Prognosis in Consumption*, London, Longmans, Green, 1865.
43 Rosenberg, *Explaining*, 266.

aetiological models, taking over by 1900. Thus, in the period 1865–1900, medical scientists moved their primary gaze from the results of disease to disease processes, and then to causes, though this sequence is best seen as additive and overlapping, rather than a series of paradigm shifts.

In the 1850s and 1860s, pathology took another reductionist turn, changing from the study of the morbid anatomy of gross lesions to cellular pathology and intimate alterations in cells and their position.[44] The creation of the 'cellular body', for all life forms from the 1830s, was critical to this reorientation.[45] The microscope was first applied to produce even finer distinctions between tissue changes, and in some cases it was possible to make these from specimens taken from the sick person.[46] Secondly, and more importantly, the microscope was used to study disease processes, either from sequences of morbid materials from different stages of a disease or from observations in experimental animals. Rudolph Virchow (1821–1904) pioneered the former and his student Julius Cohnheim (1839–84) the latter, especially in his investigations of inflammation that showed migrations of white blood cells.[47] The work of both was influential in Britain, not least because of the numbers of students and doctors who visited laboratories in Germany to learn of advanced work and to use the experimental facilities. The changes in pathology during the 1860s were reflected in T. H. Green's popular textbook of pathology, first published in 1871.[48] Green was a graduate of University College Hospital, London, who had studied in Virchow's Institute in Berlin and was Assistant Physician, Lecturer on Pathology and Superintendent of Post Mortem Examinations at Charing Cross Hospital, London. His book was structured around the assumption that there were two kinds of changes in diseased tissues and cells – *degenerative* and *inflammatory*. In fact, this gave three processes: (i) degeneration; (ii) degenerative change combined with inflammation (e.g. tumours) and (iii) inflammation. Most of the text described the many different types of degeneration and inflammation, illustrated by the changes in tissues and cells revealed by the microscope. Medical students and interested practitioners would also have referred to Lionel Beale's two guides to the use of the microscope in medicine, which went through many editions for the 1850s and remained essential handbooks for such work until overtaken by bacteriology manuals in the 1880s.[49]

Typically, Green's textbook was little concerned with the causes of pathological changes, although he did outline general principles. The origins of

44 Maulitz, 'Pathological Tradition', 179–83.   45 Bynum, *Science and the Practice*, 100, 123–6.
46 B. Bracegirdle, 'The Microscopical Tradition', in Bynum, *Companion Encyclopaedia*, 104–12.
47 R. Maulitz, 'Rudolf Virchow, Julius Cohnheim and the Programme of Pathology', *BHM*, 1978, 52: 162–82.
48 T. H. Green, *An Introduction to Pathology and Morbid Anatomy*, London, Henry Renshaw, 1871. Green noted that the other great division in pathology was between 'organic' and 'functional' disorders.
49 L. S. Beale, *The Microscope, and its Application to Clinical Medicine*, London, S. Higley, 1854; idem, *How to Work with the Microscope*, London, Churchill, 1861. Fifth and final edition in 1880.

degenerative changes were said to lie in physiological weaknesses, poor nutrition or inherited tendencies, or were prompted by injury or irritation. In many cases the origin would appear to be spontaneous, precipitated by internal forces that medical science had not, and might never, comprehend. I feel that it is worth restating the point that this situation was not seen as a problem. As we have seen, traditional physic and modern medical science had not constituted disease in causal terms, where treatment would focus on removing causes. Disease involved structural or functional perturbations, and hence treatment was in large part about positive interventions to promote repair, to restore function or to aid the regeneration of damaged structures. Only in a limited number of conditions, mostly in surgery, were interventions negative actions designed to counter processes or remove lesions. Inflammations were usually ascribed to injuries, so causes were less mysterious and many obviously came from outside of the body. Green listed four origins of inflammation: traumatic (mechanical, chemical or temperature), infective, idiopathic, and specific (as in smallpox).[50] There was much debate on the status of inflammation: Was it a normal healthy process to be encouraged, or a pathogenic process to be countered? Surgeons recognised healthy and unhealthy wound healing, producing, respectively, 'laudable pus' and infected pus.[51] The ideal form of wound healing – 'healing by first intention' – saw clean-cut tissues brought together to rejoin with little inflammation, and without serious scabbing and scarring. With open or deep wounds, where tissue had been lost or killed, inflammation seemed inevitable and was linked to the process in which new (granulation) tissue grew across the wound. The disturbance caused by the initial tissue damage, and the time taken to heal, made these wounds more prone to abnormal inflammation, mortification (i.e. degeneration) and perhaps sepsis – an infective process and an example of Green's second source of inflammation. In the 1860s, the term 'infective' was used in pathology for the internal spread of morbid cells, as in cancers, or chemical poisons, as with septic and zymotic diseases. The term 'infectious' for the person-to-person transmission of the disease, directly or indirectly, was not that commonly used, even in public health medicine, where contagion and miasmatic were the preferred terms.

Interest in the chemistry of the body had been stimulated by localised pathology, as it appeared that local lesions often produced systemic effects on the whole body by chemical means. Altering the body's chemistry through nutrition or drugs that directly changed the internal milieu, or acted indirectly by altering the rates of processes like excretion, was a major approach in therapeutics. Anaesthetics showed the potential of chemicals for local and systemic

---

50 Green based his chapters on inflammation on Sanderson's teaching as reflected in Holmes's surgical textbook. T. Holmes, ed., *System of Surgery*, 5 vols., London, Longmans, Green, 1870–71.
51 C. Lawrence and R. Dixey, 'Practising on Principle: Joseph Lister and the Germ Theories of Disease', in Lawrence, *Medical Theory*, 158–62. Only in the 1870s and 1880s was all pus remade as dangerous.

Table 1. *Comparison of Fermentation, Putrefaction, Sepsis and Zymosis*

Fermentation	Putrefaction	Septic disease process	Zymotic disease process
Seeding the liquor	*Contamination of dead matter*	Contamination of dead matter or devitalised tissues	'The manifest introduction into the system of a virus (ferment, zyme, virus, germ)'
Delay in activity	*Delay in activity*	Slow start but process accelerates	Incubation, or the virus 'lying dormant for a certain period'
Effervescence	*Decomposition*	Festering, suppuration, mortification	'The enormous increase and multiplication of the poison' giving inflammation, sweating
Rise in temperature	*Rise in temperature*	Fever, production of foul sweet smell	'The production of fever'
Exhaustion of substrate	*Destruction of organic matter*	Destruction or disintegration of tissue	Subsidence of disease and the possibility of subsequent immunity

effects, while the commercial success of chemists, druggists and heterodox medical systems, many still based on humoral models, showed the wide currency of the 'chemical body'. Septic and zymotic disease processes had been considered purely chemical, but in the 1860s many scientists, led by Pasteur, argued that they were 'vital processes'. The challenge came from new views of the nature of fermentation and putrefaction, which had been accepted as analogues, respectively, for zymotic and septic diseases. Interests in chemical explanations of diseases had led doctors to highlight similarities between the general properties of fermentation and zymotic disease processes, for example, rises in temperature, the delay in the process starting and the exponential increase in activity before the process halted (see Table 1). Indeed, the reliance on analogy meant that doctors spoke and wrote of the zymotic 'theory' of disease.

The most developed thinking on this topic was that of the German chemist Justus von Liebig.[52] Zymotic theory was rooted in Liebig's ideas of decomposition and degeneration, where disease was seen as 'a spreading internal rot, that . . . came from an external rot, and . . . could be transferred to others'.[53] The agent responsible was assumed to be a chemical and was referred to as a 'zyme',

52 W. H. Brock, *Justus von Liebig: The Chemical Gatekeeper*, Cambridge, Cambridge University Press, 1998.
53 C. Hamlin, 'Providence and Putrefaction: Victorian Sanitarians and the Natural Theology of Health and Disease', *Victorian Studies*, 1985, 28: 386.

or, more usually, a 'ferment', because of its ability to excite chemical changes or the breakdown of tissues. It is important to note that ferments are not disease entities; they are best thought of as catalysts that could, in the right bodily and environmental conditions, initiate disease processes, or, like sparks, start fires. Zymotic disease ferments were thought to arise from a number of sources. At one extreme were the noncontagious diseases, such as malaria and cholera, whose poisons arose spontaneously from rotting vegetable matter in the environment and were quite durable. At the other pole were the highly contagious diseases, such as smallpox, whose poison or virus was assumed to be short-lived, having arisen spontaneously, or been nurtured, in another animal body. Their immediate origin and affinities with animal physiologies seemed to allow such contagious ferments to act more rapidly and with greater virulence than those from vegetable or environmental sources. In fact, smallpox and other highly contagious diseases were said to be spread and caused by so-called *contagium viva*, which translates as living contagia, or, to be more historically accurate, contagia with the properties of living matter. Thus there were potential, though not necessary, continuities between explanations of disease due to contagium viva (or the older term *Contagium animata*) and those due to living germs. Septic ferments, also thought to be of animal origins, were believed to be simpler, being the breakdown products of freshly rotting tissues. Zymotic disease processes were essentially 'fluidist', with changes in the blood a major site of disturbances.

The idea of poison diffusing radially from a foci of dead tissue was accommodated to the new cellular pathology. Virchow had proposed that all disease was due to the malfunctioning of existing cells, not to the production of new and distinct diseased cells. As we will see, this commitment often led Virchow and other cell theorists to set themselves against germ theories of all types. Doctors who adopted cellular pathology to guide their work presumed that changes to cells were wrought, either by internal malfunctions (as in cancers) or by the influence of extracellular stimuli, be these derived from the internal bodily milieu or from the wider environment, as in the remote effects of epidemic conditions. Whatever their origin, morbid changes were believed to spread from cell to cell by chemical, physical or even nervous stimuli, not from the movement of old cells or the proliferation of new ones. In 1864, the Cambridge surgeon George Humphry (1820–96) explained what all this meant for septic disease:

[It] spreads not by the propagation and dissemination of germs, but by impressing upon the nutritive processes in adjacent tissues, or in other parts of the body, of a tendency to like variation of its own; that is to say, by assimilation and fermentation, rather than by germination.[54]

54 *BMJ*, 1864, ii: 184. Humphry contended that pyaemia had constitutional origins, rather than being due to accidental contamination or the diffusion of pus. Hence he favoured the open method, plus general treatment with stimulants, fresh air and cleanliness.

Humphry uses the word 'germ' here to refer to the growth of new protoplasm, cells or tissues within the body, not to an external disease agent.[55]
'Germ' was, of course, a contraction of 'germinal matter' – the seeds, spores
or other reproductive form of any organism.[56] Also, the development of
genetics in the final decades of the nineteenth century saw a growing use of
the notion of 'germ plasm' for reproductive cells, although by this time 'bacteria' had replaced 'germ' in discourses on diseases. The use of 'germ' for new
disease-matter was not uncommon in the 1860s. For example, in 1861 Horace
Dobell (1828–1917) published his book entitled *Germs and Vestiges of Disease*,
in which he argued that the (subcellular) remnants of previous diseases
remained dormant in the body as 'evasive and occult beings', and could
emerge again to reawaken the specific disease, or lurked insidiously under-
mining general health.[57] As we will see, the most developed notion on
disease-germs in the mid-1860s was the bioplasm theory of Lionel Beale,
who maintained that many diseases were due to the action of degraded protoplasmic elements formed from the protoplasm of defective or dead cells.
In other words, Beale's view was that the 'germs of disease' were produced
within the body. The sense of 'germs' as external contaminants was most commonly associated with 'fungus theories' of epidemic diseases, which had
largely failed to explain cholera in 1848–49, and to the more recent work of
Hallier on the same disease.[58] In fungal and parasitic accounts of disease, the
causative agent was, literally, the seeds, spores, eggs or adult form of another
organism, which was believed to alter the structure or function of the human
body when they settled and developed in what was for them an unnatural
milieu. That said, a large part of the attraction of the word 'germ' in the
1860s, and later, seems to have been the flexibility of its protean meanings.[59]

In public health medicine, the chemical version of zymotic theory had
been applied to four groups of diseases, as in William Farr's (1807–83) classification in 1854:

> **Miasmatic** – diffusible through air or water and producing fevers of two main
> types: those derived from the human body or animal matter, such as smallpox;
> and those derived from the earth and plant matter, such as ague (malaria).
>
> **Contagious** (Enthetic – 'introduced from without') – communicated person-
> to-person by contact, puncture or inoculation, such as syphilis or glanders.

55 J. Morris, *Germinal Matter and the Contact Theory: An Essay on Morbid Poisons, their Nature, Sources, Effects, Migrations and Means of Limiting their Noxious Effects*, London, Churchill, 1867.
56 J. K. Crellin, 'The Dawn of the Germ Theory: Particles, Infection and Biology', Poynter, *Science and Medicine*, 57–76.
57 H. Dobell, *Lecture on the Germs and Vestiges of Disease and on the Prevention of the Invasion and Fatality of Disease by Periodic Examination*, London, John Churchill, 1861. Dobell was a physician to the Royal Infirmary for Diseases of the Chest, London.
58 Pelling, *Cholera, Fever*, 147–202.
59 L. W. Sedgwick, 'A Report on the Parasitic Theory of Disease', *Transactions of the St Andrew's Graduates Association*, 1869, 116–48.

Dietetic – arising in the blood from poor diet or bad food, for example, scurvy.
Parasitic – animal and plant organisms infesting the skin, intestines and other structures of the body.[60]

Public health medicine concerned itself mainly with the first category, although the prevention of food poisoning (e.g. ergots from wheat), food contamination (e.g. tapeworms from mealy pork) and parasitic infestations (e.g. lice) were within its remit, and the extension of the Contagious Diseases Acts to control syphilis beyond garrison towns was a common plea amongst medical men in the mid-1860s.[61] The Contagious Diseases (Animals) Act, 1869, was passed to try to control epizootic diseases, such as the cattle plague and bovine pleuropneumonia, which were assumed to be passed by close contact. Contagious diseases were experienced as amongst the most specific, following a definite sequence of symptoms and pathological changes. Smallpox exemplified this, and its contagiousness was felt to be almost tangible – people felt that they could see and feel particles breaking off from pustules on the skin of fevered bodies and floating in the air. These particles were also spoken of as 'viruses', 'poisons' or 'fomites', the latter word being used both for the disease-agent itself and for anything that might be carrying it. How similar these agents were to chemical poisons was a moot point, and became more controversial as living germ theories were advanced more forcefully. Proponents of chemical ideas argued that zymes should not be considered as akin to inorganic poisons. Rather, they were best regarded as complex organic molecules that had properties such as delayed effects, followed by exponential rates of development and the mitigation of effects over time; the growth of crystals in solution was another common analogy.

Sanitary reform in the 1840s, ideologically and practically, was centred on campaigns against dirt and overcrowding. Sanitarians aimed to implement environmental improvements to remove the conditions in which epidemic and zymotic disease poisons arose and spread. In the early 1860s sanitarian beliefs about the origins of epidemics were given a new gloss by Charles Murchison's 'pythogenic theory of disease', that is, diseases generated from filth. In the mid-1860s zymotic theory remained a 'theory' in the sense that no one had isolated or determined the exact nature of any disease poison, ferment, zyme or 'dirt'. There were many claims to have isolated disease-agents – chemical, vegetable and animal – but few stood the test of critical evaluation. In the 1860s disease-poisons were generally understood to be complex organic chemicals, possibly an alkaloid (a nitrogen-based compound), capable of crystal-like 'growth'.[62] Chemists' work with organic mol-

---

60 W. Farr, *Sixteenth Annual Report of the Registrar General for 1854*, BPP, 1855 [1970], xv, 1.
61 F. Mort, *Dangerous Sexualities: Medico-Moral Politics in England since 1830*, London, Routledge Kegan Paul, 1987.
62 C. Hamlin, *A Science of Impurity: Water Analysis in Nineteenth Century England*, Bristol, Adam Hilger, 1990, 133.

ecules from living organisms pointed to their having special properties, possibly akin to living matter itself.[63] Debate in medicine, such as it was, concentrated on the physical form of ferments (gas, liquid, solid or particulate), rather than whether they were animal, vegetable or mineral. The very idea that the poison might be a living being or 'organic-germ' seemed old-fashioned, for example, a rerun of the cholera–fungus controversy, of early modern notions of 'animalcules' as the causes of disease and even back to Aristotle.[64] This was a sensitive issue, as MOsH believed that their 'practice' was 'very far in advance of theory'. They maintained that, despite knowing little or nothing about the intimate nature of disease-poisons, they knew how to reduce their spread, virulence and effects.[65] Trends in the incidence of epidemics and falls in mortality rates, despite increasing urbanisation and industrialisation, implied that something, most probably sanitary reform, had improved the health of towns since the 1840s and was continuing to do so.

The term 'miasmatic' is one of the most ambiguous terms in the history of nineteenth-century medicine. It is now associated with the idea of disease-poisons wafting around in mists, and with vague 'prescientific' thinking, often cited as a symbol of medical ignorance before germ-theory. In fact, miasmatic explanations of disease were historically quite precise and amongst the most well-grounded ideas of the Victorian period. Rather than being refuted or overturned by the adoption of 'true' germ theories of disease, the meanings of miasmas were refined until they were subsumed within a spectrum of contagious and infectious diseases. From the 1860s, the term 'contagious' was increasingly applied to 'catching' airborne diseases, transmitted directly at very close quarters (e.g. smallpox), as well as those transmitted by inoculation (e.g. syphilis) or touch (e.g. scabies). This left those diseases 'transmitted-at-a-distance' by whatever means. This large group seemed to be of two types: those where the poisons came from another person, for which the term 'infectious' began to be used; and those where the poisons came from the environment, such as malaria, for which 'miasmatic' continued to be used. The model infectious disease became typhoid fever. Its poisons or germs were believed to be carried in excremental discharges, spreading in the water supply, in food or in escaping sewer gases. However, many doctors and scientists believed that the poison or germ went through certain developmental stages outside of the body. The most influential ideas on events in this out-of-body period were those of the German hygienist Max von Pettenkofer.[66] He maintained that poisons (or germs) underwent changes in the soil, influenced primarily by groundwater levels but with other variables also

63 W. H. Brock, *Fontana History of Chemistry*, London, Fontana, 1995.
64 Pelling, *Cholera, Fever*, 146–202.
65 C. A. Cameron, 'Public health', *DQJMS*, 1869, 48: 608.
66 C. E. A. Winslow, *Conquest of Epidemic Disease: A Chapter in the History of Ideas*, 1943, Madison, University of Wisconsin Press, 1980, 311–20.

playing a determinant role. British followers of Pettenkofer, of whom there were many in public health medicine, often termed such diseases 'contagious-miasmatic'. One reason why these ideas were popular was that they offered an explanation of the common phenomenon of the spontaneous or *de novo* origin of disease outbreaks, and were congruent with the multicausal models used in epidemiology. There has been a tendency to see 'miasmatic' as a shrinking, residual category for those diseases whose precise mode of spread remained unknown, with malaria the paradigmatic case. This is unfortunate, as between the 1860s and late 1890s, when the malaria's aetiology was moulded around a parasite and vectors, doctors had specific beliefs about how the malaria poison (or germ) arose in the soil and spread in the air, in ways still thought possible for cholera and typhoid fever.[67] The belief that disease poisons, or bacterial germs for that matter, could arise *de novo* in the environment was not readily set aside.

For most public health doctors, the most important questions about the nature of disease were not about the intimate nature of pathological or physiological processes in individual bodies, but how diseases were spread into and within populations. Thus, the dominant approach for understanding disease in public health medicine was epidemiological. The practical and political questions were about how best to prevent diseases in communities, and to control outbreaks once they had started. Public health policy had been riven since the 1840s with divisions between so-called contagionist and anticontagionists.[68] The former group maintained that the prevention and control of epidemic diseases should be based on the use of quarantines and *cordon sanitaires*. The latter group, as the form of the word suggests, was primarily defined by its opposition to contagion and, above all, opposition to the use of quarantines and isolation to control epidemics.[69] However, anticontagionists had their own programme of prevention and control, which relied on environmental improvements to eradicate the conditions in which fevers could arise and spread. Anticontagionists maintained that very few diseases were contagious enough to warrant the use of such draconian measures. Moreover, they said that quarantines would not work, even for contagious diseases: first, because air-borne poisons, if not those carried in water, food, sewers or on goods, could easily cross man-made barriers; second, because poisons could arise *de novo* at any time or place, especially in unsanitary conditions and where humans were crowded together; and, third, because strict implementation could never be guaranteed because of human incom-

67 M. Worboys, 'From Miasmas to Germs: Malaria, 1850–1879', *Parassitologia*, 1994, 36: 61–8.
68 E. Ackerknecht, 'Anticontagionism between 1821 and 1867', *BHM*, 1948, 22: 562–93; R. Cooter, 'Anticontagionism and History's Medical Record', in P. Wright and A. Treacher, ed., *The Problem of Medical Knowledge: Examining the Social Construction of Medicine*, Edinburgh, Edinburgh University Press, 1982, 87–108.
69 See evidence to the *Select Committee on Cattle Disease etc.*, BPP 1864, [431], vii, 1.

Table 2. *Comparison of Contagionism and Anticontagionism, c. 1860*

	Contagionism	Anticontagionism
Model diseases	Smallpox, cattle plague	Malaria, cholera
Origin	External contamination; from a preexisting case; ultimate origin unknowable	Configuration of circumstances; de novo, spontaneous or sporadic; product of putrefaction, filth
Spread of infection	Body-to-body; regular; mostly traceable	Aerial diffusion; sporadic; body-to-body or mediated transmission possible
Infectious matter	'Virus', chemical or living agent given off by animal bodies; *contagia vivum*	Miasma, poisoned air from decaying plant sources
Cause	Single and exciting	Multiple and remote, exciting proximate, or unknowable
Conditions of infection	Direct contamination normally sufficient to produce disease	Induced 'at-a-distance'; mediated by predisposition of individuals, though direct contamination is possible
Disease process	Zymotic	Zymotic
Immunity	Prior infection most important; predisposition unimportant	Predisposition significant; bodily constitution and general health
Disease syndrome	Specific and fixed, constant	Variable and mutable, irregular
Primary method of disease prevention	Quarantine and isolation to prevent transmission virus or poison – inclusive	Environmental improvements to prevent generation and diffusion of poison – exclusive

petence and corruption. An essential point to grasp is that the supporters of the two views disagreed more about policies and politics than they did about the nature of epidemic diseases. The most bitter disputes were about whether what liberals saw as draconian state measures could be justified, or whether trusting to sanitary improvements and not attempting to keep epidemics out was negligent. Both camps agreed on the limiting cases: smallpox was accepted to be highly contagious while malaria was noncontagious, but beyond this similarities and differences were complex (see Table 2).

In terms of their pathology, aetiology and epidemiology, the great majority of epidemic diseases and zymotic fevers was neither wholly contagious nor noncontagious. Even the same disease was seen to vary in virulence and infectivity over time, across space and between communities. For example, where several cases of diphtheria appeared in a family, this was attributed either to the fact that they had all had been exposed to the same sewer gases, or that the disease had been spread from person to person or, more usually, both. As Pelling has shown, the commonest position adopted within medicine was 'contingent contagionism'; that is, the degree to which diseases were 'catching' was variable, differing between diseases and influenced by many factors, from *remote* causes, such as climate, through to *proximate* ones, such as personal predisposition.[70] With all zymotic diseases, the poison (ferment or zyme) was regarded as necessary, but not on its own a sufficient exciting cause of disease. Other factors had to be present, ranging from global variables, such as the seasons, through to inherited predispositions in the constitutions of individuals.

The notion that zymotic diseases struck 'susceptible individuals' was very important and gave meaning to the social, gender and ethnic patterns of disease incidence. While state medicine enacted laws and established agencies to remove nuisances, supply clean water, build sewage systems, reduce air pollution, drain and pave streets, prevent food adulteration and vaccinate children, it also promoted healthy, sober living. Hamlin has pointed to the moral dimension of pythogenic and zymotic theories where 'the pure was corrupted by contact with impurity'.[71] This was seen in the fact that the distribution and effects of disease-poisons were neither random nor determinant. They produced their worst effects in bodies weakened and vulnerable due to inheritance, ignorance, indifference, neglect or abuse of the laws of health and cleanliness. Over and above filth and overcrowding, these factors explained the higher incidence of zymotic diseases amongst the poor, the feckless, the dissolute, drunks, migrants and minorities, who were collectively and symbolically known as the 'Great Unwashed'.[72] Together with the well-known variations in susceptibility by age and sex, all of these factors defined the 'contingencies' of contagion. This view also offered understandings of the changing virulence of epidemics and the different properties of the same disease in different circumstances. Indeed, one of the major objections that old-style sanitarians had to the early panspermic germ theories, where the air was full of microbial life or its germs, was that the spread of disease was random, meaningless and amoral rather than patterned, salutary and moral.

The experience of cholera played a pivotal role in shaping public disease theories and control policies in the 1850s and 1860s. After the epidemic of 1848–49, the standing of anticontagionism rose due to the repeated failure of quarantines to halt the spread of the disease between countries and within

70 C. Hamlin, 'Predisposing Causes and Public Health in Early Nineteenth Century Medical Thought', *SHM*, 1992, 5: 43–70.
71 Hamlin, 'Providence', 389.
72 M. Sigsworth and M. Worboys, 'The Public's View of Public Health in Mid-Victorian Britain', *Urban History*, 1994, 21: 237–50.

them. The cholera poison had passed through quarantine barriers, and often appeared *de novo* in suitable conditions behind them. In the 1850s, a number of human as well as animal diseases were fashioned by medical and sanitary authorities to be noncontagious, and hence best prevented by general environmental and sanitary reforms rather than waiting for threats and instituting quarantines. In 1862–63, a committee of the Royal College of Physicians decided that leprosy, historically amongst the most feared contagions, was a hereditary disease and recommended that ancient leper statutes be repealed.[73] Anticontagionists saw themselves as proactive, 'inclusive' and truly preventive, while contagionists were reactive, 'exclusive' and often only offered control of established epidemics. The imperative for anticontagionists was to prevent epidemics at their source by eliminating the conditions in which poisons arose and which facilitated their elaboration and spread. Beyond this, they argued that the factors that determined the intensity and spread of epidemics were so many and conditional that narrowly focused controls could never be successful. However, in Britain in 1865 the star of contagionism began to rise, not due to changed views of cholera, which was spreading westward across Europe once again, but because of the epizootic crisis of cattle plague that reignited medical and political debates over contagion-anticontagion, and, incidentally, raised the profile of germ theories of disease.

---

73 *Lancet*, 1867, i: 17, 43–4, 189–90, 253–4. The enquiry was started in 1862 after a request from colonial officials in the West Indies on whether the incarceration of lepers was justified.

2

Veterinary Medicine, the Cattle Plague and Contagion, 1865–1890

In most historical accounts of the germ theory of disease, the 'Golden Age of Bacteriology' dawned in Germany in 1876 when Koch showed that a specific bacillus was the necessary cause of anthrax, also known as splenic fever.[1] Immunology, Jenner apart, is said to have begun four years later in France, when Pasteur produced a protective vaccine by attenuating the bacillus of chicken cholera.[2] Research on contagious animal diseases was, therefore, the source of key moments in the history of germ ideas and practices.[3] This pattern continued in virology, when in 1898 the first pathogenic animal virus identified was that of foot-and-mouth disease.[4] This chapter does not revisit these landmarks nor focus directly on their reception; rather, it discusses changes in the understanding of contagious animal diseases and their relation to disease control practices.[5] Historians have recognised the importance of animal models in the pathological researches that led to the construction of bacterial germ theories from the 1870s, however, less attention has been paid to other aspects of the relationship between animal and human medicine.[6]

---

1 W. Bulloch, *The History of Bacteriology*, London, Oxford University Press, 1938; H. A. Lechevalier and M. Solotorovsky, *Three Centuries of Microbiology*, New York, Dover Publications, 1974; P. Collard, *The Development of Microbiology*, Cambridge, Cambridge University Press, 1976. Anthrax was and is a serious disease of sheep and cattle with a high lethality. The main external symptoms are 'malignant pustules', fever and prostration, while internally it can produce pneumonia, haemorrhages and gangrene of the spleen.

2 W. D. Foster, *A History of Medical Bacteriology and Immunology*, London, Heinemann, 1970; D. J. Bibel, *Milestones in Immunology: A Historical Exploration*, Madison, WI, Science Tech, 1988, 19–23; A. M. Silverstein, *History of Immunology*, San Diego, CA, Academic Press, 1989.

3 In a footnote Winslow suggested that, 'An interesting monograph could be prepared on the early contributions of veterinary medicine to our knowledge of the aetiology of human disease'. C. E. A. Winslow, *Conquest of Epidemic Disease: A Chapter in the History of Ideas*, 1943, Madison, WI, University of Wisconsin Press 1980, 296.

4 A. P. Waterson and L. Wilkinson, *An Introduction to the History of Virology*, Cambridge, Cambridge University Press, 1978, 30–4.

5 L. Wilkinson, *Animals and Disease: An Introduction to the History of Comparative Medicine*, Cambridge, Cambridge University Press, 1992.

6 W. F. Bynum, *Science and the Practice of Medicine in the Nineteenth Century*, Cambridge, Cambridge University Press, 1993; idem., '"C'est un malade": Animal models and concepts of human disease', *JHM*, 1990, 45: 397–413.

Amongst the most important of these were the debates within veterinary medicine, and between veterinary and human medicine, on the control of contagious animal diseases. From the 1860s, unlike their medical counterparts, veterinarians accepted that most epizootics were contagious and spread by the transmission of some disease-matter – *materies morbi* or virus – from beast to beast. This position was maintained with a strong commitment to germ theories of disease, but hostility to germ practices.

The received opinion on laboratory medicine in Britain is that it was behind that in continental Europe from the 1850s. However, the response to the cattle plague and other epizootics reveals a different picture. A Royal Commission was appointed to advise the government on the control of the outbreak, and this body organised pioneering investigations into the nature of the contagia and the pathology and aetiology of the disease. It was able to draw on researchers of high repute, and their work initiated further work and debate. Amongst the many findings of the commission were John Burdon Sanderson's report that the disease was transmissible by inoculation, and Lionel Beale's claim to have identified what he termed the 'germs' of the disease.[7] Sanderson went on to become the leading researcher in the scientific investigations on the 'intimate pathology of contagion' initiated by John Simon on behalf of the Medical Department of the Privy Council, and Beale, a renowned microscopist, went on to publish two books on disease germs.[8] Simon later observed that the researches of the Royal Commission had pioneered experimental pathology in Britain and had been 'the first step of discovery'.[9] Much of the research supported by Simon's department from the late 1860s was undertaken at the Brown Animal Sanatory Institute, London, hereafter the 'Brown', which was founded in 1870 with research on animal diseases one of its main roles.[10] Interestingly, the Brown was headed by a suc-

---

7 This paralleled the auxiliary scientific investigations begun by the Medical Department of the Privy Council in 1865. Indeed, John Burdon Sanderson worked for both bodies and after 1866 carried out much of his work for the Medical Department at the Albert Veterinary College. Sanderson Papers, University College, London, Appointment diaries, 1866–9.

8 T. Romano, *Making Medicine Scientific: John Burdon Sanderson and the Culture of Victorian Science*, Unpublished PhD Thesis, Yale University, 1993; G. L. Geison, 'Lionel Smith Beale', in C. C. Gillispie, ed., *Dictionary of Scientific Biography*, New York, Charles Scribner's Sons, 1974, 539–41.

9 *Report of the Medical Officer of the Privy Council and Local Government Board*, New Series, No. 3, Report on Scientific Investigations, 1874, BPP. 1875, [C.1068], xxxi, 5.

10 G. Wilson, 'The Brown Animal Sanatory Institute', *Journal of Hygiene*, 1979, 83: 155–76, 337–52, 501–21. In 1852, Thomas Brown left some £22,000 for the establishment of an Animal Sanatory Institute that was to offer treatment for sick animals, facilities for research into animal diseases and lectures to the public. After long legal wranglings the scheme was eventually taken over by the University of London and the 'Brown', as it became known, opened as an independent agency in July 1871 with Sanderson as its Superintendent and Edward Klein his unpaid assistant. These appointments show that even before it opened, the Brown had been taken over by the metropolitan medical elite. Professor William Sharpey (1802–80) and Richard Quain (1816–98), who steered its establishment, had refused offers from the Albert Veterinary College and the RVC to house the institute, despite the fact that as well as a research facility there was an animal hospital and dispensary. The latter provided a ready supply of interesting diseases and research mater-

cession of distinguished medical men, not veterinarians: Sanderson, William
S. Greenfield, C. S. Roy (1854–97), Victor Horsley and C. S. Sherrington
(1857–1952), and for two decades enjoyed the services of the 'father of British
bacteriology', Edward Klein.[11] Contrary to Simon's assertion, no great 'discoveries' were made at the Brown on either animal or human diseases, nor
was it a catalyst for the institutionalisation of experimental pathology or bacteriology in either veterinary or human medicine. As French has shown, the
restrictions of the Cruelty to Animals Act, 1876, which in part was stimulated by metropolitan reaction to experiments at the Brown, was a major
factor in the slow development of laboratory research in Britain, as was the
linkage of medical schools to hospitals rather than universities.[12] However, I
want to suggest that there was an additional factor in the relative backwardness of British laboratory medicine, namely, that neither veterinarians nor the
government's Veterinary Department supported experimental research;
indeed, they were hostile to it. This was principally because they feared that
'research' would produce alternative methods of control that would erode the
place that veterinarians and administrative controls had established in the
administration of surveillance and policing after the cattle plague crisis of
1865–66.

VETERINARIANS AND THE CONTROL OF ANIMAL DISEASE
BEFORE 1865

In 1865, veterinary medicine was still an unreformed profession. Reformers
had sought to improve the social position and incomes of the professional by
seeking status through learning, qualification and organisation, essentially following the path set by medicine.[13] The establishment of the Royal College
of Veterinary Surgeons (RCVS) in 1844 was seen as a landmark in their campaign, but the privately owned veterinary schools refused to concede the
college any real authority on qualifications for many years. The profession
was not practically or formally unified until the passage of the Veterinary Surgeons Bill, 1881, which defined qualifications and created a register of veterinary surgeons, much along the lines of the Medical Act, 1858. However,
veterinarians had an ambivalent attitude towards medicine and the medical
profession. They acknowledged that they too practised 'medicine' and were

ial, although around ninety percent of the animals treated were horses and dogs. The research side
was shaped, therefore, largely by the interests of Sanderson, his contacts and the research contracts
that he was awarded by agencies. The main demand came from the Privy Council's Medical
Department and the RASE, with significantly no requests for research from the government's
new Veterinary Department.

11 See: W. Bulloch, 'Edward Emanuel Klein', *JPB*, 1925, 28: 684.
12 R. D. French, *Antivivisection and Medical Science in Victorian England*, Princeton, NJ, Princeton
University Press, 1975.
13 This section is based principally on I. Pattison, *The British Veterinary Profession, 1791–1948*, London,
J. A. Allen, 1983.

engaged in a similar campaign for status and occupational control, yet they were aware of their lower social standing and organisational deficiencies.[14] Veterinary surgeons were routinely subjected to attacks about their competence and learning, especially as medical men tried to distance themselves from 'horse doctors' and other quacks. In a similar vein, qualified veterinary surgeons tried to distance themselves from farriers, cow leeches, knowledgeable farmers and 'veterinary quacks'. While medical men vigorously policed the encroachment of veterinarians into human medicine, they made frequent incursions the other way. They investigated and wrote about animal diseases, and many in the lower ranks no doubt treated animals too. Investigations were justified as comparative pathology, and doctors showed their authority in their increasing use of the rhetoric and ideas of science. The usual defence of veterinary surgeons that their knowledge was practical rather than scientific counted for little against the growing power of organised medicine.

In the mid-1860s there were approximately 3,500 veterinary practitioners in Britain, of whom only thirty percent were members of the Royal College, as against forty percent who were unqualified, leaving thirty percent with other credentials.[15] Veterinary qualifications were awarded by five schools: the RVC, the Veterinary College, Glasgow, and in Edinburgh the Dick College and the New Veterinary College, with John Gamgee's new Albert Veterinary College in London struggling to gain a foothold. Teaching was predominantly practical, with an apprenticeship element common. Education, practice and income were dominated by the horse; other livestock and domestic companion animals received much less attention. Most veterinarians worked in private practice, although there was an influential group of army veterinarians who dealt exclusively with horses and the odd regimental mascot. There were, of course, a huge number of horses at that time, each representing a significant capital asset for its owner that was well worth protecting by paying for the treatment of injuries and sickness. Significant veterinary income from treating companion animals lay in the future; in perhaps less sentimental times, the 'repair' cost of most pets was higher than their 'replacement' cost. For different economic reasons, veterinary surgeons saw relatively few farm animals, for as soon as a beast showed any signs of disease it was expedient to slaughter it before its value fell or, if the disease was catching, for contagions to spread. The RVC constantly complained of the difficulty of teaching 'diseases of animals of the farm' because of the imperatives of early disposal.[16] Also, many farmers treated their own animals using traditional

---

14 R. H. Dyer, 'The Social Position of the Veterinary Surgeon', *Veterinarian*, 38, 1865, 360. Dyer claimed that medical men no longer used the tradesmen's entrance, nor did they deal with servants; whereas veterinary surgeons never got near the house, only making it to the stables, where they met grooms and estate workers.

15 Figures cited in Pattison, *Veterinary Profession*, 62.

16 *Veterinarian*, 35, 1862, 276.

remedies, or utilised a range of lay healers, as was only too evident during the cattle plague crisis.[17]

Britain's island geography and trade restrictions had given its agriculture and stock-rearing industry relative immunity from epizootics over many centuries.[18] This situation changed in the 1840s, as the repeal of protectionist legislation and improvements in the speed of transportation combined to allow diseased animals to be imported more readily.[19] In 1843, the Royal Agricultural Society of England (RASE), warning of the new dangers and the need for a better understanding of cattle diseases, had sponsored the appointment of James Beart Simonds (1810–1904) to a new Chair of Cattle Pathology at the RVC, London, and it was Simonds who became chief government advisor.[20] Outbreaks of foot-and-mouth disease and sheep-pox in 1848 confirmed fears that free-trade in livestock would bring an easier exchange of animal diseases. Both diseases were seen as 'foreign', and the government adopted a policy of 'stamping out' using legislative orders that allowed the slaughtering and the exclusion of affected beasts through quarantines and port inspections.[21] The orders were controversial as they were seen by the supporters of free-trade as a backdoor method of reintroducing protection. There was, however, little public or professional debate on the question; the outbreaks did not spread, the legislative powers were little used and the whole problem was soon overshadowed by the most serious cholera epidemic of the century, which also arrived in Britain in 1848.[22]

Throughout the 1850s and early 1860s, Simonds remained a part-time adviser to the government and continued to help monitor the threat of epizootics. His advice, based on the absence of further serious outbreaks and following the general midcentury movement against contagion and quarantines, suggested that the dangers of imported diseases had been exaggerated.[23] He led veterinary opinion to the position where certain livestock diseases, like the cattle plague, were accepted as imported, but where the great major-

---

17 Homoeopathy was strong amongst veterinarians and was used to treat the cattle plague. *Veterinarian*, 38, 1865, 792, and *BMJ*, 1865, ii, 589.
18 An epizootic is the equivalent in animal populations of a human epidemic, i.e. high morbidity or mortality due to a disease that is not normally present in a region. G. Fleming, *Animal Plagues: Their History, Nature and Prevention*, London, Chapman and Hall, 1871; T. Duckham and G. T. Brown, 'The Progress of Legislation against Contagious Diseases of Livestock: Parts I and II', *JRAS*, 1893, 54: 262–86.
19 J. Gamgee, 'Epizootics', *Veterinarian*, 1867, 40: 537.
20 I. Pattison, *A Great British Veterinarian Forgotten: James Beart Simonds*, London, J. Allen, 1989, passim.; J. B. Simonds (1810–1904), *DNB*, Suppl. 1, pp. 318–9.
21 Ministry of Agriculture Fisheries and Food (MAFF), *Animal Health: A Centenary, 1865–1965*, London, HMSO, 1965, 7–11.
22 A similar controversy is discussed by S. Hoy and W. Nugent, 'Public Health or Proctectionism? The German-American Pork War', *BHM*, 1989, 63: 198–224.
23 L. Wilkinson, 'Zoonoses and the Development of Concepts of Contagion and Infection', in A. R. Mitchell, ed., *History of the Healing Professions: Parallels between Veterinary and Human Medicine*, Wallingford, CAB International, 1993, 73–90.

ity were native diseases. Cattle plague was an extremely lethal disease that produced fever, dysentery and skin eruptions, and was thought to be native to the Steppes of Russia. In 1857 Simonds removed two other 'foreign', imported disease threats with the stroke of his pen, when, from an analysis of the history of foot-and-mouth and pleuropneumonia, he decided that these were native diseases that flared up spontaneously in certain environmental conditions.[24] The conviction that such diseases were sporadic and able to diffuse as miasmas (poisoned air) was the basis, as we have seen, of anticontagionist policies.

From the late 1850s, Simonds's expertise on epizootics and his support of anticontagionism were challenged by John Gamgee, first as principal of the New Veterinary College, Edinburgh, and then of the Albert Veterinary College. Gamgee was a strong advocate of quarantines and the control of livestock movements.[25] In the early 1860s Gamgee gained a high profile with warnings of the dangers of imported diseases and, based on European experiences, the calls he made for stronger veterinary policing at ports and within the country. As both an outsider and a challenger of veterinary orthodoxy, Gamgee found few supporters and even fewer friends amongst his professional peers. However, he did find support for his views at the first International Veterinary Congress in 1864, although this was hardly surprising as he organised the event and was one of only two, both unofficial, British participants.[26] In 1864 Gamgee's campaign inspired the introduction of two parliamentary bills that aimed to strengthen the 1848 Orders. The measures were opposed by leading veterinarians as well as by agricultural and livestock interests, who, while they might have welcomed them as a form of import control, feared for exports and the disruption of internal trade. The opposition to the measures and to Gamgee personally was spelt out in the evidence given to a Select Committee that looked into the proposals and the parliamentary debates. Predictably, both bills were defeated.[27] The vote was twelve months before the start of the great cattle plague outbreak in 1865, which decimated the British cattle herd, saw agricultural and veterinary opinion at

24 The finding was based on an analysis of tariff returns. J. B. Simonds, 'Cattle Disease', *JRAS*, 1857, 18: 201. In his biography, Pattison has vigorously denied that Simonds supported the spontaneous generation of disease, arguing that he was a confirmed contagionist. The point historically is that one could be both, regarding the origins and the transmission of disease as distinct.
25 J. R. Fisher, 'Professor Gamgee and the Farmers', *Veterinary History*, 1979–80, 1 (2): 50. See the report that Gamgee prepared in 1862 for the Medical Department of the Privy Council, *Cattle Diseases in Relation to the Supplies of Meat and Milk*, BPP 1863, xxv, 269. S. A. Hall, 'John Gamgee and the Edinburgh New Veterinary College', *VR*, 1965, 77: 1237–41. In 1864, Gamgee left Edinburgh to establish another new school in London, the Albert Veterinary College, as a direct challenge to the RVC. R. D'Arcy Thompson, *The Remarkable Gamgees: a story of achievement*, Edinburgh, Ramsey Head, 1974.
26 J. W. Barber Lomax, 'The First International Veterinary Congress', *Journal of Small Animal Practice*, 1963, 4: Suppl. 17–21. The government ignored the meeting, as did the veterinary press.
27 *House of Commons: Parl. Debates*, 173, 1864, Cols. 1740–53 and 1864, 176, Col. 1567; *Times*, 16, 21 and 27 June 1864.

every level switch to contagionism, and to call for exactly the kind of measures advocated by Gamgee.[28]

THE CATTLE PLAGUE AND VETERINARIANS

In the summer of 1865 the first government response to confirmation that the cattle plague (later called rinderpest) was prevalent in London was to use the 1848 Orders. Local authorities were asked to appoint inspectors to monitor markets, check cattle movements and, most controversially, to use the pole-axe to slaughter affected beasts.[29] Elite veterinarians accepted that cattle plague was at the contagious end of the disease spectrum and only disagreed over whether the first case had arisen spontaneously or had been imported. Farmers, breeders and rank-and-file veterinarians largely followed the tenets of anticontagionism. They assumed that cattle plague had arisen spontaneously and then spread its influence via the atmosphere. This view was expressed forcefully in their opposition to the policing of the movement of animals and to slaughtering, which they experienced as more economically damaging than the disease itself. That cholera, the exemplary anticontagionist disease, was also threatening again gave support to the idea that some malign, possibly atmospheric, epidemic influence was present in the country. Nonetheless, uncertainties over the sources of the disease and the hostility of the livestock industry made control measures difficult to implement.

Once the epizootic took hold, the government created a Veterinary Department, headed by Simonds and modelled on the Medical Department. The department was charged with collecting and collating statistics on the incidence of livestock disease and to oversee controls.[30] Within a few months hundreds of part-time inspectors had been appointed and veterinary surgeons found themselves enjoying new powers and status as local functionaries. By autumn it was clear to everyone that the epizootic was not being controlled by existing measures, as it continued to spread across virtually the whole country. The unpopularity of inspection and slaughtering, together with the economic losses borne by farmers, were powerful reminders of the initial failure to check the outbreak.[31] The developing sense of crisis, and the

28 J. R. Fisher, 'The Economic Effects of Cattle Disease in Britain and its Containment', *Agricultural History*, 1980, 54: 281.

29 The best source on the development of this epizootic are the books of press-cuttings made by Simonds. See: *The Rinderpest, Vol. I, II and III*, Historical Collection, R.V.C. Library, London. Also see: J. A. Hall, 'The Cattle Plague of 1865', *MH*, 1962, 6: 45–58.

30 MAFF, *Animal Health*, 18, 24–8.

31 See: *Veterinarian*, 1865, 38: 627, 653, 906. Initially there was support for the pole-axe as the disease was considered incurable, but later in 1865 more and more veterinarians reported cures and faith in treatment grew. Misdiagnoses and pathological confusions showed that veterinarians had little shared knowledge of stock diseases.

seeming powerlessness of the experts to do anything, damaged veterinarians in the eyes of the public and the medical profession.[32] Interestingly, there was little discussion about the dangers to human health of eating infected meat, as previous experience had shown that there was a species-barrier for the disease between livestock and humans.

During the autumn of 1865 the disease showed no signs of abating, losses mounted and the public was hit by rising meat and dairy prices. The government and veterinarians had difficulties winning support for their programme of control as it was identified with slaughtering, which was presented by critics as arbitrary, wasteful, barbaric, fatalistic and decidedly 'unscientific'. When it became clear that the control measures were not working, the government appointed a Royal Commission to collect evidence and weigh opinion on more effective measures. Significantly, its membership was predominantly medical, not veterinary.[33] This was due in part to the greater authority of medical men; but it also revealed the slenderness of Britain's veterinary resources as, apart from Gamgee, the metropolitan elite already held posts in the Veterinary Department. The commission reported quickly in November 1865, recommending stronger internal regulation of cattle movements. The government did not relish adopting such a programme in the face of opposition from landed and livestock interests, so while exhorting greater vigilance they left local authorities to implement controls. The Second Report of the Royal Commission in January 1866 made similar recommendations, gave further support to the slaughtering and put greater stress on the threat posed by the importation of diseased livestock.[34] In the same month the seeming impotence of both the medical and veterinary professions allowed the established church to strike a blow against the growing hegemony of science with a National Prayer Day, asking for deliverance from the crisis.[35] In February 1866, the government took more decisive action and introduced stricter measures that were to be more rigidly enforced. However, it was neither prayer nor the advice of the Royal Commission that brought the change; instead, it was a national lobby by livestock interests calling for stronger veterinary policing and import controls.[36] Stung by mounting economic difficulties and first-hand experience, livestock farmers and the

32 In the second half of 1865, the *Times* led a campaign that was critical of Britain's veterinarians. See: *Times*, 19 August 1865. For a defence of veterinary actions, *Veterinarian*, 1865, 38: 627, 906.

33 *First Report of the Commission Appointed to Inquire into the Origin and Nature of the Cattle Plague*, BPP 1865 [C. 3591], xxii, 1. The Commission included: Lyon Playfair, Richard Quain, MD; Bence Jones, MD; E. A. Parkes, MD; T. Wormald, Pres. of Royal College of Surgeons of London; R. Ceeley, MRCS; and C. Spooner, Principal of the R.V.C.

34 *Second Report of the Commission appointed to inquire into the origin and nature of the cattle plague*, BPP 1866, [C.3600], xxii, 227.

35 F. M. Turner, 'Rainfall, Plague and the Prince of Wales: A Chapter in the Conflict of Religion and Science', *Journal of British Studies*, 1974, 13: 46–65.

36 *Times*, 9 February 1866, 3d.

meat trade had changed from anticontagionists to contagionists in a matter of months, although they linked their new support for quarantines and slaughtering with the expectation of compensation from the state.[37]

The pursuit of stricter veterinary policing seemed to be vindicated in the late spring of 1866, when reported outbreaks and deaths began to decline.[38] How vigorously controls had been stepped up is impossible to say, although it is worth noting that over the next half-century the justification for each of the dozens of amendments made to animal disease control legislation was to remedy the weaknesses of prior legislation. Epidemiologists, like William Farr, had predicted that such a decline would occur independently of any human agency as a consequence of the natural laws of epidemics, yet this did not stop veterinarians and the government from claiming that their actions had halted the epizootic.[39] Further evidence that veterinary policing was effective came in falls of the reported incidences of two other contagious cattle diseases, pleuropneumonia and foot-and-mouth disease.[40] The cattle plague epizootic was seen in hindsight by veterinarians as a large epidemiological experiment that had taught everyone that epizootics were contagious and had vindicated the practical policies advocated by elite veterinarians against their rank and file, farmers and the fanciful ideas of medical men.

THE CATTLE PLAGUE, MEDICINE AND GERMS

The medical profession was involved in the cattle plague crisis from the outset, offering opinions on the nature, prevention and treatment of the disease.[41] There were differences within the medical profession about what to do: some argued for the application of medical measures such as vaccination, isolation in 'cattle sanatoria' and the use of antiseptics; however, elite opinion supported policing measures from the outset.[42] The main medical journals also supported slaughtering and quarantines, as writers confidently predicted that, like any other disease, the cattle plague would eventually succumb to medical control.[43] The initial basis for this was a perceived

---

37 Fisher, 'The Economic Effects', 281–2.
38 *Report on Cattle Plague in Great Britain during the years 1865, 1866 and 1867*, BPP 1867–8, [C.4060], xviii, 220. Also see: *BMJ*, 1866, i: 405, 444.
39 *BMJ*, 1866, i: 207.   40 *Veterinarian*, 1867, 40: 296.
41 A new account of this episode is given in: T. M. Romano, 'The Cattle Plague of 1865 and the Reception of "Germ Theory" in Mid-Victorian Britain', *JHM*, 1997, 52: 51–80.
42 *Veterinarian*, 1866, 39: 353. Also see: *First Report*, 145. Dr. Tripe said he spoke for the 'unanimous opinion of the medical profession that treatment would avail'. His proposed cattle sanatoria were described as 'El Dorados' in an editorial in the *Veterinarian*, 1965, 38: 627, 920. In 1865, John Simon called for cattle movements to be stopped and quarantines to be introduced. Also see: *Lancet*, 1865, ii: 212, 433. Vaccination in this context involved the inoculation of vaccinia or cowpox lymph – it was not until the 1880s that the word took on its current, wider meaning. Vaccination was justified by assumed similarities between all pox diseases.
43 *BMJ*, 1865, ii: 334, 374, 611, 662; and ibid., 1866, i: 405, 444.

similarity or equivalence between the cattle plague and diseases like small-pox. Indeed, at the turn of 1865 there was interest in the possibility that vac-cination might offer protection by exhausting the substrates in the body that supported the development of pox diseases.[44] Emerging medical authorities, such as Richard Quain (1816–98), Benjamin Ward Richardson (1828–96) and Charles Murchison (1830–79), backed by Simonds, argued for the identity of the two diseases, or at least a close family resemblance. Gamgee and Sander-son stood against this position. The dispute was about more than the patho-logical anatomy of a single disease; it was over the very nature of disease. Quain and Murchison maintained a nonontological conception, where the different pustules produced in the two conditions were due to interactions between poisons and the different skins of cattle and humans. Gamgee and Sanderson assumed that the two diseases were specific and distinct entities. An editorial in the *Medical Times and Gazette* put the case against the cattle plague being specific and ontological:

There is scarcely a disease which has not a considerable range in aspect according to the different degrees of intensity in quality or quantity of the virus, and the state of the living being upon whom it plays; hence the varying character of epidemics – malig-nant, sthenic, asthenic, fatal or mild. As the local expressions of disease depend, of course, upon the degree of development of the general condition, variations are met with accordingly, and this is an important consideration at the present time in reference to Rinderpest.[45]

Clinical experience showed that even well-defined and seemingly specific dis-eases had many variations; for example, with measles the editorial went on to say that the disease could be 'mild (as in the East) – malignant, abortive, as in *Rubeola sine catarrho*, or anomalous, as in *Rubeola notha*, and the pseudo-measles of Dr Salisbury'.

Many theories on the origin and character of the cattle plague were advanced by medical men. Richardson accommodated cattle plague within his particular zymotic model – the 'glandular theory of disease' (also known as the 'physical' or 'catalysis' theory), in which the poisons of disease were said to arise in the body and emanate from it as abnormal, chemical secre-tions.[46] There was also support for the cattle plague being a quite specific parasitic disease, which was not that surprising as liver flukes and tapeworms were more prevalent in animals than humans.[47] Beale gave credence to the parasitic theory when he reported finding entozoa in the muscles of cattle killed by the plague, although he did not say whether they were cause, effect or accidental visitors.[48] While Beale was quite open-minded early in the epi-

44 *MTG*, 1866, i: 14–15, 23; J. R. Fisher, 'British Physicians, Medical Science, and the Cattle Plague, 1865–88, *BHM*, 1993, 67: 651–69.
45 *MTG*, 1866, i: 67.   46 *BMJ*, 1870, ii: 467.   47 *Times*, 3 January 1866; *MTG*, 1866, i: 41–2.
48 L. S. Beale, 'Entozoa(?) in the Muscles of Animals Destroyed by the Cattle Plague', *MTG*, 1866, i: 57–9.

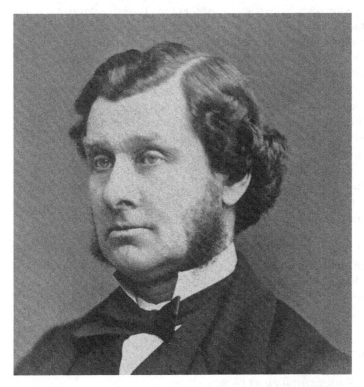

Figure 5. Lionel S. Beale in 1873 (Reproduced by courtesy of the Wellcome Institute Library, London)

zootic, his investigations for the Royal Commission became the basis for the development of his bioplasm theory of disease (see Figure 5). In the Third Report of the Commission, Beale wrote that 'living particles of extremely minute size are quite competent to give rise to all the symptoms observed'. The 'living particles' he had in mind, which he termed 'bioplasm', were the subcellular components or the degraded protoplasmic elements of diseased human cells, not independent microorganisms.[49] In other words, a particular configuration of the body had produced its own contaminants, and these could spread internally and externally as contagia.

The findings of all of the investigations made by the investigators employed by the Royal Commission were published in June 1866. This report was seen

49 J. B. Sanderson, (1828–1905), *PRSL*, B, 1907, 79: iii–xviii; Cf. *BMJ*, 1905, ii: 1481. Lionel S. Beale, (1828–1906), *PRSL*, B, 1907, 77: i: lvii–lxii. Charles Murchison, *BMJ*, 1879, i: 648–50. It was hoped by some medical men that the commission might be a precedent and model for an enquiry into cholera. *Lancet*, 1866, ii: 12.

as a model of advanced medical research. The *BMJ* commented that, 'in truth, we know of no disease affecting man, whose characters have been better studied'.[50] Sanderson's observation that cattle plague could be transmitted by inoculation was said in an editorial in the *BMJ* to be 'pregnant with consequences for medical doctrine', and was seen to give support to 'the organic living nature of the poisons of zymotic disease'.[51] Beale's finding that 'the "poison", "virus", "contagium", "materies morbi". . . . consists of very minute particles of matter in a living state, each capable of growing and multiplying rapidly when placed under favourable conditions', was also said to be highly significant for the medical profession.[52] The *Medical Times and Gazette* discussed Beale's work in great detail and reproduced his histological drawings, including illustrations of germinal matter (see Figure 6).

It is noteworthy that, from the late 1860s to the late 1870s, there were no similar illustrations of bacterial and other types of germs in medical journals, which I will argue showed a distrust of microscopy and the dictum that 'seeing is believing'. The text of the Third Report said that Beale's results had been supportive of chemical theories of zymosis and ignored his germ ideas. Beale was unhappy about this reading of his work, as he felt that his conclusion was unequivocal, namely, that the contagious particles of the disease,

consist of living matter formed in the organism of man and animals . . . . [and] bear somewhat the same relation to the germinal matter of normal cells that the pus corpuscles or cancer cells do, and therefore that the contagious germs have been derived by continuous descent from the normal germinal matter of the organism.[53]

Beale was very careful to distance himself from any idea that disease-germs consisted 'either of insect, of animalcules, or any kind of vegetable organism'.[54] Indeed, as Pelling noted, his ideas represented what most people would have understood by a 'germ theory of disease' in the mid-1860s. In Britain, similar notions had been proposed by James Morris,[55] Sanderson,[56] James

50 *Third Report of the Commission Appointed to Inquire into the Origin and Nature of the Cattle Plague*, BPP 1866, [C.3653], lix, 321; *BMJ*, 1866, ii: 42.
51 *MTG*, 1866, ii: 13–14.
52 *MTG*, 1866, i: 623–6, 625–6.
53 L. S. Beale, 'Observations on the "Granular Matter" and "Complex Albuminoid Matter"', *MTG*, 1866, ii: 658–9. At this time Beale was proposing that cholera was spread by germinal matter that detached itself from the lining of the gut. Beale wrote an appendix on the microscopy of the disease in C. Shrimpton, *Cholera: Its Seat, Nature, and Treatment*, London, Churchill, 1866.
54 *MTG*, 1866, ii: 327. L. S. Beale, *Disease Germs; Their Real Nature*, London, Churchill, 1870; idem., Beale, *Disease Germs; Their Supposed Nature*, London, Churchill, 1870.
55 J. G. Morris, *Germinal Matter and the Contact Theory: An Essay on Morbid Poisons, their Nature, Sources, Effects, Migrations, and the Means of Limiting their Noxious Agency*, London, Churchill, 1867. Morris also wrote on protoplasm in the 1870s, but his main work was in neurology.
56 J. B. Sanderson, 'The Intimate Pathology of Contagion', *Twelfth Report of the Medical Officer of the Privy Council for 1869*, BPP 1870 [C.208], xxxviii, 591; *Thirteenth Report of the Medical Officer of the Privy Council for 1870*, BPP 1871, [C.349], xxxi, 763.

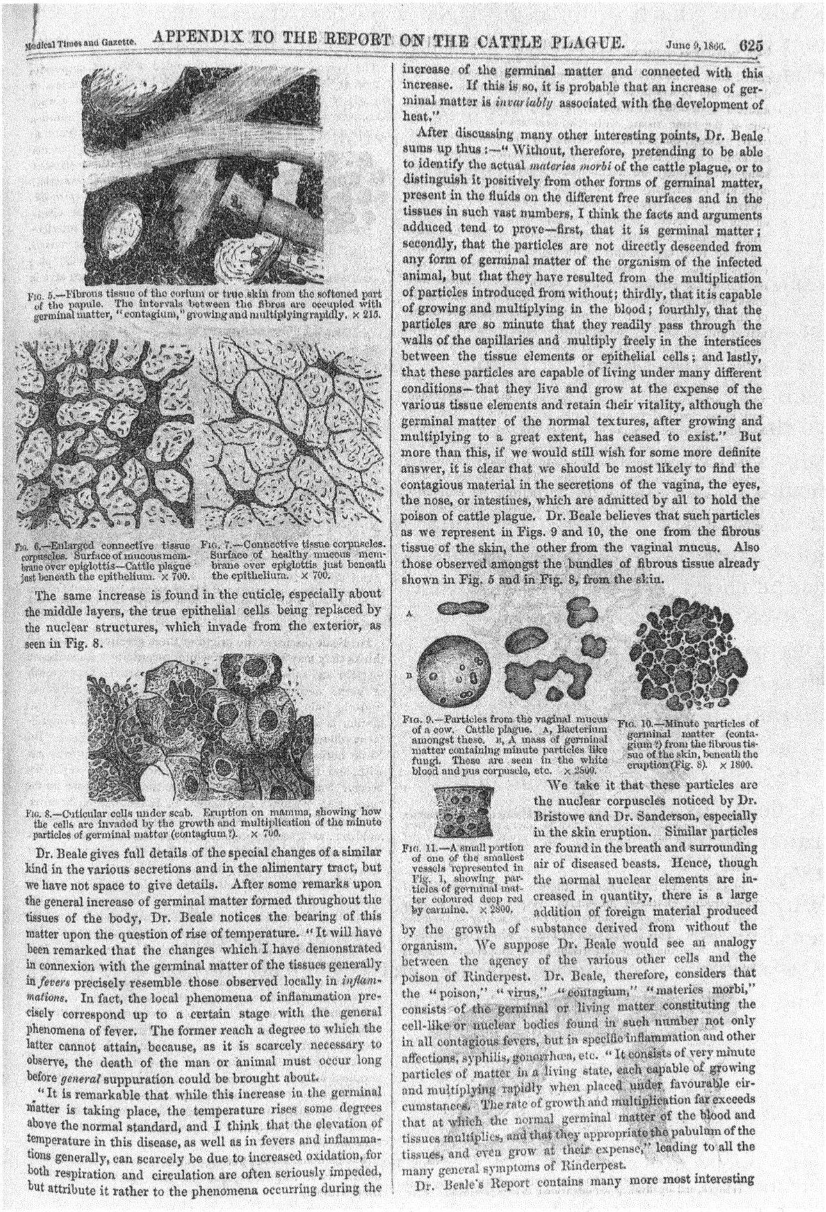

Medical Times and Gazette. APPENDIX TO THE REPORT ON THE CATTLE PLAGUE. June 9, 1866. 625

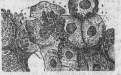

Fig. 5.—Fibrous tissue of the corium or true skin from the softened part of the papule. The intervals between the fibres are occupied with germinal matter, "contagium," growing and multiplying rapidly. × 215.

Fig. 6.—Enlarged connective tissue corpuscles. Surface of mucous membrane over epiglottis—Cattle plague just beneath the epithelium. × 700.

Fig. 7.—Connective tissue corpuscles. Surface of healthy mucous membrane over epiglottis just beneath the epithelium. × 700.

The same increase is found in the cuticle, especially about the middle layers, the true epithelial cells being replaced by the nuclear structures, which invade from the exterior, as seen in Fig. 8.

Fig. 8.—Cuticular cells under scab. Eruption on mamma, showing how the cells are invaded by the growth and multiplication of the minute particles of germinal matter (contagium?). × 700.

Dr. Beale gives full details of the special changes of a similar kind in the various secretions and in the alimentary tract, but we have not space to give details. After some remarks upon the general increase of germinal matter formed throughout the tissues of the body, Dr. Beale notices the bearing of this matter upon the question of rise of temperature. "It will have been remarked that the changes which I have demonstrated in connexion with the germinal matter of the tissues generally in *fevers* precisely resemble those observed locally in *inflammations*. In fact, the local phenomena of inflammation precisely correspond up to a certain stage with the general phenomena of fever. The former reach a degree to which the latter cannot attain, because, as it is scarcely necessary to observe, the death of the man or animal must occur long before *general* suppuration could be brought about.

"It is remarkable that while this increase in the germinal matter is taking place, the temperature rises some degrees above the normal standard, and I think that the elevation of temperature in this disease, as well as in fevers and inflammations generally, can scarcely be due to increased oxidation, for both respiration and circulation are often seriously impeded, but attribute it rather to the phenomena occurring during the

increase of the germinal matter and connected with this increase. If this is so, it is probable that an increase of germinal matter is *invariably* associated with the development of heat."

After discussing many other interesting points, Dr. Beale sums up thus :—" Without, therefore, pretending to be able to identify the actual *materies morbi* of the cattle plague, or to distinguish it positively from other forms of germinal matter, present in the fluids on the different free surfaces and in the tissues in such vast numbers, I think the facts and arguments adduced tend to prove—first, that it is germinal matter ; secondly, that the particles are not directly descended from any form of germinal matter of the organism of the infected animal, but that they have resulted from the multiplication of particles introduced from without; thirdly, that it is capable of growing and multiplying in the blood; fourthly, that the particles are so minute that they readily pass through the walls of the capillaries and multiply freely in the interstices between the tissue elements or epithelial cells ; and lastly, that these particles are capable of living under many different conditions—that they live and grow at the expense of the various tissue elements and retain their vitality, although the germinal matter of the normal textures, after growing and multiplying to a great extent, has ceased to exist." But more than this, if we would still wish for some more definite answer, it is clear that we should be most likely to find the contagious material in the secretions of the vagina, the eyes, the nose, or intestines, which are admitted by all to hold the poison of cattle plague. Dr. Beale believes that such particles as we represent in Figs. 9 and 10, the one from the fibrous tissue of the skin, the other from the vaginal mucus. Also those observed amongst the bundles of fibrous tissue already shown in Fig. 5 and in Fig. 8, from the skin.

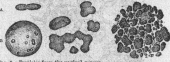

Fig. 9.—Particles from the vaginal mucus of a cow. Cattle plague. A, Bacterium amongst these. B, A mass of germinal matter containing minute particles like fungi. These are seen in the white blood and pus corpuscle, etc. × 2800.

Fig. 10.—Minute particles of germinal matter (contagium?) from the fibrous tissue of the skin, beneath the eruption (Fig. 8). × 1800.

Fig. 11.—A small portion of one of the smallest vessels represented in Fig. 1, showing particles of germinal matter coloured deep red by carmine. × 2800.

We take it that these particles are the nuclear corpuscles noticed by Dr. Bristowe and Dr. Sanderson, especially in the skin eruption. Similar particles are found in the breath and surrounding air of diseased beasts. Hence, though the normal nuclear elements are increased in quantity, there is a large addition of foreign material produced by the growth of substance derived from without the organism. We suppose Dr. Beale would see an analogy between the agency of the various other cells and the poison of Rinderpest. Dr. Beale, therefore, considers that the "poison," "virus," "contagium," "materies morbi," consists of the germinal or living matter constituting the cell-like or nuclear bodies found in such number not only in all contagious fevers, but in specific inflammation and other affections, syphilis, gonorrhœa, etc. "It consists of very minute particles of matter in a living state, each capable of growing and multiplying rapidly when placed under favourable circumstances. The rate of growth and multiplication far exceeds that at which the normal germinal matter of the blood and tissues multiplies, and that they appropriate the pabulum of the tissues, and even grow at their expense," leading to all the many general symptoms of Rinderpest.

Dr. Beale's Report contains many more most interesting

Figure 6. Part of the report in the *Medical Times and Gazette* of Lionel Beale's work for the Royal Commission on the cattle plague, showing illustrations of bioplasm. *Medical Times and Gazette*, 1866, i: 625 (Reproduced by courtesy of the Director and University Librarian, the John Rylands University Library of Manchester)

Ross[57] and A. E. Sansom.[58] Each of these envisaged a process whereby the sick threw off from their skin, exhaled from their lungs, or discharged from their bowels or bladder some 'germinal matter' (Morris) or particulate matter (Sanderson) that would graft (Ross) on to another body or infect (Sansom) another person. I will discuss these germ theories in later chapters, but for the moment I want to return to veterinarians and their developing pathological and aetiological ideas.

VETERINARIANS, CONTAGION AND THE NEW PATHOLOGY

The decline in the incidence of cattle plague and other diseases in 1866 came to be celebrated as a great landmark in the history of British veterinary medicine.[59] Veterinarians forgot their earlier disagreements and made as if they had always known that epizootics were contagious and that veterinary policing was the way to control them. As contingent contagionists they maintained that agricultural and environmental conditions determined that Britain, the most 'developed' country in the world, was not the 'home' of any major contagious disease, as the Russian Steppes was for the cattle plague and Bengal for Asiatic cholera. However, they now stressed that British livestock would always be vulnerable to imported diseases and that epizootics could, if conditions were favourable, be 'naturalised' and become native to the country. Keeping out and stamping out animal contagions became imperative, and was the aim of most of the veterinary legislation passed after 1867. The programme was enshrined in the major Contagious Diseases (Animals) Act (CD(A)A), 1869, that scheduled as imported dangers: cattle plague, pleuropneumonia, sheep-pox, foot-and-mouth disease, sheep scab and glanders.[60] This legislation was contemporary with the Contagious Diseases Acts, 1864, 1866 and 1869, which aimed to control sexually transmitted diseases in garrison towns. Why livestock legislation was given a title so similar to measures against venereal disease and prostitution is unclear, although prostitutes and campaigners against the Contagious Diseases Acts eventually turned the case around and complained that they were being treated like 'beasts of the field'.

57 J. Ross, *The Graft Theory of Disease*, London, Churchill, 1872.
58 A. E. Sansom, *The Antiseptic System: A Treatise on Carbolic Acid and its Compounds*, London, Gillman, 1871.
59 In the late 1870s and 1880s, the view in some sections of the profession was that the government and elite veterinarians were becoming complacent. This was especially the view of Fleming and expressed forcefully in the *Veterinary Journal*. See: *VJ*, 1877, 4: 189, 551; 1877, 5: 200; 1878, 6: 186, 196. However, in the longer term the assessment was much more favourable. See: J. McQueen, 'Veterinary Science', *Encyclopaedia Britannica*, 10th edition, London, 1911, p. 6.
60 MAFF, *Animal Health*, 31. It has been suggested that the 1864 Act tried to 'hide' behind Gamgee's cattle bill of the same year. However, the original medical legislation was not that controversial and the two sets of controls were based on quite different methods. J. Walkowitz, *Prostitution and Victorian Society: Women, Class and the State*, Cambridge, Cambridge University Press, 1979.

There is no doubt that the experience of the cattle plague advanced the standing of contagionism in veterinary medicine, human medicine and in wider public discussions.[61] The most widely cited medical account of contagion of the last quarter of the century, that given by John Simon in 1878, cited the 1866 epizootic as a model contagious disease.[62] According to Simon contagious diseases could be passed on via an intermediate agency or host as well as by direct contact. By this time Simon was convinced that all contagia had a common characteristic, namely, 'that in appropriate media they show themselves capable of *self-multiplication*'. Even when his 1878 essay was reprinted in Quain's *Dictionary of Medicine* in 1882, he was unwilling to say that contagia were living organisms and caused diseases, although many people read him as endorsing bacterial germ theories. The qualification that contagia needed 'appropriate media' to develop showed the importance of the continuing belief in the role of predisposing and contingent factors. Simon classed contagia as either *parasitic*, that is, independent organisms that produced disease by mechanical obstruction or draining nutritive resources, or *metabolic*, that is, 'viruses' that produced diseases by their chemical, usually poisonous effects on the physiology of those infected. The receptivity of the body was thought to be most significant with the metabolic poisons, although Simon used the metaphor of contagia as 'sparks' that needed suitable 'fuel' to develop and spread.[63] Simon's account of contagion also revealed his medical roots in pathology, especially his interest in disease processes rather than aetiology. However, he made the typical assumption that once 'contagia' or any zymotic agent established itself in the body, the disease process tended to run its course, which made disease prevention all important.

From the 1860s, through the research supported by his medical department, Simon developed a programme of investigation into the 'intimate pathology of contagion', which involved microscopy and experimental studies of contagious matter. This programme developed directly out of the cattle plague investigations and used some of the same researchers, notably Sanderson. The main aim was to determine the nature and actions of the 'active principle' of contagion, with a view to the better control of disease transmission and the possible extension of vaccination. In medicine, as opposed to surgery, this was the main context in which laboratory research on the role of germs in disease was pursued in Britain for most of the 1870s.[64]

61 J. Clarke Jervoise, *Infection, with Remarks by Miss Nightingale*, London, Vacher and Sons, 1882. Florence Nightingale's notes on this volume refer to the 'disease-germ-fetish' and 'disease-germ-hypthesis', comparing to 'the witchcraft-fetish'. She regards the hypothesis as speculative, likely to be damging to commerce and human intercourse, and to undermine all sanitary legislation.

62 J. S. Simon, 'Contagion' in R. Quain, ed., *A Dictionary of Medicine, Vol. 1*, London, Longmans Green, 1882, 294. Although published in 1882, the text was written in 1878.

63 The complexity of ideas of contagion in the early 1870s was illustrated by the discussion in Frederick Robert's textbook. F. T. Roberts, *A Handbook of the Theory and Practice of Medicine*, London, H. K. Lewis, 1873, 118–26.

64 These investigations are discussed in Romano, *Making Medicine*, 153–69.

The government's new Veterinary Department supported no comparable investigations. Elite veterinarians were sceptical of such research, not least because their collective judgement was that medical scientists had produced so little of benefit in 1865–66. George Fleming, head of the Army Veterinary Service, later editor of the *Veterinary Record* and committed contagionist, wrote of the Third Report on the Cattle Plague in 1866 that,

Regular medical men and medical critics have lauded this third report as an immense achievement of high scientific attainments. In vain have I searched through it for a single practical fact worth the paper it is printed on and which was not known to veterinary medicine.[65]

There were other attacks in the veterinary journals on the way medical practitioners had pontificated about controlling and curing cattle plague and what nonsense most of this had turned out to be.[66] Veterinarians claimed that practical, administrative measures based on experience had delivered the country from the crisis, not advanced medical ideas or research.[67] The clear species-barrier to human infection shown by the cattle plague was very useful to veterinarians in maintaining and defining their professional terrain. Thus, the number of diseases that they regarded as true zoonoses – animal diseases that can be transmitted to humans – was quite small and enabled veterinarians to deny that there was much common ground between veterinary and human medicine.

The veterinary profession had a clear interest in the state agencies and controls that developed from 1866, especially from the time of the 1869 Act. The metropolitan elite became advisers and administrators to a department of the Privy Council, while rank-and-file veterinary surgeons increasingly enjoyed the authority of acting as part-time state inspectors, posts that also brought extra income. Such was their commitment to this system that they became indifferent and hostile to the exploration of alternative control methods. Elite metropolitan veterinarians came to associate laboratory research with new methods of control that would threaten existing control measures. In 1873, G. T. Brown (1827–1906), by then chief government adviser, spoke disparagingly of the debates in surgery and medicine about the 'minute pathology of contagion' and in favour of 'whole-animal', population or epidemiological approaches[68]:

If a critic wished to secure attention to his remarks, he would carefully avoid such a commonplace statement as that which refers the extension of disease to the movement of infected animals and proceed to a discussion of the possibility of spontaneous origin, the

65 *Veterinarian*, 1867, 40: 578.
66 *Veterinarian*, 1865, 38: 780, 792, 906; 1866, 39: 353; 1867, 40: 563.
67 C. Hawley, 'The Medical Profession and the Curing of the Cattle Plague', *Veterinarian*, 1865, 38: 906–10.
68 'George Thomas Brown, 1827–1906', *DNB*, Suppl. 1, pp. 236–7.

prevalence of minute spores of fungi, atmospheric changes and the indirect conveyance of the poison by flies, birds and other quadrupeds . . . . but still the fact remains that the malady is kept in a state of activity mainly by means of the living creatures suffering from it.[69]

Simonds and G. T. Brown made inoculation experiments at the RVC in the mid-1870s, but these were whole-animal experiments that were monitored clinically and not by microscopy or pathological examinations.[70] In 1875, the RASE withdrew its grant for the investigation of animal diseases from Simonds at the RVC because he refused to make the experimental investigations of pleuropneumonia that they sought.[71] Sanderson, who took over the investigations, then found his work hampered by the Veterinary Department's refusal to relax regulations so that infected cattle could be moved to his laboratory. Indeed, it was reported that Simonds had remarked that, 'there was nothing more to be discovered with reference to important diseases'.[72] The veterinary elite had moved to an extreme contagionist position where they were nervous about having any infected animals and hence any contagia at all in the country. Through the 1870s their standard response to other livestock disease threats was to suggest that they be added to the schedule of the 1869 CD(A)A and be subject to administrative control.[73] When the cattle plague arrived again in 1877, the government appointed another advisory group, this time a Select Committee on the Cattle Plague and the Importation of Live Stock. The title confirms how the problem of livestock diseases was seen as one of external contamination of the British herd; indeed, policy was said to be guided by the 'importation theory of disease'. Unlike the Royal Commission in 1866, the Select Committee was content to receive verbal and written evidence on the administration of existing legislation and the particular experience of this epizootic. They did not support pathological or any other experimental investigations.

An idiosyncratic, but none the less important example of the influence of the importation theory can be seen in the career of John Gamgee after the 1865–66 crisis. The cattle plague and its consequences were not, as might be expected, used by Gamgee to further his career in veterinary medicine and pathological research. He did make further investigations of epizootics in North America, but his energies were increasingly directed to the development of refrigerated meat storage. He had not abandoned the fight against imported livestock diseases; rather, he had chosen to pursue

69 *JRAS*, 1873, 34: 449.
70 *JRAS*, 1874, 35: 269, 459.
71 The grant was transferred to Sanderson at the Brown Institute. *JRAS*, 1876, 37: viii.
72 *VJ*, 1876, 2: 73.
73 Thus, there were at various times proposals to add rabies, swine plague (also known as pig typhoid and hog cholera), anthrax, sheep pox, glanders and even tuberculosis.

it by other means. His aim was to replace the trade in livestock with that in 'refrigerated meat'. Gamgee believed that epizootic diseases could be controlled only by a total ban on livestock trade, as he was convinced that veterinary inspection and policing would always be liable to maladministration and evasion. He saw the best hope in replacing the trade in livestock, which could carry living contagia, with one in 'deadstock', which could not.

That veterinary thinking structured around the health of the livestock economy rather than diseases of organs and tissues was illustrated by an occasional feature on 'Pathological Contributions' that appeared in the *Veterinarian* in the 1870s. This reported, not the latest findings from the postmortem room or laboratory, but the statistical returns to the Privy Council Veterinary Department of the number of animals dying of epizootics or slaughtered under legislative orders.[74] The data indicated the waxing and waning of scheduled diseases in the national herd. The reports were also used to show how a single infected animal could be the source of a national epizootic, reinforcing the perception of the vulnerability and fragility of the livestock economy. There were obvious parallels, if not direct linkages, between this view and the weakness of British agriculture in general at this time and its vulnerability to imports.

VETERINARIANS AND GERMS

From the mid-1870s germs and bacteria became a regular topic for reports at meetings of regional and other veterinary medical associations.[75] To the surprise of those who introduced the subject, opinions in the meetings were generally favourable. Veterinarians were persuaded of the living germ theory of disease despite there being many competing views on the nature and action of germs, and before practical demonstrations with microscopes and cultures became routine. Indeed, in the 1870s many investigators, including Sanderson, assumed that microscopy was unreliable and rested the case for germs on analogies. Despite the uncertainties, veterinarians found germ theories of disease congenial for two main reasons: first, germs were moulded to support their ideas on the control of epizootics; and, second, they were remade to be congruent with prevailing pathological models in veterinary medicine. Thomas Greaves, a regular speaker on germs at veterinary meetings in the late 1870s, made germs the agents of the contagious diseases

---

74 For example see: *Veterinarian*, 1879, 52: 26, 92. Many issues in the 1870s and 1880s contained this feature.

75 George Fleming, the editor of the *Veterinary Journal*, was a supporter of germ-theory and an authority on actinomycosis and tuberculosis. The content and editorial policy of his journal was markedly different from that of its rival, the *Veterinarian*, in its support of germ-theory and the reporting of bacteriology. In 1877 there was extended discussion of Koch's work on anthrax. See: *VJ*, 1877, 4: 118, 349, 451.

that the profession had to control.[76] The powers of propagation of living germs were like those of a single infected beast entering the country – both could spread and multiply. This 'fact' was said to reinforce the need for the most stringent quarantine and inspection measures, and for always erring on the side of safety.[77] As important was the ability to contrast specific germs with the vague 'something-in-the-air' ideas of anticontagionists that had left Britain open to epizootics before 1865. Support for germ theories was also associated with rejection of the spontaneous generation of disease, which still had wide support amongst veterinarians and had been an obstacle to introducing quarantine measures earlier. Germs were also readily accommodated within two pathological models that were more common in veterinary than human medicine – parasitic and dietetic diseases.[78] Parasitic diseases were more prevalent in domestic and farm animals than in humans, so when Greaves referred to germs as vegetable parasites and microparasites his audience would have been familiar with the idea of diseases having external and even single causes. Veterinarians also treated many more dietetic diseases; hence the assumed pathogenic action of germs through chemical poisons had an obvious parallel in dietary poisons. That said, Greaves still stressed the receptivity of the affected animal to parasitic agents and poisons, and did not see germs as all-conquering invading agents.

While provincial veterinarians discussed and generally endorsed bacterial and other germ theories of disease, the metropolitan elite continued to be sceptical towards emergent germ practices. In particular, they were unsympathetic to the work of the Brown Animal Sanatory Institute as a place 'for really original research in great questions of pathological research and comparative hygiene'.[79] Through the 1870s Sanderson, Klein and Greenfield studied a number of animal diseases, including anthrax, but their main work was on human diseases.[80] The superintendents in the 1880s worked on animal diseases, notably Roy's investigation of pleuropneumonia, which was supported by the BMA, and Horsley's work on rabies.[81] The first major

76 For example, in 1878, Thomas Greaves (Manchester) spoke on 'Germs' to the Liverpool, Yorkshire, Central and Midland Counties Veterinary Medical Associations: *VJ*, 1878, 6: 53, 366; 1878, 7: 52, 350; 1879, 9: 1–7. Also see review by J. H. Steel, 'Principal Facts Hitherto Ascertained Concerning Bacteria', *VJ*, 1879, 9: 156, 238.

77 G. Fleming, *A Manual of Veterinary Sanitary Science and Police*, London, Chapman and Hall, 1875, *passim*.

78 T. S. Cobbold, 'Address at Opening of R.V.C., 1879–80 Session', *Veterinarian*. 1879, 52: 761. Also see: G. T. Brown, 'Animal Parasites', in C. E. Shelley, ed., *Transactions of the Seventh International Congress on Hygiene and Demography*, London, Eyre & Spottiswoode, 1891. John Farley has argued that the links between 'worm theories' and germ theories were weak. My argument in the volume overall is that this assessment is mistaken. Cf. J. Farley, 'Parasites and the Germ Theory of Disease', *Milbank Quarterly*, 1989, 67: 50–68.

79 Quoted in: W. D. Tigertt, 'Anthrax: William Smith Greenfield, MD, FRCP, Professor Superintendent, The Brown Animal Sanatory Institute', *Journal of Hygiene*, 1980, 85: 415.

80 Anon. 'W. S. Greenfield', *EMJ*, 1919, 23: 258.

81 C. S. Roy, 'The Pathological History of Epizootic Pleuropneumonia', *VJ*, 1880, 10: 1, 176.

'discovery' to emerge from research at the Brown was in 1874, when Klein 'caused much sensation in scientific circles' by announcing that he had found the germs of two diseases – those for typhoid fever in humans and for the pox in sheep.[82] Neither 'discovery' stood the test of peer evaluation, and Klein was forced to retract when Creighton found that both the supposed 'micrococci' of typhoid and his 'mycelial growths' in sheep-pox were only 'some albuminous or kindred material' – an artefact of his preparation methods.[83] In 1877 Klein reported that swine fever in pigs was caused by a bacillus, although he did not publish a description of the organism until several years later.[84] These findings were subsequently challenged by no lesser figure than Pasteur in 1882.[85] Whether we think that Klein was unlucky or lacking skill does not really matter; what did matter was the damage done to the credibility of research on the intimate pathology of contagion amongst already sceptical veterinarians and certain medical practitioners too. Klein's 'errors' were used by elite veterinarians to defend animal diseases from the encroachments of medical and pathological experts. *The Veterinarian*, edited by Simonds and G. T. Brown, was very severe on Klein and other researchers. This led Fleming's rival *Veterinary Journal* to defend its publication of Klein's work in 1877, saying that those 'who exalt over such mistakes as those of Klein . . . are likely to drive us back to the age of farriery'.[86]

John Tyndall attempted to elevate Klein to the status of microbe hunter as part of his campaign against spontaneous generation, and for the reform of medicine.[87] Klein's results were the product of an established research programme in microscopic pathological anatomy and histology. They were the type of findings presaged by the reports of microscopic organisms being associated with disease since the 1860s, and more recently with Obermeier's description in 1872 of a spirilla in the blood of patients with relapsing fever. Other investigators had deduced the presence of germs by chemical and

82 This episode is discussed in greater detail in Chapter 4. But see T. Lauder Brunton, 'Dr. Klein and the Pathology of Small-pox and Typhoid Fever', *Practitioner*, 1875, 14: 5–10. Also see: *Centrallblatt fur der Medin. Wissen.* 1874, 692, 706. E. Klein, 'Research on the Smallpox of Sheep', *PRSL*, 1874, 22: 388–91.

83 C. Creighton, 'Note On Certain Unusual Coagulation Appearances Found in Mucus and other Albuminoid Fluids', *PSRL*, 1877, 25: 140–4; E. Klein, 'Note on the Mycelium Described in my Paper on the Smallpox of Sheep', *PRSL*, 1877, 25: 259–60.

84 E. Klein, 'Enteric or Typhoid Fever of the Pig', *Supplement to the Sixth Annual Report of the LGB, containing the Report of the Medical Officer of Health for 1876*, BPP 1878, [C.1608], xxxvii, Pt. ii, 455; E. Klein, 'Infectious Pneumo-Enteritis in the Pig', *Supplement to the Seventh Annual Report of the LGB, containing the Report of the Medical Officer of Health for 1877*, BPP 1878, [C.2130–1] xxxvii Pt. ii, 403; E. Klein, 'The Bacteria of Swine Plague', *Journal of Physiology*, 1884, 5: 1–13.

85 L. Pasteur, 'Sur le rouget, ou mal rouge de porcs', *Comptes Rendus*, 1882, 95: 1120–3.

86 G. Fleming, 'The Part Played by Minute Organisms in Disease', *VJ*, 1877, 4: 118–20; I. Pattison, 'Major-General Sir Frederick Smith and James Beart Simonds: "A veterinarian destroyed"', *VR*, 1984, 114: 657–8.

87 A. Adam, *Spontaneous Generation in the 1870s: Victorian Scientific Naturalism and its Relationship to Medicine*, PhD Thesis, C.N.A.A., 1988.

experimental methods, for example, Chaueau's work on vaccinia and Sanderson's isolation of 'sepsin'.[88] However, all of these methods were, in the words of an editorial in the *Veterinary Journal* in 1877, 'prone to error'.[89] Historians have suggested that this changed with Koch's work on anthrax, published in 1876, which introduced methods that allowed the germs of disease to be observed more easily and for causative relations between germs and disease to be demonstrated. Matters were not that clearcut at the time. In the late 1870s, Koch's results were viewed as sceptically as other germ claims, and their potential was only thought to be 'very great, if they are found to bear the test of further experience and observation'.[90] In 1877, Professor William Williams, New College, Edinburgh, took on Tyndall, Davaine, Koch and others maintaining that anthrax originated spontaneously, citing epidemiological rather than laboratory evidence.[91] More generally, those who accepted a role for bacillary germs and those who did not all agreed that 'circumstances and surroundings', and diet had to be taken into account.[92] In Britain, anthrax was not that serious a problem in livestock and was not scheduled as contagious; hence Koch's work did not attract much attention in veterinary circles. If anything, it had more relevance to medicine, where its occupationally linked human form – Woolsorters' disease – was studied by doctors in the West Riding.[93] Germ theories seemed much more significant for scheduled diseases, and it was the purported germs of rabies, glanders and tuberculosis that were most reported in veterinary journals from the late 1870s.[94] The accounts of the development of germ ideas presented to veterinary audiences looked to British and French research rather than Germany, so the lineage of work on germs ran through Tyndall, Sanderson and Lister, to Pasteur, Chauveau, Davaine and Lemaire.[95]

Throughout the 1870s laboratory and clinical research on animal diseases had made use of inoculation to study two issues: first, to determine which diseases were contagious and to what degree; and, second, to explore the value of protective inoculation from other diseases and modified contagia. The latter was stimulated by reports that many farmers had protected their stock against bovine pleuropneumonia by inoculating them with pustular matter from the tail of diseased animals, in practices that sought to emulate Jenner's procedures. However, the staff of the Veterinary Department saw the development of preventive inoculation as a threat to administrative control and possibly to the department itself. They returned to the familiar theme of the lessons of cattle plague and the failure of vaccinations and laboratory

88 See Chapters 3 and 4.   89 *VJ*, 1877, 4: 118–20.   90 Ibid., 349.   91 Ibid., 237.
92 *Veterinarian*, 1880, 53: 846.
93 *Lancet*, 1880, i: 778, 819, 926; J. Spear, 'The "Woolsorters' Disease" or Anthrax Fever', *TESL*, 1875–81, 4: 277–300.
94 *VJ*, 1878, 6: 34, 53–5, 190.
95 *VJ*, 1878, 6: 52; 1879, 8: 46–74.

studies. Such hostility was no doubt one factor in the decision of the Veterinary Department in 1875 to prohibit the movement of beasts to the Brown.[96] However, Sanderson found other ways to evaluate inoculations and concluded, in his inimitably equivocal manner, that the policy of stamping out disease should remain, but called for further investigations of inoculation. The Veterinary Department welcomed the first of his recommendations and used it as ammunition against the vociferous proinoculation claims being made, principally in Scotland, by James Rutherford and his supporters. Supposedly following methods developed empirically, and pioneered in New Zealand, there was a vocal lobby for this new preventive strategy. However, the Veterinary Department recommended that the research should not be supported.[97] They argued that such work might be appropriate for the countries of Continental Europe, where long land frontiers and political problems made legislative solutions difficult, but the island geography of Britain made policing and stamping out the best answer to all contagious animal diseases.[98]

Sanderson had been working since the late 1860s on smallpox vaccination, and his research on pleuropneumonia was an extension of this. He hoped that inoculation studies would answer an important question about the effects of transmission of contagious matter: did virulence increase or diminish with each successive transmission? After the publication of Koch's studies of anthrax in 1876, Sanderson took up the bacillus as an experimental agent. It was relatively large, easy to see and manipulate, and always present in the blood of infected animals. He began experiments from which he reported that the properties of the bacillus were altered by its passage through the rat.[99] Prior experience with inoculations of contagious matter had shown that successive inoculations could lead either to 'exalted' or 'diminished' virulence. While this phenomenon was explored by Pasteur with fowl cholera, Sanderson and then his successor, William Greenfield, worked with anthrax. On 5 June 1880, one month before Toussaint announced the first anthrax vaccine in France, Greenfield wrote that he had been:

led to the conclusion that the poison [of anthrax] becomes progressively less virulent with successive generations of artificial cultivation. I have thus been able to obtain a modified virus, which when inoculated produces less severe symptoms, and appears to be partially protective against future more severe attacks.[100]

96 *Veterinarian*, 1879, 52: 351. These recommendations were dismissed by Rutherford and his allies as mere laboratory findings and insignificant when compared to the experience of the measures in herds at home and abroad.
97 *VJ*, 1879, 9: 14, 410.
98 C. A. Cameron, 'Report on Public Health', *DJMS*, 1877, 64: 526–49.
99 J. B. Sanderson, 'Report on Experiments on Anthrax Conducted at the Brown Institution, February 18 to June 30, 1878', *JRAS*, 1880, 41: 267.
100 The issue of priority is discussed in Tigertt, 'Greenfield', 415–20. *Lancet*, 1880, i: 866. On Pasteur's work see: G. L. Geison, 'Louis Pasteur', in Gillispie, *Dictionary of Scientific*, 392–98. On Pasteur's work at Pouilly-le-Fort, see: G. L. Geison, *The Private Science of Louis Pasteur*, Princeton, NJ, Princeton University Press, 1995, 145–76.

When Pasteur announced his fowl cholera vaccine in October 1880, the Paris correspondent of the *Lancet* observed,

We have drawn attention to the chief features of Mr Pasteur's communication . . . to point out that its most important fact has been already anticipated by one of our own investigators in the same field . . . . Dr Greenfield.[101]

At the end of the following year, after the display at Pouilly-le-Fort, Greenfield himself commented that Pasteur had used 'a precisely similar method, and with results fully confirming those which I published more than a year ago'. Graciously, he rejoiced in Pasteur's success, but claimed some priority for England. What is important about this episode is not the priority dispute, which never happened, but the relative neglect of Greenfield's work in Britain. Greenfield later said that this was due to the fact that the work was not developed due to the lack of funding and the difficulties created by the vivisection laws. In this context, it was significant that in 1881 Greenfield, who was medically qualified, moved to a medical post as Professor of Pathology at Edinburgh.[102] Also, it is no surprise to find that the Veterinary Department showed no interest in his work, and that his successor at the Brown, C. S. Roy, worked on the heart and only investigated anthrax on a visit to South America.

Little was heard of anthrax again in Britain until it was added to the CD(A)A in 1886. By this time, the previously sceptical G. T. Brown had become interested in the bacillus and planned to undertake his own experimental work on its longevity in the soil. However, the absence of the disease and hence the bacillus from Britain led him to abandon his project. He was seemingly unwilling to sanction the importation of the organism or infected animals from abroad, even for his own research. Undaunted, he pursued the inquiry by other methods, principally from 'the facts of the history of the disease in the United Kingdom'; in other words, he published an explanation based largely on administratively generated data.[103]

The question of inoculation against pleuropneumonia remained an issue because Rutherford did not give up his fight for its trial and acceptance.[104] In the 1880s he gained the support of Professor Williams and the subject became a bone of contention between the two veterinary colleges in Edinburgh, with Tom Walley and John M'Fadyean of the rival Dick College vigorously opposing any alternative that weakened administrative control and

101 *Lancet*, 1880, ii: 750–2.
102 W. S. Greenfield, 'Pathology, Past and Present', *Lancet*, 1881, ii: 738–41, 781–6. Also see: W. S. Greenfield, 'Report on an Experimental Investigation of Anthrax and Allied Diseases, made at the Brown Institution', *JRAS*, 1881, 42: 30–44.
103 *Annual Report of the Agricultural Department on Contagious Diseases Inspection and the Transit of Animals for 1885*, BPP 1886, xix, [C.4703], 6.
104 T. Walley, 'Thrashing out the Pleuro Question', *VJ*, 1889, 37: 280–5.

stamping out.[105] The 'Pleuro Question', as it became known, reached a peak in 1887–88 and the government sought a resolution by the appointment of a Departmental Committee.[106] The committee was also asked to report on whether, following the identification of the causative *Tubercle bacillus* and the growing acceptance of contagion, tuberculosis should be added to the CD(A)A. This aspect of the committee's work will be discussed in Chapter 6, but at this stage it should be noted that the committee contained no scientists, and was full of people with a vested interest in the current system. Again the committee did not support experimental investigations to help them with their assessments.

Most of the oral and written evidence collected on pleuropneumonia was against inoculation and in favour of the continuation of control through the CD(A)A.[107] In fact, the authors of the report were worried lest research might undermine the Act:

We consider that if it should be deemed necessary or desirable that further experiments should be conducted, they should be commenced on the clear understanding that the investigation is undertaken entirely in the interests of science, and without any reference to the measures proper to be adopted for the extinction of the disease.[108]

Very significant was the evidence of John M'Fadyean, who was then emerging as a leading veterinary authority in the new science of bacteriology. The following exchange took place when he was questioned by G. T. Brown:

Brown: You think, in reference to the possible discovery of the organism of pleuropneumonia, it would be advantageous to have experiments set on foot?
M'Fadyean: No, I do not see that more than an indirect interest might attach to it. No great benefit would result from a knowledge of the specific organism of pleuropneumonia if inoculation cannot be used as a means of eradicating the disease.
Brown: If you got rid of the disease you would not care about the organism?
M'Fadyean: Well, as a matter of pathological curiosity I should like to possess as many specific organisms as possible.
Brown: But on no other ground?
M'Fadyean: No.[109]

Thus, in 1888, even a committed bacteriologist like M'Fadyean was led to conclude that his interest in pathology was secondary to the interests of disease control. Once again experimental veterinary pathology and

105 *VJ*, 1887, 24: 33, 86, 197; ibid., 1887, 25: 209, 380, 415–36. I. Pattison, *John McFadyean: A Great British Veterinarian*, London, J. A. Allan, 1981.
106 *Report of the Departmental Committee appointed to inquire into Pleuropneumonia and Tuberculosis in the United Kingdom*, BPP 1888, [C.5461], xxxii, 267.
107 See editorial in *JCPT*, 1888, 1: 234, 276. New Pleuropneumonia Orders were passed by Parliament in 1888.
108 *Departmental Committee . . . Pleuropneumonia*, 64.
109 Ibid., p. 449 (paragraphs 4996–8).

bacteriology was not being neglected in veterinary medicine; it was being deliberately avoided.

VETERINARIANS, 'BACTERIOLOGY' AND 'IMMUNOLOGY'

As long as the veterinary elite consciously avoided germ research, there were few opportunities for rank-and-file veterinarians to learn about or take up experimental studies, despite their ideological commitment to bacterial germ theories and contagion. It is worth noting that antivivisection sentiment was strong in the profession and the Cruelty to Animals Act, 1876, was more restrictive on veterinary research than it was on medical.[110] However, it was not just laboratory work that veterinarians eschewed; they had little interest or need for the most famous of all germ practices – antiseptic surgery – despite having to deal with wounds that were usually dirty and had to heal in the most insanitary conditions.[111] That said, horses, dogs and livestock seemed not to suffer from wound sepsis, a fact that was variously attributed to the properties of their skins and tissues, their open-air existence or their habituation to filth and dirt. Antiseptic techniques were covered in veterinary textbooks and lectures by the 1880s, but only in relation to dressings, or as a means of securing cleanliness, not as a system of surgical practice. The main priorities in veterinary operations were how to tether the animal, and how to avoid losing instruments inside the animal. Oiling instruments to prevent rusting was given priority over sterility, and one textbook advised veterinarians undertaking operations to find a soft place for the animal to lay during an operation, such as 'a dung-heap covered by straw'.[112]

As noted in G. T. Brown's planned investigation of anthrax, the rising tide of bacteriology eventually infiltrated Britain's elite veterinarians. In 1886, twenty years after the cattle plague investigations and the start of laboratory

---

110 H. E. Carter, 'The Veterinary Profession and the R.S.P.C.A.: The First 50 Years', *Veterinary History*, 1989–90, 6 (2): 68–70. The three veterinarians who gave evidence to the 1875 Royal Commission on Vivisection were not enthusiastic about the practice. The Cruelty to Animals Act, 1876, specified that veterinary experiments could only be performed 'under anaesthetic and with a view to the advancement of veterinary science', that is, not for physiological demonstration. *Report of the Royal Commission on the Practice of Subjecting Live Animals to Experiments for Scientific Purposes*, BPP 1876, [C.1397], xli, 1. Cf. G. Fleming, 'Vivisection and the Diseases of Animals', *Nineteenth Century*, 1882, 11: 468–78.

111 In 1877, one veterinarian wrote of antisepsis passing 'almost into disuse'. *VJ*, 1877, 5: 9. Also see: *VJ*, 1879, 9: 37, 122; *Veterinarian*, 1879, 52: 376. Antisepsis was regarded as a technique of wound dressing, not an operative procedure. It should be noted that relatively few veterinary operations were performed at this time.

112 G. Fleming, *A Textbook of Operative Veterinary Surgery*, London, Baillière, Tindall and Cox, 1884, 4–8 Professor McQueen's lectures at the RVC in the 1890s did emphasise the need for antiseptic precautions as well as dressings, although the emphasis was still on the latter. Lecture Notes, H. P. Standing, 1894, and W. N. Thompson, no date (1894), Historical Collection, RVC, London.

researches by the Medical Department, the Veterinary Department finally commissioned its first experimental investigations. However, these were not aimed to advance veterinary knowledge as such, but to defend veterinary science against the encroachments of medical researchers, and one researcher in particular – Edward Klein. One result of the acceptance of bacterial aetiologies for infectious diseases was a growing interest in how bacteria spread. The passive diffusion of germs in air and water was favoured in the 1860s and 1870s, but in the 1880s attention was increasingly turning to specific points of passage and means of transmission, especially active carriage. Historians have discussed the ways in which flies and vermin became implicated as vectors, but contemporaries also worried about farm and domestic animals as sources and carriers, for example, the spread of typhoid fever via cow's milk and diphtheria by cats.[113]

The specific context of the Veterinary Department's move into experimental research was one such instance – an outbreak at Hendon in Middlesex of infection that seemed to have been caught from cows. This prompted the Medical Department to ask Klein to investigate the problem, and he reported that it was due to a previously unrecognised disease of cattle – which he rather unimaginatively called the 'Hendon Disease'.[114] He suggested that this was a form of scarlet fever, not previously recognised by veterinarians, that in certain conditions was communicated to humans. The veterinary elite was outraged by Klein's incursions into veterinary medicine and his 'discovery' of a common disease that they had previously failed to recognise. To defend the profession's honour and terrain, and the species barrier between human and animal diseases, the Veterinary Department employed E. M. Crookshank, who was none other than Lister's bacteriologist at King's College Hospital, London, to make a fresh investigation.[115] The choice was significant, for Crookshank and Klein were metropolitan rivals for the leadership of the 'British school of bacteriology'. Crookshank quickly reported that the 'Hendon Disease' was cowpox, not scarlet fever. The veterinary press applauded his work and its vindication of veterinary expertise; one report stated that 'no more absolute refutation of an error has ever

113 G. Sims Woodhead and J. M'Fadyean, 'Notes on the Microparasites of Domestic Animals', *Veterinarian*, 1886, 59, 591. On milk see: *BMJ*, 1883, ii: 591, 744. *BMJ*, 1879, i: 48, 148; *BMJ*, 1890, i: 1081, 1259; G. Turner, 'Report on the Experience of Diphtheria, Especially its Relations to Lower Animals', *Supplement to the Sixteenth Annual Report of LGB, Containing the Report of the Medical Officer for 1886*, BPP 1887, [C.5171], xxxvi, 619. Turner reported evidence of diphtheria in pigeons, chickens, swine, horses and cats.

114 L. G. Wilson, 'The Historical Riddle of Milk-borne Scarlet Fever', *BHM*, 1986, 60: 321–42.

115 Crookshank's career was changed by this episode. At King's he had a prestigious appointment working with Joseph Lister and William Watson Cheyne, running London's largest bacteriology course and main bacteriological laboratory. His researches on Hendon disease led him to inquire into the nature of cowpox and then to work on veterinary bacteriology. He adopted heterodox positions on vaccination and became a marginal figure. E. M. Crookshank, *The History and Pathology of Vaccination*, Vol. I, London, H. K. Lewis, 1889.

been made'.[116] An indication of what was at stake was that, despite the disease having long disappeared, Crookshank's report was rushed out in a special publication in the summer of 1888, rather than awaiting inclusion in the Veterinary Department's annual report at the end of the year.[117] Overall, Klein's work was so discredited that his reasonable claims to have identified a streptococcus closely associated with, if not the cause of, scarlet fever remained unacknowledged.[118]

Crookshank was retained as bacteriologist to the Veterinary Department and undertook other studies of animal diseases, though only those outside of the remit of the CD(A)A, such as actinomycosis and tuberculosis.[119] In 1888 he gave the first lectures on bacteriology at the RVC, assisted by Horsley and William Watson Cheyne, the latter also from Lister's department at King's College. In the same year laboratory work in bacteriology was introduced.[120] Surprisingly, this was many years ahead of practical bacteriology becoming routine in the medical curriculum.[121] This innovation undoubtedly came from Crookshank and Cheyne, who were already running similar extramural courses at King's College Hospital, London. It seems that the veterinary elite was quite happy for details of germs and how to observe them to be disseminated, but still saw no connection between the new science of bacteriology and the improvement of stamping out policies. In 1888, G. T. Brown observed that the minute character of swine fever was of scientific interest, but 'from the sanitary police point of view it is of not much consequence'.[122] This was not how matters seemed in France, where Pasteur and his associates had produced vaccines against fowl cholera, anthrax, swine erysipelas and, most famously, rabies.[123] The latter had brought Pasteur national fame and had raised expectations of the potential of laboratory medicine to prevent and cure human and animals diseases. So, what was the reaction to this in Britain?

Rabies was a zoonose that concerned both veterinarians and medical practitioners. Its control had been debated in the late 1870s, when the issues were the by now familiar ones of did the disease arise spontaneously, or always

116 *VR*, 1888–89, 1: 301. M'Fadyean referred the Power and Klein's work and another claim about Diphtheria in animals as 'absurd'. *JCPT*, 1888, 1: 239.

117 G. T. Brown, *Report on Eruptive Diseases of the teats and udder in cows in relation to Scarlet Fever in Man*, BPP 1888, [C.5481], xxxii, 1.

118 Wilson, 'The Historical Riddle', 338–42. *Lancet*, 1887, i: 1193; 'Report by Dr Klein on the Etiology of Scarlet Fever', in *Sixteenth Annual Report*, Appendix B, 367–414.

119 *Annual Report of the Agricultural Department of the Privy Council on Contagious Diseases, etc., for 1888*, BPP 1889, [C.5679], xxvii, 3. Appendix.

120 *Veterinarian*, 1888, 61: 713.

121 *Lancet*, 1894, ii: 487. The establishment of courses and laboratories for practical instruction in London teaching hospitals lagged behind provisions in the provinces and in Scotland.

122 *Annual Report of the Agricultural Department of the Privy Council on Contagious Diseases, etc., for 1887*, BPP 1888, [C.5340], xxxiii, 7. Experiments were abandoned at the RVC because of the cost and the absence of a vivisection licence.

123 R. Dubos, *Pasteur and Modern Science*, New York, Anchor Books, 1960, 123.

come from a prior case? Was rabies a specific disease at all? Could the disease be controlled by quarantines as a prelude to stamping out?[124] The disease, with the fearful symptoms of 'lock jaw' and hydrophobia and its association with ferocious, salivating dogs attacking innocent people, came to symbolise public fears about the spread of germs and the communicability of animal diseases to humans.[125] Public fears waxed and waned with the overall inci-dence of the disease and awareness of cases through the press. There was alarm in 1877 when the annual death toll reached an all time high of seventy-nine and again in the mid-1880s. This time the government's response was to propose adding the disease the CD(A)A to allow the regulation of dogs coming into the country and the destruction of affected beasts.[126] These mea-sures came into effect at almost the exact moment when Pasteur announced his treatment for humans bitten by rabid dogs in the summer of 1885.[127] This innovation attracted huge public and medical attention, but went largely unreported in the veterinary press.[128] In 1886, Victor Horsley, who was uniquely qualified, being both Superintendent of the Brown and a surgeon at the National Hospital for Epilepsy and Nervous Diseases, and at Univer-sity College Hospital, led a government-sponsored enquiry into Pasteur's work.[129] Horsley successfully repeated Pasteur's work and the Brown subse-quently offered a diagnostic service for the whole country.[130] However, neither the Brown nor the National Hospital developed the treatment, nor did either supply rabies vaccines to the medical profession. Also, neither the government nor private charity took up and sponsored the innovation as elsewhere in Europe, where the innovation was the basis for the establish-ment of the Pasteur Institutes. In the 1880s and 1890s, the small number of rabies cases in Britain had to travel to Paris for treatment, with the delay and expense that entailed. The government decided that, in Britain, rabies was to be controlled in the same way as other contagious animal diseases – it was to be stamped out and kept out. Quarantines on imported dogs were insti-tuted and, in the short term, muzzling orders were made and stray dogs were rounded up and destroyed. Control began in London and was eventually

---

124 T. Watson, 'The Abolition of Zymotic Diseases, *Nineteenth Century*, 1877, 1: 380–96; W. Acland, 'Rabies and Hydrophobia', *VJ*, 1878, 6: 34. Amongst other methods suggested was a tax on dogs to discourage irresponsible owners, enforced by destroying untaxed dogs. Also see: J. K. Walton, 'Mad Dogs and Englishmen: The Conflict over Rabies in Late Victorian England, *VH*, 1978–9, 12: 3–26.

125 H. Ritvo, *The Animal Estate: The English and Other Creatures in the Victorian Age*, Cambridge, MA, Harvard University Press, 1987, 167–202.

126 *VJ*, 1887, 24: 183.

127 Geison, *Private Science*, 177–256.

128 L. Wilkinson, 'The Development of the Virus Concept as Reflected in the Corpora of Studies on Individual Pathogens. 4. Rabies', *MH*, 1977, 21: 30.

129 S. Paget, *Sir Victor Horsley: A Study of his Life and Work*, London, Constable and Co., 1919.

130 V. Horsley, 'On Rabies: Its Treatment by M. Pasteur, and on the Means of Detecting it Suspected Cases', *BMJ*, 1889, i: 342. Also see: G. Fleming, *Pasteur and His Work: From an Agricultural and Veterinary Point of View*, London, William Clowes, 1886.

extended to the whole country. It was so successful that by 1902 rabies had been stamped out. The hidden cost of this successful policy was the neglect of the opportunities to develop sophisticated new pathophysiological technologies, and to capitalise on the potential of Pasteur's work to advance the institutionalisation of experimental medicine.

For two decades after the cattle plague crisis of 1865–66, elite British veterinarians created and sustained a distinct conception of livestock pathology that was concerned with the national herd and whole animals. Their main concern was with the threat 'foreign' contagious diseases posed to the British livestock industry. They supported administrative control measures that sought to keep out and stamp out any and every epizootic that threatened the country. This policy was facilitated by Britain's island geography and the fact that it also offered a degree of economic protection to the livestock industry. However, the veterinary elite developed this policy to further their interests and those of the wider profession. Having been converted to contagionism by the experiences of 1865–66, in the 1870s veterinarians at all levels welcomed the support that germ theorists gave to contagionism and exclusive disease control policies, though it did not matter to them whether germs were chemical poisons, Beale's bioplasm, ferments, bacteria or *materies morbi*, or whether their nature remained unknown. In certain ways the 'importation theory' that underpinned animal disease control policies was analogous to bacterial germ theories of disease in medicine. Both explained disease in terms of 'foreign' or 'external' agents that invaded an otherwise healthy system, eventually disrupting or destroying its normal functioning. In medical discourses, the infective agents were 'germs', the system the human body, and the process was infection. With epizootics, the agents were diseased cattle, the system was the livestock economy, and disease was spread by importation. The main difference was that veterinarians claimed to have a proven and superior means of controlling and eliminating epizootics, namely, stamping out. This contrasted with the limited means that medical investigators had to combat contagious diseases in individuals or populations.

The policies and practices associated with stamping out took British veterinary medicine on a trajectory quite distinct from that developing in human medicine. Indeed, there were conflicts when the two met practically, or in the new subject of comparative pathology. Elite veterinarians developed an antipathy to laboratory researches, which increasingly became the symbol of the new scientific medicine and the reformed medical profession. Thus, despite the early institutionalisation of veterinary research at the Brown, experimental medicine was eschewed by elite veterinarians, both because research laboratories might be foci for contagia to spread and because they feared that experimental work on therapeutics or prophylaxis would allow the adoption of inferior, meliorist control policies, like preventive inoculation. Thus, while germ theories of disease were widely used by veterinarians, the kinds of germ practices that developed in medicine, from antisepsis through to vaccination, were not. This orientation was congruent with the distinct identity that veterinarians were developing, which saw their professional legitimation and advancement in terms of the authority of the state and not science. The alternative trajectory of veterinary medical development with regard to epizootic diseases identified here is not entirely original; it was recognised, perhaps inadvertently, a quarter of a century ago in a centenary history of the animal health in Britain. This did not contain the expected and seemingly obligatory list of dates and discoverers of the germs of the main diseases; instead it listed, over six pages, the 'Acts, Orders and Regulations' of administrative control.

3

Germs in the Air: Surgeons, Hospitalism and Sepsis, 1865–1876

Germ-theory first came to the attention of medical practitioners in the controversies over antiseptic surgery that began in Britain in the late 1860s. The story of this development has been told many times and in Britain is largely about the work of one man – Joseph Lister.[1] Lister's greatness and fame are attributed to the fact that he made surgery safe and 'scientific', basing his clinical innovations on principles derived from Pasteur's germ theory of fermentation and putrefaction. Moreover, it is said that while his practices changed many times, he always remained faithful to the principles of germ-theory.[2] From my point of view there are two immediate problems: first, there was not a single germ-theory, and, second, any germ-theory was open to a number of interpretations and could generate many principles. Thus, claims, like Lister's own in 1869, repeated many times since, that germ-theory uniquely dictated the new antiseptic surgery are problematic.[3] More troubling still, I support those historians who recently have shown that Lister and his supporters changed their principles many

---

1 G. T. Wrench, *Lord Lister: His Life and Work*, London, T. Fisher Unwin, 1915; R. J. Godlee, *Lord Lister*, Oxford, Clarendon Press, 1924; W. Watson Cheyne, *Lister and His Achievement*, London, Longmans Green, 1925; H. C. Cameron, *Joseph Lister: The Friend of Man*, London, Heinemann, 1948; F. F. Cartwright, *Joseph Lister, the Man Who Made Surgery Safe*, London, Weidenfeld and Nicolson, 1963; R. B. Fisher, *Joseph Lister, 1827–1912*, New York, Stein and Day, 1977. The history of surgery has recently been reviewed by C. Lawrence, 'Democratic, Divine and Heroic: The History and Historiography of Surgery', in C. Lawrence, ed., *Medical Theory, Surgical Practice*, London, Routledge, 1993, 1–47.

2 L. Granshaw, '"Upon this Principle I Have Based a Practice": The Development of Antisepsis in Britain, 1867–90', in J. V. Pickstone, ed., *Medical Innovation in Historical Perspective*, London, Macmillan, 1992, 17–46. As early as 1874, Sampson Gamgee noted that the practice had undergone many changes, but that the theory had been 'adhered to with unflinching fidelity'. *Lancet*, 1874, i: 51. In 1880, William MacCormac (1836–1901) also noted that 'The theoretical basis on which the antiseptic method rests remains unchanged through all the manifold changes in detail'. W. MacCormac, *Antiseptic Surgery*, London, Smith Elder 1880, 101. MacCormac was seemingly converted to Listerism after experiences in the Franco-Prussian War and championed Listerism at St. Thomas's Hospital, London. Also see: N. J. Fox, 'Scientific Theory Choice and Social Structure: The Case of Joseph Lister's Antisepsis, Humoral Theory and Asepsis', *History of Science*, 1988, 26: 367–97. Fox terms the hygienic-constitutional approach 'humoralism', a term I find unhelpful.

3 *BMJ*, 1869, i: 302.

times.[4] Lister's role as the leading champion of germ theories within surgery means that his name and those of his followers loom large in this chapter, though I set his ideas and work in the context of wider surgical uses of germ theories and practices.[5]

This chapter begins with an account of surgeons' understanding and management of wounds and sepsis in the 1860s. Next, I discuss the 'hospitalism' crisis of the late 1860s as the main context in which germ theories were first propounded in the surgical literature. In the wake of the cattle plague and initial veterinary antipathy to laboratory medicine, Lister became one of Britain's leading germ theorists, a position that he shared with Lionel Beale, Charlton Bastian and John Tyndall. The presence of Bastian and Tyndall highlights a previously neglected context for the development of germ ideas in surgery, namely, the British spontaneous generation debate, which I consider next. I then look at the spread and use of Lister's ideas and innovations, with particular emphasis on the changing relations between antiseptic practice and the principles elaborated from developing theories about germs and their action. Finally, I review the state of surgical opinion on wound sepsis in the mid-1870s and suggest that Lister's methods had gained more converts than his theory. A decade after the introduction of Listerism, most surgeons continued to use a variety of wound management procedures and assumed a chemical rather than a germ model of septic infection.

SURGERY, WOUNDS AND SEPSIS IN THE 1860S

In the 1860s surgeons mainly treated wounds from injuries and accidents, although some of their work derived from medical conditions that produced sores, fissures and fistulas. Elective operations were few, so wound treatments were largely concerned with repairing or reuniting already damaged tissues. Wound sepsis, which many historians tell us was a great drag on surgery at this time, was only occasionally mentioned in reflections on surgical practice. This may have been due to an understandable reluctance to admit difficult problems, but hospital records confirm that sepsis was often confined to individuals and that serious epidemics were sporadic. That said, sepsis was a particular threat, especially following deep injuries, after amputations, in military surgery and when epidemic conditions 'settled on' hospitals.[6] When single patients were affected, sepsis was regarded as just another complication that surgeons' had to manage, like blood loss and shock. When septic fevers

4 C. Lawrence and R. Dixey, 'Practising on Principle: Joseph Lister and the Germ Theories of Disease', in Lawrence, *Medical Theory*, 153–215.
5 Lawrence and Dixey have recently shown that Lister's ideas on the pathology of wound infection did change between 1867 and 1883, and that, largely unacknowledged at the time or since, Lister and his followers moved from a germ theory of putrefaction to one of infection in the early 1880s. Lawrence and Dixey, 'Practising on Principle', 186–205.
6 *Lancet*, 1853, ii: 79.

affected a ward or wing of a hospital, the problem was as much political as medical, requiring decisions on closing wards and halting admissions. After 1850, many surgeons suggested that the incidence of septic infections was rising and they looked back to the days when all wounds healed quickly and cleanly.[7] There is some modern evidence to support this view, and it is certainly plausible that a deterioration in the state of wounds and their contents was coincident with industrialisation and urbanisation.[8] Certainly, more accident victims were treated in the casualty departments and surgical wards became overcrowded and insanitary.

Sepsis literally meant 'to make rotten' and was synonymous with the production of foul, stinking wounds and sloughing off dead flesh. The process was assumed to be analogous with putrefaction and understood only to take place in dead or devitalised tissue. However, once decomposition set in, surgeons believed that chemical breakdown products (septic poisons) could spread their toxic effects to adjacent and distant tissues. Generally, well-nourished and healthy tissues were assumed to be able to counter septic poisons, but in sufficient concentrations and over a long duration even healthy tissues might weaken and succumb. There were four main types of septic disease: (i) erysipelas, a spreading infection of the skin; (ii) gangrene, a rapidly disseminating decay of muscle and bone; (iii) septicaemia, general blood poisoning, and (iv) pyaemia, when abscesses (pockets of infected pus) formed in different parts of the body. None of these conditions seemed wholly specific; their severity, duration and outcome was unpredictable, depending on many factors, from the extent of any initial injury through to the general health of the patient. Blood and tissues could decay very quickly indeed, as in septicaemia and hospital gangrene, or sepsis could endure for months, as with boils on the skins. A historical discussion of septic diseases also requires sensitivity to changing uses and meanings. For example, septicaemia now refers to an infection in the blood by bacteria, yet in the 1860s its origins were thought to be internal, lying in defective nutrition, or the loss of vitality in tissues due to structural abnormalities that affected the circulation. Such sources were spoken of as 'autogenesis', 'endogenous', 'spontaneous' or '*de novo*', and are illustrative of the physiological conception of disease.[9] Most septic diseases involved the blood in some way, which again reinforced their interiority. However, surgeons believed that septic poisons could escape from the body, to be carried by air, water or touch to other bodies, where they could initiate sepsis if they found a nidus in dead or devitalised tissues. However, spread by contagion, or what would now be termed cross-

7 *Lancet*, 1855, ii: 1; *BMJ*, 1860, 980.
8 E. D. Churchill, 'The Pandemic of Wound Infection in Hospitals', *JHM*, 1965, 19: 390–413; D. J. Hamilton, 'The Nineteenth Century Surgical Revolution – Antisepsis or Better Nutrition?', *BHM*, 1982, 56: 30–40.
9 On idiopathic pyaemia, see *MTG*, 1863, i: 96; ii: 204; 1864, ii: 29, 55.

infection, was thought to be relatively uncommon. Most septic conditions were assumed to arise internally and spontaneously in damaged tissues, with the effect of external causes largely indirect, for example, general epidemic conditions lowering a person's vitality or the cold weakening circulation. Like most other clinicians, surgeons did not pay much attention to the causes of disease. At one level they were obvious, say, in injuries or sores, but generally they were assumed to be so many and in the past that they did little to help with the surgeon's main priorities – diagnosis, prognosis and treatment.

The treatment and management of all kinds of wounds, septic or otherwise, was central to surgical practice, and each surgeon had his own ideas and techniques.[10] Many methods were highly individualistic, but there was a general presumption that wounds healed well, and sepsis was avoided, if the vitality of tissues and local circulation were maintained. This is what happened in the ideal form of repair – 'healing by first intention' – where cleanly cut tissues were brought together to rejoin with little or no inflammation. There was much debate on the status of inflammation: was it a 'normal' healthy process to be encouraged, or a pathogenic process to be countered? Or, were there different types and intensities of inflammation – some healthy and some unhealthy?[11] With open or deep wounds, especially where tissue had been lost or had died, healing took longer and involved new granulation or scar tissue growing across the wound. The time factor, as well as the prior damage, made these wounds prone to intense inflammation, mortification and sepsis. Thus, the main question for surgeons faced with such wounds was what practical plan to use to reduce inflammation, to prevent sepsis starting and to control the process once it was under way? The answers usually involved a judicious mixture of treatments to encourage healthy inflammation and counter abnormal inflammation (e.g. poultices, cold water dressings and ointments), plus measures that maintained vitality and aided the natural healing powers of the body (e.g. cleanliness and dietary). If and when a wound became septic, more vigorous methods were used, such as the excision of affected tissues, cautery (burning the tissue with a hot iron) and the application of powerful 'antiseptic' agents. In 1853, Golding Bird recommended applications of 'undiluted nitric acid or caustic potash' to destroy gangrenous sloughs and 'prevent the absorption of septic matter into the constitution'.[12] Bird also administered stimulants and tonics in the hope that these would strengthen the patient's tissues from within and enable them to counter the poisons. In the 1860s, any measures that countered or suppressed the poisons

10 S. Gamgee, *BMJ*, 1867, ii: 355–6, 561–2.
11 The definitive discussion of inflammation was by John Simon in Holmes's textbook. J. Simon, 'Inflammation', in T. Holmes, ed., *System of Surgery*, London, Longmans Green, 1870, 1–113.
12 *Lancet*, 1855, ii: 1. He also used vinegar, lime juice and iodine.

of septic infection, local and external, constitutional and internal, might have been termed 'antiseptic'.[13]

'SOMETHING IN THE AIR': SURGEONS AND HOSPITALISM

Sepsis and septic fevers would probably have remained a technical problem for surgeons had not sanitarians, like William Farr, statistician to the Registrar General who was aided and abetted by Florence Nightingale, transferred the rhetoric and prescriptions of the sanitary movement from the urban environment and the 'Great Unwashed' to urban hospitals and their patients.[14] In the 1860s these critics claimed that voluntary and state hospitals were failing in their primary mission 'to do the sick no harm'.[15] The main determinants of the 'crisis' were said to be the location of hospitals, their size and overcrowding, which together produced the great evils of smell, dirt and poor ventilation. As elsewhere, sanitarians focused on places and populations – hospitals and their patients – and with a broad class of fevers – terming the four main septic infections 'hospital diseases'. After allowing for seasonal and other variations, hospital mortality levels were said to be intolerable, especially in comparison to those in private practice. A small number of surgeons, notably James Young Simpson (1811–70), added their voice to the criticism and helped construct a malaise known as 'hospitalism'.[16]

The 'hospitalism crisis', which began in the early 1860s, hit a crescendo in 1869, becoming an intraprofessional dispute. Simpson made a concerted attack on existing hospitals and called for them to be either relocated, rebuilt, run along more hygienic lines or all of these.[17] This was an issue for many

---

13 The following antiseptics were mentioned as useful in the treatment of pyaemia in 1867: charcoal poultice, solution of carbolic acid, chlorine, chlorinated soda, chloride of zinc and escharotic mineral acids. *Lancet*, 1867, i: 203.

14 J. Farr, 'Miss Nightingale's "Notes on Hospitals"', *MTG*, 1864, i: 186–8, 491–2, and J. S. Bristowe and T. Holmes, 'The Hospitals of England', *Sixth Report of the Medical Officer of the Privy Council on the State of Public Health, 1863*, BPP 1864, [3416], xxviii, 1. Also see: Granshaw, 'Upon this Principle', 18–20; A. J. Youngson, *The Scientific Revolution in Victorian Medicine*, London, Croom Helm, 1979, 164–71. On Farr's wider work and ideas on disease: J. M. Eyler, *Victorian Social Medicine: The Ideas and Methods of William Farr*, Baltimore, MD, Johns Hopkins University Press, 1979. On Florence Nightingale's work on infectious diseases: C. E. Rosenberg, 'Florence Nightingale on Contagion: The Hospital as Moral Universe', in C. E. Rosenberg, ed., *Healing and History: Essays for George Rosen*, New York, SHP, 1979, 116–36.

15 J. H. Woodward, *'To Do the Sick no Harm': A Study of the British Voluntary Hospital System until 1875*, London, Routledge Kegan Paul, 1974; R. Lambert, *Sir John Simon, 1816–1904, and English Social Administration*, London, McKibbon and Kee, 1963. The definitive statement of the hospital reformers was: J. Y. Simpson, *Hospitalism: Its Effects on the Results of Surgical Operations*, Edinburgh, Pentland J. Young, 1869.

16 For a review of the hospitalism debate, see: J. E. Erichsen, *Hospitalism and the Causes of Death After Operations and Surgical Injuries*, London, Longmans Green, 1874.

17 James Simpson was at this time Professor of Midwifery at Edinburgh and was also championing 'stamping out' smallpox. J. Y. Simpson, *Proposal to Stamp out Smallpox and other Contagious Diseases*, Edinburgh, Edmonton and Douglas, 1871.

inner-city institutions, for example, the campaigns to move the Manchester Royal Infirmary to the suburbs, and the controversy over the resiting of St Thomas's in London.[18] Elite physicians and surgeons were divided, though most closed ranks to defend what had become a vital area of professional activity. Surgeons argued that hospital mortality was affected by many factors besides sanitary conditions, for example, admission criteria, the nature and severity of the patient's illness or injury, their general health and constitution and wider epidemic influences.[19] Statistics and other evidence were traded and the controversy rumbled on into the 1870s, fading away as hospital mortality levels improved and the star of sanitarianism waned. The contribution of sanitary improvements to falling hospital mortalities is unknown, but the verdict in 1876 of William Cadge (1822–1903), surgeon at the Norwich and Norfolk Hospital, is interesting. He said that the improvements at his hospital were due to two secondary factors, building improvements and the adoption of antiseptics, but the principal gains had come from the employment of a qualified matron and the way she had created a more hygienic and moral environment in the wards.[20]

While surgeons firmly rejected any simple sanitary analysis of hospital mortality, they found no difficulty in supporting calls for better hygiene, greater cleanliness and the improvement of the healing environment.[21] There were, however, differences between the interests and perspective of surgeons and sanitarians. Surgeons' work focused on individual bodies and their afflictions, not hospitals and patient populations. However, the 'crisis' and the wider influence of anticontagionism led surgeons to ponder the possible role of air in the spread hospital diseases. Surgeons had no great difficulty with the idea that 'something-in-the-air' was associated with certain cases of septic diseases, and with the occasional hospital epidemic. Indeed, surgeons would like to have known the nature of septic poisons, but were happy to continue with their empirically derived antiseptic and anti-inflammatory methods. It was left to chemists, who were more interested in the poisons of zymotic diseases, to pursue the matter. Robert Angus Smith (1817–84), William Crace-Calvert and other chemists had analysed the air of towns and hospitals and found higher levels of organic compounds, but were able to identify only a few possible septic substances.[22] The absence of a consistent dose-effect for the supposed chemical, septic poison, was puzzling. After all, the tiniest septic

18 L. Granshaw, *St Thomas's Hospital, London 1850–1900*, unpublished Ph.D. Thesis, Bryn Mawr College, 1981, 110–90; G. Goldin, 'Building a Hospital of Air: The Victorian Pavilions of St Thomas's Hospital, London', *BHM*, 1975, 49: 512–35.

19 Holmes stated that most deaths after amputations were due to prior injuries or hospital conditions, not the effects of the operation as such. *BMJ*, 1866, ii: 683. Also see: J. Paget, 'The Risks of Operations', *Lancet*, 1867, ii: 1, 33, 151, 219.

20 *BMJ*, 1876, i: 502–4.

21 On pyaemia : Fergusson, *MTG*, 1863, i: 96; 1863, ii: 107, 407; 1864, ii: 179; 1866, ii: 234.

22 *MTG*, 1860, i: 463.

wound might lead to massive and fatal disease, as in the pin-prick dissection injuries that often killed medical students and doctors; yet, very deep wounds sometimes healed sweetly. However, if septic poisons were capable of 'multiplication', then it was possible that they were living entities, or involved molecules so complex that they had the properties of life. That said, Angus Smith saw no need to choose between chemical and biological agents, as several different entities might be involved, for example, gases, vapours, effluvia, exanthemata (pathogenic material given off by the sick), cells and other organised bodies, or their germs.[23]

The role of nonchemical agents in hospital diseases was first discussed explicitly by a surgeon, Thomas Spencer Wells (1818–97), in an address to the BMA in August 1864.[24] Wells spoke in the context of the hospitalism debate, which he linked with one of 'the most recent discoveries in physiological chemistry' – Pasteur's ideas on germs, fermentative change and disease.[25] He reported the suggestion that living organisms played a role in fermentation and putrefaction, and hence in sepsis. Wells used many terms for these microorganisms: 'microscopic beings', 'cryptogamic vegetables and infusorial animalcules', '*Monads, Bacteria and Vibriones*', and 'inferior beings'.[26] In France, Trousseau had linked such 'inferior beings' to puerperal fever. Wells now extended this to sepsis and offered a range of possible pathological models:

Applying the knowledge for which we are indebted to Pasteur of the presence of organic germs which will grow, develope (*sic*), and multiply, under favourable conditions, it is easy to understand how some germs find their most appropriate nutriment in the secretions from wounds, or in pus, and that they so modify it as to convert it into a poison when absorbed – or that the germs after development, multiplication, and death, may form a putrid infecting matter – or that they may enter the blood and develope themselves, effecting in the process deadly changes in the circulating fluid.[27]

The practical consequence for Wells was that surgeons should apply antiseptic substances on and into wounds, and dose patients with sulphites in the hope that these would 'modify the fluids and tissues [of the body]

23 J. M. Eyler, 'The Conversion of Angus Smith: The Changing Role of Chemistry and Biology in Sanitary Science, 1850–1880', *BHM*, 1980, 54: 216–34.
24 Sir Thomas Spencer Wells qualified at Trinity College, Dublin, and St. Thomas's. He then worked in the Navy, before a period with Magendie in Paris and on the Marquis of Northampton's expedition to Egypt. In 1851 he settled in London. He edited the *Medical Times and Gazette* between 1851 and 1858, worked in the Crimea in 1853–54, and gained his first hospital appointment at the Samaritan Free Hospital for Women and Children in 1854. He gained fame from the late 1850s, with Thomas Nunn at the Middlesex, as an ovariotomist. It was said that he drew confidence for this operation from his Crimean experience, where he had found the peritoneum tolerant to injury. T. S. Wells, *The Revival of Ovariotomy and its Influence on Modern Surgery*, London, Churchill, 1884.   25 *BMJ*, 1864, ii: 385.
26 T. S. Wells, 'Some Causes of Excessive Surgical Mortality after Surgical Operations', *BMJ*, 1864, ii: 384.   27 Ibid., 386.

. . . so as to render its organic constituents more able to resist the putrid fermentation'. In conclusion, he warned against exaggerated expectations from these measures and trusted that no one would 'neglect those leading principles of sanitary science which govern the size and construction of hospitals, or . . . attention which should always secure the most scrupulous cleanliness and purity'. The reports of the discussion of this paper show that these ideas provoked no great reaction; most comments were about the role of hospital conditions. Those discussants who mentioned organic germs saw them literally as 'seeds', recommending that steps be taken to ensure that any 'spores . . . be got rid of' and that 'bandages containing sporules be burnt'. Otherwise, Wells's audience seems to have understood his remarks as typical speculation about the nature of septic processes, and believed that organic germs, if they existed, were ferment-like or acted by producing chemical poisons.[28]

The next British surgeon to discuss airborne organic germs was Joseph Lister (see Figure 7), in his now famous paper, 'On the Antiseptic Principle in the Practice of Surgery'. This paper was read at the Annual Meeting of the BMA in Dublin on 9 August 1867 and published on 21 September 1867.[29] This paper followed publications earlier in the same year on the techniques of using carbolic acid dressings for treating compound fractures.[30] Lister began his August paper uncontroversially by confirming his adherence to a chemical account of septic poisoning: 'the great principle that all the local inflammatory mischief and general febrile disturbance . . . are due to the irritating and poisonous influence of decomposing blood and sloughs'. His next step was more controversial; he said that decomposition in wounds was 'brought about by the influence of the atmosphere'. Here he was entering an ongoing dispute between those surgeons who recommended leaving wounds open and exposed, and those who advocated covering them with poultices and all manner of dressings. The former saw oxygen as a boon to healing while the latter feared its power to inflame. Lister argued that oxygen was irrelevant; rather, the key factor was the flora and fauna of the atmosphere. He had adopted Pasteur's view that living organisms produced putrefactive changes and argued that 'the septic property of the atmosphere depended . . . on minute organisms suspended in it, which owed their energy to their vitality'. The assumption that air contained many microorganisms, a position termed 'panspermism', was just as contentious as the idea that minute organisms produced sepsis. Lister was not rejecting chemical theories of sepsis; rather, he was adding

28 See comments of Routh and Thudichum. *BMJ*, 1864, ii: 195.
29 J. Lister, 'On the Antiseptic Principle in the Practice of Surgery', *Lancet*, 1867, ii: 353–7, 668–9. Also in *BMJ*, 1867, ii: 246–8.
30 J. Lister, 'On a New Method of Treating Compound Fractures, Abscess, etc.', *Lancet*, 1867, i: 336–9, 357–9, 387–9, 507–9: ii: 95–6.

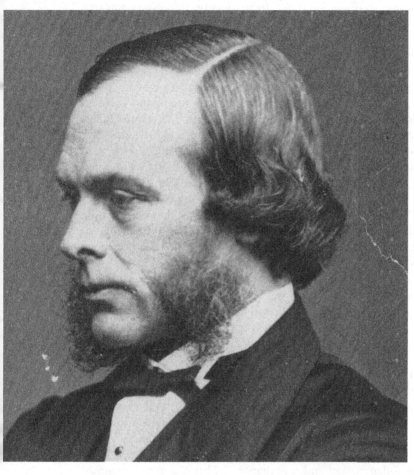

Figure 7. Joseph Lister (Reproduced by courtesy of the Wellcome Institute Library, London)

to them the idea that independent living organisms produced the poisons. The important pathological and practical point made by Lister was that the root cause of all septic mischief came from outside the body, and did not originate in wounds from the spontaneous breakdown of tissues. Thus, Lister advised that wound management should rest on the assumption that 'decomposition in the injured part might be avoided without excluding the air, by applying as a dressing some material capable of destroying the life of the floating particles'. The material he favoured and championed was carbolic acid, which had been used for many years by surgeons in various ways, but had recently become available in purer form due to improved industrial processes.[31]

Lister preferred to call his methods 'antiseptic surgery', but the term 'Listerism', coined by his contemporaries, is more useful as it distinguishes his specific methods from general antiseptic measures.[32] Listerism was designed to counter sepsis in the wound, first by 'the destruction of any septic germs which may have entered the wound', and then by attempting 'to guard effectually against the spreading of decomposition into the wound'. This description highlights that Lister was treating already infected wounds. The article overall was mainly devoted to the details of new dressings, which were presented as something of a panacea. As well as halting sepsis, they promoted healthy suppuration or 'laudable pus', acted as a mild anaesthetic and prevented wounds from throwing off putrid exhalations and septic particles (exanthemata).[33] With this latter point, Lister was directly addressing the issue of 'hospitalism', as he went on to say that his methods reduced the incidence of pyaemia, hospital gangrene and erysipelas. The details of Lister's carbolic acid treatment were further elaborated on in other papers in 1867 and 1868. Each time he cited Pasteur's germ-theory as his inspiration. A largely implicit assumption at this time, but one that was very important subsequently for Listerism, was that sepsis could not occur in healthy tissues, which led Lister to believe that the normal, healthy body was germ-free.

Echoing points recently made by Granshaw, and Lawrence and Dixey, I want to stress the unexceptional nature of many aspects of Lister's initial publications. Although he grandiosely announced a new 'principle', his writing was characterised by detailed descriptions of dressings and other technicalities. The reaction to his work shows that most surgeons took cognisance of only his plans for wound treatment and ignored its theoretical justification. Indeed, he offered little elaboration of Pasteurian germ-theory at this early juncture, and his thinking continued to rely heavily on his own long-standing ideas on inflammation and suppuration.[34] That Lister had proposed a technical rather than a theoretical innovation was evident when Listerism was listed under headings such as 'Surgical Novelties' and 'Hospital Efficiency', topics on which there were always numerous proposals.[35]

31 F. Crace Calvert, *On Protoplasmic Life and the Action of Heat and Antiseptics Upon It*, Manchester, W. H. Clegg, 1873. Also see: J. K. Crellin, 'The Disinfectant Studies of Frederick Crace Calvert', in *Die Vortrage der Hauptversammlung der Internationalen Gesellschaft fuer Gemeinchte der Pharmacie*, Stuttgart, Wissenschaftliche Verlaysyesellschaft MBH 1966, 61–7.

32 *BMJ*, 1867, ii: 305.

33 *MTG*, 1866, i: 97. On Lister's ideas on inflammation and suppuration, see: Lawrence and Dixey, 'Practising on Principle', 162–71.

34 J. Lister, 'On the Early Stages of Inflammation', *PTRSL*, 1858, 2: 645–702.

35 *BMJ*, 1867, ii: 293; *BFM-CR*, 1870, 45: 443–50; 46: 54–74. Granshaw notes that the *Lancet* indexed most references to Lister's work under 'Carbolic Acid' until the mid-1870s. Granshaw, 'On this Principle', 22–3.

In the late 1860s many surgeons seem to have tried Listerism. However, they reported finding difficulties in translating his words into action, and in affording the materials and the extra time that his dressings required. Those who visited Glasgow and learned firsthand seemingly had the most success. The picture that emerges from the literature is that those surgeons who found an obvious general advantage adopted Listerism wholesale. However, most surgeons found marginal benefits with certain procedures, and hence they used Listerism selectively, or adapted it to their existing repertoire. Many surgeons used Listerism for nongerm reasons. Eben Watson told the Glasgow Medico-Chirurgical Society in May 1869 that he used carbolic acid because it helped tissues coagulate, harden and resist the action of oxygen in the air.[36] Other surgeons found that there was no benefit, ignored Listerism and continued with their existing methods. The only surgical technique that Listerism overtly challenged was the 'open treatment', where the drying, seasoning and scabbing of wounds emulated nature's ways.[37] Despite citing advanced science, deploying elaborate techniques and using industrial chemicals, Lister also claimed that his methods were 'natural'. After all, it was unnatural for the body's surface to be broken and for alien beings to enter the normally germ-free body, so anything that countered these was restoring a state of nature.

If Listerism was congruent with much surgical theory and practice, what set it apart and led it to be so widely discussed in the late 1860s and early 1870s? It would be both presentist and historically inaccurate to say that this was because Lister was proposing a revolution in surgery. Such a view depends on a particular interpretation of the history of surgery that was created by Listerians after 1880.[38] The controversies that Lister's work generated have to be explained. To do this, the views of contemporary critics and agnostics have to be taken symmetrically with those of Lister and his supporters. The first challenge Lister faced was that his methods were unoriginal.[39] Antiseptic chemicals were already widely used in surgery and medicine and, moreover, the French surgeon Lemaire had already pioneered the use of carbolic acid with septic wounds.[40] The major practical objection was that Listerism was complicated, time-consuming and expensive, which reinforces my point about the perceived technical character of his

36 E. Watson, 'On the Theory of Suppuration, and the Use of Carbolic Acid Dressings', *GMJ*, 1869–70, 2: 133–4. Lister's methods had been seen as 'sealing with carbolic acid' and were seen as analogous to James Simpson's method of acupressure – both closed the wound to air. *BMJ*, ii: 1867, 293.
37 *Lancet*, 1864, ii: 141. The pathological reasoning here was that exposure countered inflammation by cooling tissues and that the oxygen in the air promoted the formation and growth of new, replacement tissue; this was said to be nature's way and was vindicated by the absence of sepsis from wounds in animals.
38 Lawrence and Dixey, 'Practising on Principle', 162–71.
39 *Lancet*, 1867, ii: 444; *BMJ*, 1867, ii: 305.
40 Editorial, 'Carbolic Acid Treatment of Wounds', *BMJ*, 1869, ii: 269–70.

work.[41] He was also attacked for not waiting longer to publish his results, as it still remained open whether his success was independent of the cycle of hospital epidemics. In terms of the hospitalism issue, Lister was read as saying that the hygienic reform of hospitals was unnecessary because the only thing that mattered was the cleanliness and protection of the wound. Critics were able to paint Listerism as retrograde, perpetuating the surgeon's gaze on the 'local' and 'external', confirming that their work was manual rather than mental, and ignoring the wider health of the patient and medical treatments.[42]

What set Lister's speculation about germs apart from, say, that of Spencer Wells in 1864, was the manner in which he linked them to claims to have invented a very superior practice. Lister tacitly denigrated other wound management methods and questioned the competence of the surgeons who used them. A standard response to such arrogance was to ask why Lister was so exclusive and denied his patients the benefit of other tried and tested methods, including alternative antiseptic methods and medical treatments that helped the body resist septic poisoning. John Reid of Glasgow would have spoken for many when, in 1869, he observed that, 'like most surgeons, he had treated wounds in many different ways, and he invariably found that the rapidity with which a wound healed depended on the state of the system of the patient'.[43] In the same year, Thomas Nunneley (1809–70) of Leeds General Infirmary spoke of the value of antiseptic remedies 'as applied to the constitutional condition, and not to extrinsic circumstances'.[44] Lister discussed the underlying 'principle' of his methods quite sparingly at the outset and saw no need to speculate on the nature of the germs causing sepsis, though there is no doubting his belief that they were living organisms. In 1868, he wrote that, 'without a belief in the truth of that theory, no man can be thoroughly successful in the treatment' and a year later told surgeons that they had to follow 'its details such as the germ-theory dictates'.[45] In 1869 he said that 'the germ theory of putrefaction is the pole-star' and in the following year observed that the proper practice of his methods required 'a conviction of the truth of germ theory'.[46] This tactic did not work to his advantage. Most surgeons thought that their work should be guided by experience not theory.[47] Nunneley warned 'how theory influences practice, and how readily

41 *BMJ*, 1869, i: 301. In the decade or so before Lister's publications surgeons had put great stress on simple methods. See: W. Paget, *MTG*, 1862, i: 146; 1863; T. S. Wells, *MTG*, 1863, i: 96.
42 Granshaw, 'On this Principle', 22–7.   43 *GMJ*, 1869–70, 2: 135.   44 *BMJ*, 1869, ii: 153.
45 J. Lister, 'An Address on the Antiseptic System of Treatment in Surgery', *BMJ*, 1868, ii: 53–6, 101–2, 461–3, 515–7; Cf. *BMJ*, 1869, i: 302. Also see: Thomas Jones, *BMJ*, 1869, ii: 227; G. F. Elliott, *BMJ*, 1870, i: 488–9. A number of surgeons claimed that their use of carbolic acid was based on other principles, for example, to exclude oxygen or to neutralise chemical ferments. *BMJ*, 1870, i: 361.
46 J. Lister, 'Further Evidence Regarding the Effects of the Antiseptic Treatment on the Salubrity of a Surgical Hospital', *Lancet*, 1870, ii: 287–9, 288.
47 *BMJ*, 1869, ii: 227, 281, 523; 1870, ii: 407.

even able men are liable to be led away by hasty conclusions'. He went on
to warn that medicine's past was littered with 'false theories, on every imag-
inable topic, supported by every kind of evidence'.[48] The general point is
clear: Lister, like anyone else wishing to develop or use any germ-theory, had
a serious problem simply because in medicine 'theory' was associated with
speculation, not high order principles.[49]

While objecting to theory per se, critics were happy to draw on other
'theories' of sepsis as it suited them, especially what were seen to be the less
speculative ideas of Benjamin Ward Richardson (1828–96) and John Hughes
Bennett (1812–75).[50] Richardson, a metropolitan physician, sanitarian and
temperance campaigner, had his own version of the dominant chemical
theory – 'the glandular theory' – where poisons were created in the body
and could spread in bodily secretions. He had first spoken against the
Pasteur–Lister germ-theory in 1867, but in 1870 he made one of the most
influential and long quoted assaults at the Medical Society of London.[51] He
was no disinterested observer of surgical methods, having in 1867 promoted
his own new method of wound treatment – styptic colloid – a chemical that
was antiseptic and contracted tissues, forming a barrier that excluded air and
prevented the release of glandular poisons.[52] Richardson argued that Lister's
germ-theory depended entirely on analogy and that the existence of disease-
germs had not been proved. He maintained that living germ-theory was
completely contrary to clinical experience, which showed that most patients
survived fevers, an impossible condition if these diseases were due to the body
being invaded by parasite-like organisms that could multiply at a prodigious
rate. If disease-germs had the powers supposed, he felt that the struggle for
existence with humans cells would lead to a situation where 'the life of the
universe would come to consist of germs alone'.[53] Put another way, he was
saying that the Pasteur–Lister germ-theory of disease could not explain
health. He went on, in mocking tones, to say that 'Either the "germs" have
what vitalists would call an elective, or patients must be credited with a repel-
lent power, or we must take refuge in that last refuge of the baffled, an idio-
syncrasy, to regulate their action.'[54] Lastly, and very significantly, given the
claims of Lister and other germ theorists to be at the cutting edge of medical
science, he objected that germ-theory promised to take medicine 'back to

48 *BMJ*, 1869, ii: 155.
49 For a defence of the theory, see: J. Morris, *Germinal Matter and the Contact Theory: An Essay on Morbid Poisons, their Nature, Sources, Effects, Migrations and Means of Limiting their Noxious Effects*, London, Churchill, 1867, 5–6.
50 A. S. MacNalty, *A Biography of Sir Benjamin Ward Richardson*, London, Harvey and Blythe, 1950; B. W. Richardson, *The Poisons of the Spreading Diseases*, London, Churchill, 1867.
51 B. W. Richardson, 'The Medical Aspect of the Germ-Theory', *MTG*, 1870, ii: 510–12, 539–41. Also see: *BMJ*, 1870, ii: 566–7, and *Lancet*, 1870, ii: 607, 643–4. Richardson's address in 1867 was reported as having delivered a coup de grace to germ-theory.
52 B. W. Richardson, 'Styptic Colloid', *MTG*, 1867, i: 383–5, 409–10.
53 *Lancet*, 1870, ii: 633–4.   54 *EMJ*, 1867–68, 8: 1098.

the ante-medieval, if not the Deluge; for as it is that these germs are entities, so the products – the diseases – must also be entities – manifestly a
retrograde step in science'.[55]

Richardson's contention was that physiological conceptions of disease were
more congruent with cellular pathology and Bernardian physiological medicine. John Hughes Bennett, Professor of the Institutes of Medicine and
Senior Professor in Clinical Medicine at the University of Edinburgh, argued
against germs as the cause of sepsis in a lecture to Edinburgh surgeons in
January 1868. In an address entitled 'The Atmospheric Germ Theory', he said
that his own researchers and those of other histologists were 'totally adverse'
to panspermism. However, Bennett had abandoned cellular pathology and
confirmed his support for spontaneous generation, saying that 'new life
springs from the molecular death of pre-existing tissues and organisms'.[56] This
raised the stakes a great deal, for if living organisms (or their germs) were
involved in sepsis, then something quite profound was happening in putrid
wounds, namely, the spontaneous generation of life.[57]

SPONTANEOUS GENERATION AND GERM-THEORY

The extent to which Lister's ideas and practice were part of the British spontaneous generation debate, which ran almost a decade behind the more
famous French debate of the 1860s, has not been sufficiently acknowledged
by historians of medicine or science.[58] The controversy in science was
between those who maintained that life forms, however small, were ancestral
and always came from preexisting life, and those who maintained that new
life forms, especially microbial life, was always being created from nonliving
matter. The positions were complex, and do not neatly divide between vitalist versus materialists, religious versus nonreligious scientists, and biologists
versus physical scientists. The debate itself came to focus on the interpretation of experimental results, particularly what happened to organic fluids kept
in sealed glass flasks. However, speaking in 1871, Professor George Rolleston
(1829–81) said that the debate had 'Professor Lister on one side, and Professor Bastian on the other'.[59] Charlton Bastian, then Professor of Pathological

55 *BMJ*, 1870, ii: 566.
56 J. Hughes Bennett, 'The Atmospheric Germ Theory', *EMJ*, 1867–68, 13: 810–34.
57 J. E. Strick, *The British Spontaneous Generation Debates of 1860–1880: Medicine, Evolution and Laboratory Science in the Victorian Context*, Unpublished PhD Thesis, Princeton University, 1997, 48–59,
71–75; *EMJ*, 1867–68, 8, 1098.
58 Exceptions are: Strick, *British Spontaneous Generation*, passim; A. E. Adam, *Spontaneous Generation
in the 1870s: Victorian Scientific Naturalism and its Relationship to Medicine*, PhD Thesis, C.N.A.A.,
1988; J. K. Crellin, *Spontaneous Generation and the Germ Theory (1860–1880): The Controversy in Britain
and the work of F. Crace Calvert*, MSc dissertation, University of London, 1965; J. Farley, *The Spontaneous Generation Controversy from Descartes to Oparin*, Baltimore, MD, Johns Hopkins University
Press, 1977.
59 *MTG*, 1870, ii: 403.

Anatomy at University College Hospital, London, himself stated that Lister 'strongly relies for proof of germ theory' on experiments with boiled fluids in bottle-neck flasks.[60] Amongst the biographers of Lister, only Cuthbert Dukes has recognised this point explicitly, with his suggestion that in the early 1870s dressing a wound with carbolic gauze was the equivalent to Pasteur sealing a flask containing organic fluids – both were wasting their time if decomposition could occur *de novo* without contamination.[61] Rolleston was correct in identifying Bastian as the champion of spontaneous generation, a position that he occupied throughout the 1870s. However, he was wrong about Lister.[62] He was only a protagonist by implication, and after 1871 Lister chose to avoid the matter altogether. He left the fight to others, notably John Tyndall, William Roberts and John Burdon Sanderson, and did not speak out again, even when it became clear that the position of living germ theories of disease was at stake. To promote his antiseptic system with surgeons, Lister seems to have taken the tactical decision to decouple his practice from the intense controversies that grew up around germ theories and spontaneous generation.

Lister had effectively entered the debate over spontaneous generation when he announced in 1867 that he had based his new system of wound treatment on Pasteur's germ theory of putrefaction, and on panspermism. In the mid-1860s, Pasteur had been involved in a politically charged debate in France over spontaneous generation.[63] He had maintained that the decomposition of pure organic fluids in a flask occurred only when they were contaminated by the air and its panspermic life. He attempted to show, using scrupulous methods of cleanliness and experimental exactness, that if a flask remained sealed no decomposition occurred. His main opponent, Félix-Archimède Pouchet, attempted to demonstrate the opposite – that decomposition was possible without contamination. Pouchet declared that panspermism was an unwarranted and unnecessary assumption, and that any life forms present in decomposing fluids were the result of decomposition and were not its cause.

Spontaneous generation in the late 1860s referred to two phenomena: *biogenesis* (what Bastian termed *heterogenesis*) – living organisms forming

---

60 *BMJ*, 1871, ii: 403.
61 C. Dukes, *Lord Lister, 1827–1912*, London, Leonard Parsons, 1924.
62 H. Charlton Bastian, (1835–1915) 1862 University College, London (UCL); 1867 Prof. of Pathological Anatomy, UCL; 1878 Physician UCL; 1887–98 Prof. of the Principles and Practice of Medicine. His major works on spontaneous generation were: *The Modes of the Origin of Lowest Organisms*, London, Macmillan, 1871; *The Beginnings of Life*, London, Macmillan, 1872; *Evolution and the Origin of Life*, London, Macmillan, 1874; *Studies on Heterogenesis*, London, Williams and Norgate, 1904; *The Nature and Origin of Living Matter*, London, Fischer and Unwin, 1905; *The Origin of Life*, London, Watts, 1911. There is also an unpublished biography: M. Rang, *The Life and Work of Henry Charlton Bastian, 1835–1915*, London, UCH Medical School Library, 1954.
63 G. L. Geison, *The Private Science of Louis Pasteur*, Princeton, NJ, Princeton University Press, 1995, 110–42.

from dead or devitalised organic matter, and *abiogenesis* (what Bastian termed *archeobiosis*) – living organisms forming from inorganic matter – seen to be a rarer phenomenon.[64] In the 1860s, the subject was controversial because of its association with materialism and evolution. Supporters of spontaneous generation assumed that the creation of life had been continuous and was still happening. They did not reserve it for the distant past and perhaps not the agency of the Almighty. Many of those who supported evolutionary ideas thought that spontaneous generation was a necessary element of any account of transmutation; after all, life had to have originated some time. Others, including Darwin, pushed the origin of life so far back in time that it was beyond the reach of science.[65]

During the summer of 1869, the *British Medical Journal* published seven articles on 'The Origin of Life' by Bastian, which reviewed the debates between heterogenists and panspermists, concluding unsurprisingly against the latter.[66] In August, Nunneley had observed at the Annual Meeting of the BMA that any organisms in wounds were 'the result and not the cause of putrefaction'.[67] Lister was at his most combative at this time, so it was no surprise that in November of that year he included mention of spontaneous generation in an address on the germ theory of putrefaction.[68] He claimed that the doctrine had been 'chased successively to lower and lower stations in the world of organised beings' and was a refuge for ignorance that the march of science had shown to be 'gratuitous and uncalled for'. He asked why lower organisms had evolved so many different means of reproduction (sexual, asexual, segmentation and division) if they could spring spontaneously out of ordinary matter. However, he presented the origin of 'vibrios' as a secondary issue. Lister saw his main task to be persuading surgeons of the truth of panspermism and that putrefaction was due to germs, not to oxygen or chemicals alone. To make his point he relied on analogies, reports of experiments and clinical experience. He was unable to use microscopy to display his germs, or to set out definite models of how tiny vibrios could upset the physiology of large mammals, other than to speculate on their likely exponential powers of reproduction and the known powers of chemical poisons.

Having simmered in the scientific and medical press through the 1860s, an open debate on spontaneous generation erupted in January 1870, following

64 Strick, *British Spontaneous*, Ch. 2–4. The terms 'biogenesis' and 'abiogenesis' were those that Thomas Huxley championed and which gradually replaced the other, older terms.
65 Darwin followed the spontaneous generation debate and was initially an admirer of Bastian. Strick, *British Spontaneous*, Ch. 2–4.
66 H. C. Bastian, 'The Origin of Life', *BMJ*, 1869, i: 312–3, 569–70; ii: 157–8, 214–5, 270–2, 473–4, 665–6.
67 T. Nunneley, 'Address in Surgery', *BMJ*, 1869, ii: 154.
68 J. Lister, 'Introductory Lecture on the Causation of Putrefaction and Fermentation', *BMJ*, 1869, ii: 601–4.

a lecture by John Tyndall on 'Dust and Disease'.[69] Tyndall was Superintendent of the Royal Institution, London, a physicist, controversialist and senior 'public scientist'.[70] He was a leading advocate of scientific naturalism and was active in attempts to professionalise British science, which in turn led him to support moves for the reform of medical education to include experimental science. In his lecture, Tyndall reported that light beam experiments had shown the presence of minute particles of organic material in ordinary air, thereby supporting panspermism. He then controversially linked his findings to Pasteur's germ theory of fermentation, Budd's ideas on contagia and zymotic diseases, and Lister's germ explanation of septic diseases into a single germ theory. Already, on 1 January 1870, Lister had published another provocative paper, this time on the effects of his 'Antiseptic System' on the hygienic conditions in surgical wards, in which he argued that his treatment prevented the spread of sepsis between patients.[71] In his address, Tyndall boldly suggested that dust particles were the carriers of disease-germs or germs themselves.[72] His lecture received critical notices in the medical press.[73] However, Tyndall was not daunted by warnings to keep out of medical matters. Three months later he wrote to the *Times* to recommend 'the germ theory of disease' to doctors and the wider public.[74] His letter drew a spirited response from Bastian, who replied that the poisons of epidemic and septic diseases were chemicals, that these could arise *de novo* in the body, and that any germs found associated with disease had spontaneously arisen in tissues at or near their death.

Bastian, Hughes Bennett and others who supported the doctrine of the spontaneous generation of germs did not deny that these entities were associated with disease. However, they continued to favour chemicals as the agents of zymosis and sepsis, and even as the catalysts that produced germs as the result of disease processes. Like Lister, they too relied on the persuasive power of analogies, reports of experiments and appeals to clinical experience. On the first of these, matters were complicated by having to take a position on other germ theories, notably Dobell's occult notion and Beale's idea that disease-germs

69 J. Tyndall, 'On Dust and Disease', *Proc. of the Royal Institution of Great Britain*, 1870, 6: 1–14. The talk was first reported under the title: 'Dust and Haze', *Nature*, 1870, 1: 339–42, and in the medical press under the same title. Tyndall reprised his argument in June 1871 in a lecture on 'Dust and Smoke', *Nature*, 1871, 4: 124–8.

70 F. M. Turner, 'John Tyndall and Scientific Naturalism', in W. H. Brock et al. eds., *John Tyndall: Essays on a Natural Philosopher*, Dublin, Royal Dublin Society 1981, 169–80.

71 J. Lister, 'On the Effects of the Antiseptic System of Treatment upon the Salubrity of a Surgical Hospital', *Lancet*, 1870, i: 4–6, 40–42.

72 Lister had noted in his Introductory Lecture in 1869 that, 'if a ray of sunlight were to shoot through this room, we should see the sunbeam peopled with motes'. Lister, 'Introductory Lecture', 602.

73 Editorial, 'Dust and Disease', *Nature*, 1870, 1: 327; 'Dust and Spray', *MTG*, 1870, i: 125, 149, 166,

74 J. Tyndall, 'Professor Tyndall on filtered air', *Times*, 7 April 1871, 5; H. C. Bastian, 'The Germ Theory of Disease', Ibid., 13 April 1871, 4; J. Tyndall, 'The Germ Theory of Disease', Ibid., 21 April 1871, 8; H. C. Bastian, 'The Germ Theory of Disease', Ibid., 22 April 1871, 5.

were degraded or altered protoplasm. This latter process was widely seen by some as a form heterogenesis, especially as cells were said to undergo a degenerative transformation to create bioplasm.[75] Yet Beale, as a committed vitalist, quickly distanced himself from the materialist implications of spontaneous generation, saying that he was proposing the formation of *altered* life, not *new* life. Beale, like Bastian and many others, saw the major weakness of Lister's system to be its exclusive emphasis on the external causes of sepsis and the denial of any possibility of internal and *de novo* origins.[76] Nonetheless, Beale endorsed Listerism, though with a different rationale for its success, namely, that carbolic acid worked by checking the development and growth of bioplasm.[77] One of Beale's followers, A. E. Sansom, was an even greater enthusiast for carbolic acid and 'the antiseptic system' than Lister, promoting it as a panacea.[78] Beale was soon eclipsed as an authority of germs, despite his alignment with advanced scientific opinion in opposing spontaneous generation, the publication of three volumes on disease germs and extensive lecturing on the subject.[79] He had his followers in medicine but failed to create a research school; crucially, his theories were not taken up by continental researchers and they remained uniquely English, even metropolitan. His disease-germs were physicians' germs, generated internally and with internal effects. If different diseases had produced recognisably distinct types of bioplasm, then Beale's ideas might have been useful in diagnosis, but bioplasm remained undifferentiated, and thus of little clinical use and a poor resource for establishing a research programme based on histological methods. His cause was helped by the fact that most people found him very difficult to work with.

REACTIONS TO LISTERISM AND GERM-THEORY

While Listerism became synonymous with the germ-theory of disease in the eyes of many surgeons, a more common response was to separate Listerian

75 L. S. Beale, *Bioplasm: An Introduction to the Study of Physiology and Medicine*, London, Churchill, 1872.
76 The fifth verse in a poem entitled, 'Antisepticism: a Fytte', in the *Edinburgh Medical Journal* in October 1875 made the point as follows:

As to putrescence – this was the old view,
    And unconverted sceptics still it hold
That is decaying matter – quite of new
    And *suâ sponte* – germs themselves unfold
In varied forms: as maggots, mites, mildew,
    Bacteria, and in short all kinds of mould;
But LISTER says: This mischief without doubt
Comes but from pre-existent germs without.

EMJ, 1875, 21, 377
77 L. S. Beale, *Disease Germs, Their Nature and Origin*, London, Macmillan, 1872, 280–92.
78 A. E. Sansom, *The Antiseptic System: A Treatise on Carbolic Acid and its Compounds*, London, Henry Gillman, 1871.
79 L. S. Beale, 'The Nature and Origin of Contagious Disease Germs, *BMR*, 1872, 1: 31–4.

practice from its theoretical inspiration. Supporters of Lister's methods as well as his opponents adopted this tactic. In May 1870, George F. Elliott, Physician to Hull Infirmary, suggested that Listerism would be more extensively used if it had not been directed against a 'hypothetical entity'.[80] In August of the same year, William Heath, in his Address in Surgery to the BMA Annual Meeting, complained that Listerism had not been given a fair chance because it had been 'identified in the minds of the profession with one particular method, one special agent and one peculiar theory of disease'.[81] He said that its principles should be put to one side so that judgements could be made on its comparative success against other forms of treatment.[82] While favourably disposed, Heath was not prepared to be as exclusive as Lister; he felt that the success of any wound treatment would ultimately be secondary to 'the state of the system of the patient'.[83] The Manchester surgeon Edward Lund (1823–98), an early provincial convert to Listerism, explained 'antisepticity' without any mention of germs. He stated that Listerism prevented the 'autoinoculation' (absorption) of the 'excreta of wounds' – in other words, it prevented poisons infecting the body.[84] Also, many surgeons who found Listerian dressings valuable continued to attribute their success to nonantiseptic factors, for example, the way dressings excluded or filtered air, and the effects of carbolic acid in hardening tissues.[85]

Lister first soft-pedalled on germ 'theory' with a surgical audience in his Address in Surgery to the Annual Meeting of the BMA in August 1871. He began with an account of his recent experiments on germs, in which he referred to a 'few facts' and went on to say that he wished 'to avoid all doubtful disputations' as to the theoretical basis of the treatment – no doubt a reference to spontaneous generation.[86]

Following this he told his audience that believing in germs was not that important after all:

I do not ask you to believe that the septic particles are organisms. That they are self-propagating, like living beings, and that their energy is extinguished by precisely the same agencies as extinguish vitality . . . is certain. . . . But if any one, in spite of these facts prefer[s] to believe that the septic particles are not alive, and to regard the vibrios invariably present in putrefying pus or sloughs as mere accidental concomitants of putrefaction, or the results, not the causes, of the change, with such a one I, as a practical

---

80 *BMJ*, 1870, i: 488–9.   81 *BMJ*, 1870, ii: 165.   82 Also see: J. More, *Lancet*, 1870, ii: 845.
83 *GMJ*, 1869–70, 2: 135.
84 E. Lund, *Antisepticity in Surgery*, Manchester, J. E. Cornish, 1872. Lund was Surgeon at the Manchester Royal Infirmary and Professor at Owen's College.
85 In his revisions to Paget's lectures on surgical pathology, William Turner suggested that antiseptic dressings acted like a scab and excluded air. J. Paget, *Lectures on Surgical Pathology*, 3rd edition, London, Longmans Green, 1870, 170. Also see: *BMJ*, 1870, ii: 407. John Rose Cormack attributed Lister's success to 'general medical and hygienic treatment . . . rather than the niceties and complexities of his special system'. *BMJ*, 1873, ii: 257.
86 J. Lister, 'The Address in Surgery [Antiseptic treatment of Wounds]' *BMJ*, 1871, ii: 225–33, 225.

surgeon, do not wish to quarrel. Nor do I enter upon the question whether spontaneous generation can take place at the present day upon the surface of our globe.[87]

It has been suggested that Lister was being disingenuous here, yet this was his consistent position until 1877.[88] It is well known that Lister, unlike Tyndall, did not relish controversy. He was aware of the widespread attacks on germ-theory in medicine and surgery, and he knew only too well that he had made little headway in converting his immediate colleagues, let alone surgeons nationally.[89] His followers came especially from amongst young, provincial doctors and those trained in Glasgow. In addition, by 1875 there was a small band of apostles of his creed, who I have termed Listerians. These were Lister's assistants and former students, for example, William Watson Cheyne and John Chiene, who became public champions of mainstream Listerism.

Surgeons' dislike of theory led to Pasteurian germ-theory being discussed more fully in public health medicine and pathology than in surgery.[90] Bastian discussed surgical diseases as part of wide-ranging review of theories of disease in an introductory address to students at University College Hospital in October 1871.[91] On this occasion his targets included disease specificity and the idea that diseases were entities, as well as the theories of Pasteur and his followers. He adopted the common aetiological stance that two conditions were required for any disease – an internal constitutional peculiarity and an external exciting cause; the latter was only very rarely a sufficient condition on its own. Bastian was content that most septic and epidemic diseases were explained by chemical poisons, the only exceptions being those caused by parasites. As examples of parasitic diseases Bastian cited Pasteur's work on silkworm disease and, interestingly, Davaine's studies of anthrax. Bastian's pathology lectures at University College began with diseases caused by large animal parasites and worked down to smaller, fungal organisms. It should be noted that Bastian himself was an authority

---

87 Ibid., 227. In June 1871, Lister was reported as explaining his methods without mentioning germs directly, saying that in his treatment 'We do not exclude the gases of the atmosphere at all, but adopt efficient means to destroy the energy of its floating ferments.', J. Lister, 'On Some Cases Illustrating the Results of Excision of the Wrist for Caries', *EMJ*, 1871–2, 17: 144–50, 150.

88 Fox, 'Scientific Theory', 377. Fox makes this point in relation to comments made by Lister in 1883 and relates the consistency of his position from 1871.

89 John Wood (1825–1891), in his Address in Surgery to the BMA's Annual Meeting in 1873, described as a 'half-believer' in antisepsis, discussed the practice , but referred his audience to the work of Burdon Sanderson and Wilson Fox for information on germs. *BMJ*, 1873, ii: 196. Wood was joined by Lister at King's College, London, in 1877. Wood favoured subcutaneous methods and became a convert to later Listerian practices. Also see: *BMJ*, 1874, i: 446.

90 Cf. Richardson, 'Medical Aspects'; A. E. Sansom, 'On Putrefaction, Fermentation and Infection', *Lancet*, 1870, ii: 671; J. Hogg, 'The Organic Germ Theory of Disease', *MTG*, 1870, i: 659–61, 685–7.

91 H. C. Bastian, 'Epidemic and Specific Contagious Diseases: Considerations as to their Nature and Mode of Origin, *BMJ*, 1871, ii: 400–9. Bastian likened germ-theory to homoeopathy and phrenology.

on nematode worms.[92] It was against the paradigm of parasitic diseases that he found Pasteurian germ-theory wanting, especially the fact that most parasitic diseases led to death, whereas zymotic and septic diseases did not. From these and other assumptions he proposed a complex classification of 'Communicable Diseases', including septic ones (see Table 3).

He classified septic diseases as conditions of the blood 'caused and propagated by chemico-physical agencies' that either developed spontaneously or came from other bodies. He claimed that no surgeon had any doubt that in most cases septic diseases arose *de novo*; indeed, he suggested that they were readily and easily produced.[93] The different septic diseases were described as 'but different modes in which this morbid process repeats itself in certain constitutions and under certain conditions'. Only at the end of his talk did he mention spontaneous generation, when he suggested that 'in a body at or near death changes in the blood might . . . assume such a character as to lead to the evolution of Bacteria', linking this to a plea against 'any narrow or exclusive theories'. Although he never put it in these terms, he was reacting against certain features of Tyndall's scientific naturalism, mostly its monotheism, but also its reductionism and authoritarian suppression of alternative ideas.

Bastian became one of the leading British medical experts on germs in the 1870s, not least because of his expertise on spontaneous generation. He took on nonmedical interlopers, such as Tyndall and Pasteur, and articulated views that were widely held across medicine and surgery. He spoke on the subject at almost every major medical or surgical discussion of germs in the 1870s. He opened the major debate on germ-theory at the Pathological Society of London in 1875; he replied to Lister's first lecture in London on fermentation in 1877; and he was again the first to reply to Lister's address at the International Medical Congress in 1881. His authority was such that, in 1877–78, the French government set up another commission to adjudicate on his differences with Pasteur.[94] As late as 1882, Bastian wrote the entries on 'Germ Theory' and 'Bacteria' in Quain's *Dictionary of Medicine*.[95] There is no paradox in this, for he never denied their existence or their association with disease, simply that they caused disease.

Unlike Bastian, Lister never wrote a systematic account of germ-theory or bacteria for a reference work or textbook.[96] After 1871, his publications in

92 W. D. Halliburton, Lecture Notes, 1880–81, MS 269. Western Manuscripts, Wellcome Institute Library.

93 Bastian quotes Sir William Jenner: 'We know that the zymotic element which produced contagious pyaemia may be generated in the frame of man de novo.' *Practice of Medicine*, London, 1872, 56.

94 Adam, *Spontaneous Generation*, 124–31.

95 'Debate on the Germ Theory of Disease', *TPSL*, 1875, 26: 255–345. R. Quain, *Dictionary of Medicine*, London, Longmans Green, 1882, 98–9, 532–3.

96 He wrote the entry on amputation in the first edition of Holmes' textbook of surgery (1862) and contributed on the same topic and anaesthetics in the second in 1871. T. Holmes, *A System of Surgery*, London, Longman Green, 1871, 480–504, 592–653.

Table 3. *Communicable Diseases*

	Parasitic diseases	Tissue diseases	Diseases of the blood (principally)	
Pathology		Diseases of internal formed tissues and of mucous membranes	Diseases of the blood (principally)	
Pathogenesis	*Many capable of arising de novo*	*All inoculable and capable of arising de novo*	*All contagious and capable of arising de novo*	*Contagiousness either absent, little marked, or more of less virulent; all probably capable of arising de novo*
Disease	External (cutaneous) surface Internal (mucous) surface Closed (serous) cavities Tissues of organs or parts. (*Psorospermiae, Cysticerci, Nematoids*, etc.) Blood (*Bacteridia*) in 'Malignant pustule', *Psorospermiae* in 'pébrine', etc.)	Fibro-plastic growths Cancerous growths Tubercular growths Syphilis Gonorrhoea Purulent Ophthalmia Diphtheria and Croup	Erysipelas Puerperal fever Surgical fever Pyaemia Hospital gangrene Rabies	Rheumatic fever a. Dengue b. Sweating sickness Intermittent fever a. Remittent fever b. Yellow fever Summer diarrhoea – Cholera – Dysentery – Influenza – Mumps – Relapsing fever – Typhoid fever – Typhus fever Plague – Varicella – Hooping cough – Measles – Scarlet fever – Small-pox
Epidemiology		Principally sporadic	Principally endemic	Often epidemic
Cause	Caused and propagated by the presence of self-multiplication of living units	Caused and propagated by chemico-physical agencies, and not by the multiplication of living units		

H. C. Bastian, 'Epidemic and Contagious Diseases: Considerations as their Mode of Origin', *BMJ*, 1871, ii: 407.
Note that Bastian regards 'bacteria' as parasites; that cancer and tuberculosis are included because they are 'communicable' within the body; that septic and zymotic diseases are linked because they were diseases of the blood; and that every disease is capable of arising *de novo*.

medical journals concentrated on the details of antiseptic treatment and tended to mention germ-theory only in passing.[97] Indeed, he did not publish much at all in national medical journals until 1875, when he produced a series of articles on recent improvements in antiseptic surgery, including the first full details of the spray that he had introduced in 1871.[98] This innovation became a major technical obstacle to the acceptance of Listerism and also, tellingly, its icon. The spray pumped a mist of carbolic acid solution over the site of the operation, aiming to kill panspermic life and cover surfaces that might harbour germs, such as the wound itself and the surgeon's hands and instruments. The spray was time-consuming to set up and the concentration of the carbolic acid used had to be carefully controlled, as even low dilutions burned surgeons' hands and patients' flesh. The spray made operative surgery messier, more expensive and was the element of Listerism that was reputedly most often omitted, even by dedicated Listerians. While Lister maintained his silence on germs with his fellow surgeons, they saw the spray as the physical embodiment of panspermism and germ-theory. Its emblematic importance should not be underestimated. It styled Listerism as an ideal type of *cordon sanitaire*, with border measures aimed against airborne invaders, followed up by sanitary cleansing at ground level with carbolic washes, gauzes, putties and special catgut. Full protection was secured, and problems from a second aerial wave of germs were thwarted, by the creation of a defensive line of carbolic dressings. The analogy of germs with invaders needs to be qualified because, in line with panspermism, germs were not so much active invaders, but essentially passive beings, like seeds, that literally floated around and dropped into wounds.

When the BMA visited Edinburgh in 1875, Lister's work was the focus of attention, though, significantly his major contribution was two demonstrations on his wards.[99] Lister's Edinburgh colleague, James Spence (1812–82), who was known to doubt both Lister's methods and theories, gave the main Address in Surgery.[100] Spence claimed that he was just as successful as

---

97 *Lancet*, 1874, i: 51. Sampson Gamgee, a surgeon and brother of the veterinarian, also noted that theory and practice were kept separate, even on the wards. Nonetheless, he was critical of submission to 'a fixed theoretical preoccupation' and believed that the 'facts themselves' showed that Pasteur's theory, while true, was incomplete. Lister's publications between 1871 and 1875 were: J. Lister, 'On . . . Excision of the Wrist', *EMJ*, 17, 1871, 144–50; 'On a Case of Rupture of the Axillary Artery', *EMJ*, 1871, 17: 829–31; 'Cases of Omental Hernia', *EMJ*, 1873, 20: 69–73; 'A Case of Rodent Ulcer', *EMJ*, 1874, 20: 268–70; 'Cases Illustrating Antiseptic Management', *EMJ*, 1874, 20: 556–7.

98 Lister, 'Address', 1871, 227. It is somewhat ironic that Lister initially used a spray-making device developed for the administration of anaesthesia by that arch opponent of germ-theory, Benjamin Ward Richardson. On full Listerian procedures see: J. Lister, 'On Recent Improvements in the Details of Antiseptic Surgery', *Lancet*, i: 1875, 365–7, 401–2, 434–6, 468–70, 603–5, 717–9, 787–9.

99 J. Lister, 'Demonstrations of Antiseptic Surgery', *EMJ*, 1875–76, 21: 195–6, 481–7.

100 *BMJ*, 1875, ii: 197, 204.

his colleague in preventing and managing wound sepsis, but by other methods. After the meeting, Lister wrote up the details of the demonstrations that he had given for publication, relegating the following comments to a footnote:

If anyone chooses to assume that the septic material is not of the nature of living organisms, but a so-called chemical ferment destitute of vitality, yet endowed with a power of self-multiplication equal to that of the organism associated with it, such a notion, unwarranted though I believe it to be by any scientific evidence, will in a practical point of view be equivalent to a germ theory, since it will inculcate precisely the same methods of antiseptic management. It seems important that this should be clearly understood, because it appears to be often imagined that authors who are not satisfied by the strict truth of germ theory, but substitute for it some other hypothesis, invalidate antiseptic practice, which I must repeat, is not affected in one tittle by this theoretical discrepancy.[101]

Two points were being made: never mind the theory – try the practice; and, that all current theories of sepsis 'dictate' the similar methods of management. Listerism was apparently so successful in the field that ideas derived from the laboratory could be suspended.

Yet it was reported by those who visited his wards in the early 1870s that Lister 'adhered with unflinching fidelity' to Pasteur's germ-theory. His continuing faith was evident in his on-going research on fermentation and germs, his correspondence with Pasteur and the articles he published in non-medical journals, such as the *Quarterly Journal of Microscopical Science* (*QJMS*), *Nature* and the *Transactions of the Royal Society of Edinburgh*.[102] The *Quarterly Journal* was the major forum for publication on germs, monads and 'microphytes' in the early 1870s, and it was mainly through its pages that British readers were able to keep up with domestic, German and French work on microbes in botany, zoology and medicine.[103] In the early 1870s, Lister pictured germs as very simple organisms whose form and physiology was largely determined by the milieu in which they found themselves. He supposed, as did many others, that there might be just one type of pathogenic germ, and that its different effects resulted from the conditions in which it developed.

101 *Lancet*, 1875, i: 435. In surgical demonstrations given to the BMA in Edinburgh in August 1875, Lister was content simply to assert that septic ferments existed and left it to the audience to decide if they were living organisms or not. Lister, 'Demonstrations' 195–6.

102 J. Lister, 'On the Germ Theory of Putrefaction and Other Fermentative Changes', *Nature*, 1873, 8: 212–4, 232–3; idem., 'A Further Contribution to the Natural History of Bacteria and the Germ Theory of Fermentative Changes', *QJMS*, 1873, 13: 380–408; idem., 'A Contribution to the Germ Theory of Putrefaction and other Fermentative Changes, and the Natural History of Torulae and Bacteria', *TRSE*, 1875, 27: 313–44.

103 'Bacteria and their Relations to Putrefaction and Contagia', *QJMS*, 1872, 12: 207–10. Also see: L. Kern, *Deutsche Bakteriologie im Spiegel englischer medizinischer Zeitschriften, 1875–1885*, Zurich, Juris Druck and Verlag, 1972.

In wounds, germs would develop septic properties, in an inflamed throat diphtheric properties and in the soil, perhaps choleraic properties. This view met one of the commonest objections to germ theories, namely, the seemingly absurd requirement that there could be many different types of such tiny and very simple organisms, with each able to produce specific effects. Lister's support for the idea that germs were mutable or pleomorphic confirmed his allegiance at this time to Pasteur and Nageli, and against Ferdinand Cohn's presumption of fixed bacterial species.[104]

Lister's own private laboratory work was very much in the style of Pasteur and the concurrent spontaneous generation debate. He worked primarily with infusions of organic materials in flasks and test tubes, like a chemist, rather than with the microscope and vivisection methods being used by pathologists and physiologists. In a 1873 publication he made an aside on the spontaneous generation debate, saying that while his experimental work had not been designed to test the phenomenon, his results 'afforded the strongest possible evidence against it, and in favour of the germ theory of fermentative changes'.[105] Lister's tactic of pursuing research on fermentative changes and germ theories in one context, and antiseptic treatment in another, had important consequences. It meant that Pasteurian germ-theory was not disseminated directly amongst surgeons; rather, it was represented by practices. Whether surgeons would have become significant germ theorists or manipulators is a moot point. Even if they had been readily convinced of the reality and role of germs in sepsis, their primary interest would probably have been the best means of their destruction, not to cultivate and study them.

In experimental biology and medicine, in Britain and elsewhere, there was significant elaboration of the character and actions of vibrios of all kinds after 1871. Microscopists, using improved instruments and techniques, were able to fashion accounts of the life histories of 'monads'. The visual presentation of germs remained relatively unsophisticated, especially when compared to efforts put into portraying cellular changes. The lack of interest on this technical front was largely due to the fact that the simplicity of germs and pleomorphism meant that structure was assumed to be relatively unimportant. The microscope and inoculation experiments began to show constant conjunctions between certain microorganisms and specific diseases, for example, rod-shaped organisms with anthrax and spirilla with relapsing fever. However, lack of agreement on the classification of microbial life and on standard procedures meant that results were difficult to replicate. There were many claims and counterclaims; hence, very few 'monads' were widely accepted as constantly associated with specific diseases, let alone as causes. There was, however, a steady botanisation of 'monads', first through the revelation

104 W. Bulloch, *The History of Bacteriology*, London, Oxford University Press, 1938, 171–206.
105 Lister, 'A Further Contribution', 382.

of life cycles and growth patterns, then the agreement that most 'monads' were bacteria and that bacteria were plants and, finally, this led to greater interest in form and classification, a development that was aided by the increasing number of scientists following Cohn's ideas of fixed species of bacteria.

Developments around the different germ theories had little impact on surgical discourses on sepsis before 1875, as most surgeons continued to assume that they were managing a chemical phenomenon. To a degree, Listerism reinforced this view as it too relied on a neutralising chemical agent. I discuss the elaboration of putrefactive germ-theory within surgery in Chapter 5, so at this point I simply want to note some of the experimental work that could have been used in debates about germs and sepsis. As early as 1871, Bastian had highlighted studies that showed 'vibrios' present in healthy tissues, and that inoculations of the blood and secretions of animals with sheep-pox did not always lead to disease.[106] Potentially the most significant British work on wound sepsis was published in the Annual Reports of the Medical Officer to the Privy Council. In 1872, Sanderson reported, in direct contradiction to Lister, that the accidental airborne pollution of wounds by septic, bacterial germs was not a common occurrence and that 'infection with bacteria is effected solely by contact with dirty surfaces (skin, instruments or vessels)'.[107] Of course, septic disease-germs could have been something other than 'bacteria'. Sanderson articulated the common assumption that the sources of septic inflammatory disease were distinct from those of zymotic diseases: the former coming from animal sources, the latter from plants and fungi. His point was that vegetable germs (or their spores) might arrive by air; animal germs had to be carried in moisture, or be directly and quickly communicated, because they were more fragile. Sanderson had also worked on the question of whether boiling necessarily killed germs. That they proved durable might have led to further questions of their vulnerability to chemical antiseptics.[108]

The distinction between septic and zymotic diseases, which became fundamental in Britain during the 1870s, was less important elsewhere, notably in Germany, where Cohn's notion that all disease-causing germs were specific and that every infective disease would be associated with a particular species of bacteria was gaining ground. In general, bacterial germ theories enjoyed greater promotion and support in continental Europe than in Britain, though they were controversial everywhere. This disposition of support meant

---

106 Bastian, 'Epidemic', 403. J. B. Sanderson, 'On the Intimate Pathology of Contagion', *Twelfth Annual Report of the Medical Officer of the Privy Council for 1869*, BPP 1870, [C.208], xxxviii, 229–56.

107 *QJMS*, 1872, 12: 208.

108 H. C. Bastian, 'Dr Sanderson's Experiments and Archeobiosis', *Nature*, 1873, 8: 485; idem, 'On the Temperature at which Bacteria, Vibriones and their Supposed Germs are Killed when Immersed in Fluids or Exposed to Heat in a Moist State', *PRSL*, 1873, 21: 220–32.

that the principles of Listerism were more widely accepted on the continent than in Britain, which in turn meant that Listerians abroad were working with the grain of advanced medical science rather than against or outside it. However, the support that Lister received from the continent was a mixed blessing. Chauvinistic attitudes were only too evident in remarks by British surgeons. They observed that their French and German neighbours would, of course, have found Listerism useful on the battlefield when they had been reduced to warfare in 1870, and would continue to find it valuable in peacetime in their dirty, ill-ventilated hospitals. The implication was that superior British surgery, practised in cleaner, airier hospitals, did not need such elaborate precautions and 'exclusive' treatments. The achievements in medical science of these countries was recognised and accepted but was contrasted with Britain's clinical prowess, superior sanitary arrangements and lower national mortality levels.

'A CHAOS OF CONFLICTING OPINIONS'

The state of surgical thinking on septic phenomena and their control in the mid-1870s was evident in a series of meetings in London in 1874 and 1875. Although there were fewer Listerians in London than elsewhere, the debates at these meetings saw strong opinions expressed on all sides and show the range of opinions amongst British surgeons. The first debate was at a Clinical Society of London meeting on pyaemia in the spring of 1874, where 'a chaos of conflicting opinions' was reported. There was hardly any direct mention of germs as chemical theories continued to hold sway.[109] The hospitalism debate was still alive, just, but attention concentrated on the pathogenesis of pyaemia as revealed by clinical experience.[110] Thus, the main issue was, did pyaemia arise *de novo*, or did it arise after the body was contaminated by some external poison? If the origins of septic poisons were internal, were the sources localised or general? If their origins were external, then how did they spread and enter the body? These questions were posed around the practical issue of how surgeons could avoid or control the disease. The main speaker was William Savory (1826–95), a consulting surgeon at St Bartholomew's Hospital, London, and his conclusions were clear – pyaemia was due to a chemical poison that formed 'within the body itself' and then passed into the blood stream.[111] Thereafter, and on limited occasions, it might escape and start the process in another body.

109 'Debate on Pyaemia' *BMJ*, 1874, i: 146, 234–40, 306–11, 324–5, 380–6.
110 T. Holmes, 'Pyaemia in Hospital and Private Practice', *BMJ*, 1874, i: 269–70; ii: 142–5.
111 Reputedly, Savory always cut a curious figure. His cockney background led him to drop his H's (e.g. 'ernias and 'ealthy conditions) and he was said never to laugh. Yet he was a dominating, old-school anatomical surgeon at St. Bartholomew's, a former colleague of George Callender and Holmes Coote (1817–72), and friend of J. Whitaker Hulke (1830–95) and Frederick Pavy (1829–1911).

Few dissented from Savory's basic model, though the ever equivocal Sanderson wanted to allow for external 'hospitalism' effects and the internal generation of a poison.[112] The discussion of the issues was long and involved, but the most influential contribution was by William Callender (1830–78), also a surgeon at St Bartholomew's. Like many speakers, he concentrated on his own treatments and revealed his pathological ideas only in passing. His so-called 'simple methods' of wound management, which involved washing and cleanliness, had been canvassed as a distinctive metropolitan alternative to Listerism, being preventive, curative and more effective.[113] Callender stressed that the drainage of wounds was necessary to remove acrid, irritating and poisonous substances. However, he was eclectic in his techniques, recommending antiseptic agents, ventilation and the isolation of wounds – all measures where the primary aim was to halt the internal spread of poisons. He assumed that any pyaemic abscesses were so deep seated that they could not be the source of contagion between patients.[114] His central point was that surgeons did not only have to deal with the wound and the local diffusion of poisons, they also had to try and aid healing from *within* the body. In other words, they had to help 'the constitutional progress of the patient' by building up their ability to counter poisons through diet, tonics and other medical measures. Only Jonathan Hutchinson (1828–1913), working from a Beale-inspired model of pus-contagion, prioritised the control of cross-infection from secretions and exanthemata by the isolation of patients. He too wanted wounds to be free from irritation and draughts, and for patients' general health to be improved.[115] Interestingly, the only explicit mention of germs in the whole debate was by Bastian, who reported bacterial organisms being spontaneously produced in the fluids of a pyaemic patient.[116] One commentator noted that, 'Among the London authorities . . . the germ-theory was at such a discount that not one could be found to advance it or even allude to it. . . . But there was no such cold shade over the chemical doctrine of putrefaction'.[117]

A major discussion of germ theories took place a year later at the Pathological Society of London in April 1875.[118] The published report referred to

---

112 *BMJ*, 1874, i: 383.
113 In 1873, Callender had spoken on the 'Isolation and treatment of wounds' to the BMA and directly challenged Listerism with his own methods of hygiene. *BMJ*, 1873, ii. 256–7. On Callender see: *BMJ*, 1879, ii: 715–6; *St. Bartholomew's Hospital Gazette*, 1879, 15: xli–xlvii.
114 *BMJ*, 1874, i: 306–7.
115 J. Hutchinson, 'The Hospital Plagues', *BMJ*, 1874, i: 161–3. Hutchinson was Consulting Surgeon at the London Hospital. He served on the Royal Commissions on Smallpox and Fever Hospitals in 1881 and Vivisection in the period 1890–96. He was a friend of Hughlings Jackson, with whom he explored philosophical interests. H. Hutchinson, *Jonathan Hutchinson: Life and Letters*, London, Heinemann, 1946.
116 *BMJ*, 1874, i: 483–4.
117 *BFM-CR*, 1874, 54: 1–16, 15.
118 'Debate on the Germ Theory of Disease', *TPSL*, 1875, 26: 255–345.

'this obscure but important topic', but the meeting itself told a different story as the animated discussions extended over three sessions and were widely reported in the medical press. That the main address was by Bastian shows again the importance of spontaneous generation in medical discourses on germs at this time. Bastian divided his address, which was largely an attack on Pasteur–Lister germ theories, into separate discussions of (i) germ theories of septic diseases and virulent inflammations, and (ii) germ theories of specific contagious fevers. This distinction had been used by Sanderson in lectures in the winter of 1875 on 'Organic Forms in Connection with Contagious and Infectious Diseases', though he focused on zymotic diseases and said little about sepsis.[119] Sanderson's only observation was that any septic organisms were affected by their environment, whereas contagia were specific and more fixed; in many ways this was typical Sanderson, having it both ways with pleomorphism in septic disease and fixed-species in contagious diseases.

Drawing on the previous year's Clinical Society discussions, Bastian began by arguing that the preponderance of isolated cases of pyaemia, together with the well-known fact that the disease could occur without any abrasion to the body's surface, supported its internal origin. Bastian spoke of the spontaneous generation of germs in pyaemic patients as being quite common. He then adopted one of his most familiar and effective tactics, turning his opponents' words against them, which was not difficult with Sanderson. Thus, Sanderson's uncertainties over whether contagious mixtures, supposedly containing germs, could withstand boiling were fully exploited. Bastian also noted with relish Sanderson's recent observations 'that air is entirely free of living microzymes' and that healthy blood is germless. An important difference between Bastian and Lister had been over whether germs could survive in healthy tissues without causing disease. Bastian now suggested that Lister had moved closer to his own position with the notion that germs were pleomorphic. He saw this as amounting to accepting their spontaneous transformation (or transmutation), if not generation.[120] Perhaps he had no quarrel with Lister after all, as both could agree that putrefactive processes in wounds, and hence the production of poisons, ought to be reduced to a minimum:

Such a notion . . . may, however, be acted upon by the adoption of the antiseptic system of treatment (or by free exposure of wounds and frequent removal of secretion), quite

---

119 J. B. Sanderson, 'Organic Forms in Connection with Contagious and Infectious Diseases', *BMJ*, 1875, i: 69–71, 199–201, 403–5, 435–7. T. Romano, *Making Medicine Scientific: John Burdon Sanderson and the Culture of Victorian Science*, Unpublished PhD Thesis, Yale University, 1993, 153–80.

120 The remark of Lister that was used by Bastian was, 'it is not essential to assume a special virus [of hospital gangrene] at all, but that organisms common to all the sores of the ward may, for aught we know, assume specific properties in the discharges long putrefying under the dressing'. 'Debate on', 267.

independently of the question whether mere organic *débris* may act as ferments, and also quite independently of the further question whether the poisons so engendered in wounds are living entities or complex compounds not endowed with the attributes of living matter.[121]

Thus, Bastian was also willing to separate theory and practice, though there was no doubting his commitment to principles that were quite at odds with those of Lister.

The published account of proceedings records ten replies to Bastian's address, half from surgeons. Other contributors included Sanderson, Charles Murchison and Thomas Maclagan, author of a book on *The Germ Theory* published in 1876.[122] The leading surgeon to speak was Jonathan Hutchinson, who accepted that germs were the means by which specific and zymotic fevers spread from person to person, yet he remained wedded to a physico chemical account of sepsis.[123] Hutchinson had a Quaker background, like Lister, was on the scientific wing of surgery, being Secretary to the New Sydenham Society from 1859 to 1907, and had developed interests in the infective character of syphilis and leprosy. He typified a growing surgical and medical view that Listerism, Callender's methods and his own traditional anti-phlogistic system were all anti-inflammatory and all successful in careful hands. This was because each surgeon, in their different ways, made wounds clean, halted sepsis, controlled inflammation and improved the healing power of the patient's constitution.[124]

The main support for Listerism and its principles came from Knowsley Thornton, a surgeon at the Samaritan Hospital and a colleague of Spencer Wells. Thornton started from the 'absolute facts' of wound sepsis being due to the 'outward cause' of the germs of bacteria and other low forms of life,[125] though he quickly took the discussion into new territory, asking why germs did not cause problems for the ovariotomists who routinely opened and exposed the abdomen. His answer was that ovariotomists avoided sepsis, not by any special technique or system, but because of the inherent vitality of the healthy tissues of the abdomen, which prevented the germination of organisms. This, he said, 'I originally learnt from Professor Lister'. This surprised many surgeons who regarded Lister's methods as wholly based on combating external germ pollution and ignoring constitutional consider-

121 Ibid., 276.
122 T. J. Maclagan, *The Germ-Theory Applied to the Explanation of the Phenomena of Disease*, London, Macmillan, 1876. Maclagan was Physician to the Dundee Royal Infirmary, though his contribution centred on a defence of Listerian practice. He explained this in terms drawn from German work on contagia as parasites rather than putrefactive germs or ferments.
123 This theory supposed that the type of tissue in which inflammation occurred and pus corpuscles were produced was specific, and that the spread of lesions to contiguous tissues, distant parts of the body via the vascular system and transplantation to another individual as similar processes. 'Debate on', 306–8.
124 *Lancet*, 1875, ii: 743.   125 'Debate on', 312–3.

ations. Was Thornton correct in suggesting that 'vital resistance' was an integral part of Listerism? The answer to those who had worked with Lister was yes, but to those who had learned of his ideas and work second-hand and through its technologies it was no. Their perception was that everything was external and that germs were all-powerful.

In his address, Bastian argued that Listerians had assumed that the 'germs of putrefaction and the germs of disease are living organisms of similar nature', suggesting that, unlike himself, they did not distinguish between septic and zymotic diseases.[126] As I will show in Chapter 5, between 1881 and 1883 Listerians claimed that the distinction between septic and zymotic diseases, putrefaction and infection, had always been central to his system, though I would go along with Bastian and say that direct references to this distinction are hard to find in the early 1870s.[127] Nonetheless, a case could be made, for example, that it was implicit in the idea of the germlessness of healthy tissues and the distinction between (septic) germs and *contagium viva*. In 1870, Lister had written on the self-healing of healthy tissues due to their vitality:

The injured tissues do not need to be 'stimulated' or treated with any mysterious specific; ALL THAT THEY NEED IS TO BE LEFT ALONE. Nature will take care of them: those which are weakened will recover, and those which have been deprived of vitality by injury will serve as pabulum for their living neighbours. [capitals in original][128]

In this context, 'living neighbours' refers to other cells, though in infected tissues those neighbours could have been other disease-germs. Why this aspect of Listerism was not, and has not, been widely recognised goes back to the initial presentation of Listerism as an innovation in wound treatment and from surgeons' general reluctance to engage with its 'theory'. The elaborate dressing and management regimes, together with the sore hands of the surgeon, certainly suggested that Listerism had little regard for the vitality of living tissues. Lister's own surgical work and the cases he chose to illustrate his methods were largely reparative and reconstructive cases (i.e. the treatment of already damaged or dead tissue), not operative surgery that required working through and on healthy, living tissues.[129] The association with Tyndall's 'Dust and Disease' ideas, the spray and Lister's strategic position as an opponent of spontaneous generation would all have magnified the importance of external polluting agents as the main factor in the prevention and

126 *BMJ*, 1871, ii: 403.
127 A notable exception is Lawrence and Dixey, 'Practising on Principle', 177–9. They identify four components to Lister's germ theory of pathogenesis c. 1875: (i) only living organisms could produce putrefaction; (ii) a belief in pleomorphism (i.e. that septic organisms could change their form and action influenced by the external environment); (iii) the alteration of benign into pathogenic organisms in unhealthy wounds (pleomorphism in action); and (iv) an assumption that germs could not invade healthy tissue (vital resistance).
128 J. Lister, 'Remarks on a Case of Compound Dislocation, *Lancet*, 1870, i: 404–6, 440–3, 512–3, 440.
129 For comments on the limited range of Lister's surgical work, see: *BFM-CR*, 1974, 54: 6.

treatment of septic diseases.[130] Lister himself did little to combat this impression. He made no public attempts to distance the properties of his septic germs from what might be called the 'germification' of *contagium viva* and zymotic poisons in public health medicine.

Concurrent with the Pathological Society debate was a series of meetings at the Obstetrical Society of London on puerperal fever.[131] Puerperal fever was a septic, infective disease that affected women after childbirth and was widely understood to be contagious to some degree.[132] It was also one of the illnesses where physicians and general practitioners encountered traumatic septic disease. The debate is worth considering briefly for what it reveals about wider attitudes to sepsis and how marginal germ ideas were elsewhere in the profession. The issue of the contagiousness of puerperal fever was long running and had been sharpened in the mid-1870s by a court case where two midwives had been prosecuted for 'manslaughter by infection'.[133] There were obvious fears that similar charges might be brought against medical practitioners. If the statements made at the meeting are any guide to practice, the case certainly encouraged the use of any number of antiseptic precautions (anything from Condy's fluid to Turkish baths) and isolation of sufferers, though contagion was seen to be a highly contingent phenomenon.[134] Senior metropolitan figures, like Hutchinson, Callender and Wells, spoke in the debate and took the opportunity to restate their wider views of disease-agents.[135] While the role of germs and bacteria was discussed, 'theory' was seen to be a peripheral issue; the main task was how to prevent the disease poisons arising in the first place and, if that failed, how to combat them. The conclusions of the meeting were clear. Puerperal had two possible origins: i) *autogenetic* – arising within the patient: and ii) *heterogenetic* – imported from without. Autogenesis was the primary origin, and contagion was secondary. Practically, the problem was not the doctor infecting the parturating woman, as her contaminating the doctor's hands and clothing and starting the spread of the infection. The practical result was that obstetricians had to adopt measures that protected the lying-in woman from 'the formation of poisonous materials in her own system, and which secured her isolation from all contagion from without'.[136] There was no imperative to choose between these competing accounts, especially as all might have some element of truth, nor any great imperative to know the nature of the

130 See comments of Knowsley Thomson, a former student of Lister. 'Debate on', 313.
131 T. Spencer Wells, 'On the Relation of Puerperal Fever to the Infective Diseases and Pyaemia', *Transactions of the Obstetrical Society*, 1875, 17: 90–130. Also see: *BMJ*, 1875, i: 501–3, 517–22, 643–8.
132 On debates in the 1860s, see: G. P. Parsons, 'The British Medical Profession and Contagion Theory: Puerperal Fever as a Case-Study', *MH*, 1978, 22: 138–50; A. Bashford, *Purity and Pollution: Gender, Embodiment and Victorian Medicine*, London, Macmillan, 1998, 63–84. Cf. I. S. L. Loudon, *Childbed Fever: A Documentary History*, New York, Garland, 1995, xliv–liv, 89–108.
133 *BMJ*, 1875, i: 547–8, 642.   134 Ibid., 646.   135 Ibid., 648.
136 W. O. Priestley, *Transactions of the Obstetrical Society*, 1876, 18: 51.

'poisonous material or contagion' as doctors had confidence in their improving antiseptic and hygienic measures.

One final indication of surgical opinion on germs was given in a discussion on antiseptic surgery that developed unexpectedly at the Clinical Society in London in October 1875, when the discussion of a paper by Callender on the use of salicylic acid as an antiseptic shifted to a wide-ranging discussion of antisepsis. Listerism was now portrayed as an elaborate technology – not only dressings and the inconvenient spray, but of drainage tubes, carbolised ligatures and other fussy details, all of which brought added time and expense.[137] The whole tenor of the discussion was to damn Listerism with faint praise. The surgeons who spoke suggested that it had been a stimulus to greater cleanliness, to better wound management techniques and to improved after-care of the patient, but that its moment had now passed.[138] Its great, and largely incidental benefit, had been to show 'what may really be done by attending to the ordinary rules of practical surgery'.[139] Thus, they suggested that elements of the system were worth retaining, though much of the detail could now be abandoned for simpler procedures.[140] The separation of theory and practice was maintained. One of many editorials in the *Lancet* explained, 'The germ theory may be perfectly well founded; but nine surgeons out of ten do not care whether it is or not, as long as they cure their cases and reduce their mortality to the lowest possible degree'.[141] A later statement was blunter, saying that 'It would be difficult to name more than one or two who are thorough-going believers in the theory, and there are scarcely more who strictly carry out the practice'.[142] If equally good results could be obtained with the open treatment, simple cleanliness, Listerism or whatever, then it was not surprising that most surgeons found it difficult to accept that the air was 'darkened with disease-producing germs' and that the spray and the other details were essential.[143] The prospects for Listerism were less bleak elsewhere. In almost every hospital there were followers as well as sceptics, especially in Glasgow and Edinburgh, where exemplary practice had been available for all to see and learn from.

137 *Lancet*, 1875, ii: 562, 628–9, 737–9. It was reported that the use of Lister's system in London had declined; Ibid., 565.
138 Ibid., 565–6, 597–8, 743–4. Also see: S. Messenger Bradley, *Lancet*, 1876, i: 768–9, *BMJ*, 1875, ii: 769. In 1875, Mr. Barwell certainly wanted 'to simplify Lister's method'. *BMJ*, 1875, ii: 629.
139 Ibid., 598.
140 *BMJ*, 1875, ii: 769. In 1875, Mr. Barwell certainly wanted 'to simplify Lister's method'. *BMJ*, 1875, ii: 629.
141 *Lancet*, 1875, ii: 397. Also see Timothy Holmes, editor of the influential *System of Surgery*, who said that, 'He himself had used Lister's method for some years, and the more he used it the higher did his opinion of it become. . . . He did not believe in Lister's *theory* – i.e. with regard to germs, – as it did not seem to be sufficiently proved by the evidence . . .' (italic emphasis in the original), 628.
142 Ibid., 743.   143 *Lancet*, 1875, ii: 597.

Germ theories of putrefaction and sepsis had some support in surgery by the mid-1870s. However, almost a decade after Lister had announced his principle and practice, all surgeons continued to favour chemical theories of sepsis. However, Listerians combined this with the idea that germs produced the poisons. Non-Listerian surgeons were not conservative or blinkered; rather, they found the new germ ideas wanting as the sole explanation of the origin, nature and results of septic infections. Indeed, the Pasteur–Lister germ-theory had only one senior champion within surgery, and even he did not promote his principles that strongly after 1871. Thus, surgeons were left to mull over conflicting reports from laboratories and clinics. The absence of convincing and consistent microscopic demonstrations meant that germs remained 'theoretical', whereas chemicals seemed to have a physical reality. Lister's attempts to persuade surgeons to think about the body as analogous to a flask of pure organic fluid in a spontaneous generation experiment were unconvincing. Surgeons found no compelling reasons to believe that the body was only corruptible by external agencies; their experience and their understanding of sepsis told that such sepsis had many sources, including internal *de novo* origins. If anything, surgeons became less worried about exposing internal tissues and organs to the air as safer surgery, which was based on an inclusive mix of methods, gained ground. What they did worry about were arrogant Listerians who were so confident that they used narrowly based, 'exclusive' methods.

There were many technical obstacles to the adoption and diffusion of Listerism as a practice for controlling and killing germs. Unfortunately for Listerians, the spray – the best known and in the event least useful part of his system – was the physical embodiment of the most disputed elements of Pasteur–Lister germ-theory – panspermism and the external origins of sepsis. The integrity of Lister's system was also undermined by the fact that almost all of the numerous wound management techniques used by surgeons were, or could be, termed 'antiseptic'. Worse still, many of the procedures claimed by different schools were similar and were readily presented as alternative ways of achieving the same end – cleanliness. Those who advocated bacterial germ theories presented the aetiology of sepsis as one where exciting causes seemingly had complete supremacy over predisposing ones, or, as we might have put it – the 'seed' was everything. However, the idea that living tissue, the human soil, was germless and, indeed, resistant to the action of septic germs was an integral though largely unstated assumption amongst Listerians, though little appreciated outside.

Although a Listerian surgeon's practice may have been little different from that of the non-Listerian, his emerging ideology and professional orientation certainly was distinct. The non-Listerian surgeon saw the origin of sepsis as largely beyond his control, which meant that his role was to try to modify a preset pattern of morbid changes by helping the patient's body counter the internal spread of infective poisons.[144] Prior injuries, the peculiarities of the individual patient's constitution and a host of other contingent factors limited the surgeon's responsibilities. Against this, the ideal Listerian surgeon was proactive, less fatalistic and took upon himself greater obligations. With preinfected wounds, from injuries and prior disease, Listerians aimed to halt the effects of injurious germs and prevent further contamination; if they acted early and with precision, then most wounds were treatable. With wounds from elective operations, Listerians assumed that septic disease was avoidable and that any failures were the surgeon's responsibility.[145] Once Lister's special system was in place and maintained, then the body's vitality and inherent purity would restore health and order. It is at this level that we can see that Listerians did not construct germs as all-powerful agents. Septic germs were portrayed as relatively weak, unless the body was injured or unhealthy, a consideration that was to loom large in surgeons' wider accommodation with bacterial germ theories and new theories and practices in public health.

144 S. Messenger Bradley, *Lancet*, 1876, i: 768.
145 *Lancet*, 1875, ii: 744. An editorial talks of Listerism making the surgeon 'the custodian of the wound'. Holmes also acknowledged the value of the surgeon himself dressing wounds. Ibid., 628.

4

'Something Definite to Guide You in Your
Sanitary Precautions': Sanitary Science, Poisons
and *Contagium Viva*, 1866–1880

In public health medicine, germ theories of disease were not shaped
around a symbolic practice like antisepsis, nor did they have a high-profile
champion, like Joseph Lister. Also, while surgeons were able to concentrate on a single group of septic diseases, Medical Officers of Health (MOsH)
had to try and prevent a large number of zymotic diseases that had variable properties and posed distinct medical and social problems. Public health
authorities in Britain were mostly decentralised and not medically oriented,
a situation that gave MOsH considerable autonomy from government
and professional authority, though not necessarily from local political and
administrative forces. In these circumstances, it is not surprising to find
diverse policies and ideas in public health; indeed, there were a variety of
views and practices about almost every epidemic and zymotic disease. At
the national and international levels, attempts were made to develop
common policies, especially with politically important diseases, such as
cholera and smallpox. At the local level, and especially with local problems, MOsH often used their relative autonomy to pursue their own
projects, based on their own experience and ideas. Through the publications
of the Medical Department, Simon tried to lead opinion, and from the
early 1870s key writers and researchers attracted followers, notably Edmund
Parkes, William Budd, Max von Pettenkofer, Alfred Carpenter, Edward
Klein, and, in India, Timothy Lewis and D. D. Cunningham. However,
the social pressures that came from epidemic crises, and the uncertainties
around the best methods of prevention and control, meant that there was no
lack of interest in new theories of disease and methods of prevention. Indeed,
the audience for new ideas and practices in public health was not only
medical, as officials and lay people on boards of health had an interest and
say in policy.
   The development and spread of germ theories in public health medicine in Britain has been understood to have been at best uneven, and
certainly slower than in France and Germany. One of the most influential
historical discussions, by Lloyd Stevenson, argued that there was a strong

antipathy to bacteriology and laboratory medicine in British public
health.[1] Stevenson termed this position the 'Sanitarian Syndrome', as it was
based on a continuing commitment to the 1840s Chadwickian programme
of removing filth, promoting cleanliness and playing down the value of
medical intervention.[2] Stevenson built up his symptomatology from the
writings of three medically trained sanitarians: Benjamin Ward Richardson
(1828–96), George Wilson (1848–1921) and William Collins (1859–1946);
however, he left open any periodisation and just how representative the syndrome was of the beliefs of MOsH and the profession overall.[3] In this chapter
I show that antipathy to medical science was not a major facet of public
health medicine before 1880; discussion up to then was of germ theories,
not bacteriology, and laboratory medicine was a resource in debates about
zymotic diseases, but its practitioners lacked clear authority. Nonetheless, I
suggest that by the end of the 1870s the proponents of germ ideas had already
begun indirectly to reshape sanitary science, technology and policy. Thus, I
place the incorporation of living germ theories and practices into public
health at an earlier date than suggested in many recent studies, which have
emphasised the 1880s and 1890s, the coming of bacteriology and the use
of laboratory science by MOsH to improve their professional standing.[4] I
do not say that the views of germ theorists were dominant by 1880, only
that they had changed the terms of debate on prevention with a number
of important diseases. This supports my overall point about the spread of
germ ideas and practices in medicine being additive and adaptive, rather
than a series of conflicts between competing, incommensurable paradigms.
There were two key issues in public health in the late 1860s and 1870s,
around which the meanings of germ theories of disease were debated. The
first was their value for understanding the sources of epidemics, especially
the vexed question of their *de novo* or spontaneous origins; the second was
their value in understanding how to prevent the spread of zymotic diseases
once they were established in an area or community. The practical question
was what balance to make of 'inclusive' measures, mainly environmental

1 L. G. Stevenson, 'Science Down the Drain: On the Hostility of Certain Sanitarians to Animal
  Experimentation, Bacteriology and Immunology', *BHM*, 1955, 29: 1–26.
2 C. E. Rosenberg, 'Florence Nightingale on Contagion: The Hospital as a Moral Universe', in
  C. E. Rosenberg, ed., *Healing and History, Essays for George Rosen*, New York, Science History
  Publications, 1979, 116–36.
3 A. S. MacNulty, *A Biography of Sir Benjamin Ward Richardson*, London, Harvey and Blythe, 1950;
  Also, *DNB*, Suppl. 3, 1901, 297; *BMJ*, 1896, ii: 1612; *Lancet*, 1896, ii: 1575. On George Wilson, see
  Obituary notices, *BMJ*, 1921, ii: 675, and *Lancet*, 1921, ii: 877.
4 D. Porter, 'Stratification and its Discontents: Professionalisation and Conflict in the British Public
  Health service, 1848–1944', in E. Fee and R. Acheson, eds., *A History of Education in Public Health:
  Health that Mocks the Doctors' Rules*, Oxford, Oxford Medical Publication, 1991, 83–113. Also see:
  J. Raymond, 'Science in the Service of Medicine: Germ Theory, Bacteriology and English Public
  Health, 1860–1914', Paper presented to the *BSHS-HSS Conference on Science in Modern Medicine*,
  Manchester, April 1985.

improvements, and 'exclusive' measures that aimed to stop disease-agents spreading to and from people.[5]

This chapter begins with an account of the ideas and institutions of public health medicine in the 1860s, especially the character of sanitary science. The main body of the chapter is devoted to discussions of three of the most important diseases facing public health workers in this period: cholera, small-pox and typhoid (or enteric) fever. These diseases cover the spectrum of public health diseases, from the highly contagious (smallpox) through to the misasmatic (cholera). Typhoid fever occupied an intermediate and by no means fixed place on the contagious to noncontagious spectrum. Typhoid fever was a local problem, whereas epidemics of smallpox and cholera were national, even imperial, matters. I explore the changing understanding of each disease amongst sanitarians and MOsH, together with how the emergent germ aetiologies and pathologies were formed and used practically and rhetorically. Most historians agree that the aims and programme of public health professionals narrowed over the period 1865–1900, from 'inclusive' to 'exclusive' programmes. I suggest that the deployment of living germ theo-ries was a major factor in shaping and legitimating this change, and that this influence was important before 1880 and the arrival of bacteriology.

PUBLIC HEALTH MEDICINE

The organisation of public health changed markedly in the early 1870s. Following on from the Royal Sanitary Commission, 1866, new Public Health Acts were passed in 1872 and 1875. In central government, the Medical Department was moved from the Privy Council, where it enjoyed a degree of autonomy, to the more political Local Government Board, precipitating John Simon's resignation. Locally, the Acts required the appointment of MOsH in the newly created sanitary districts, leading to a rise in the number of posts in England and Wales, from 50 in 1870 to 825 by 1876.[6] Special post-graduate diploma courses in state medicine were inaugurated in 1870, although the qualification did not become mandatory for new appointments until 1892.[7] At the same time, the state medicine or hygiene component in ordinary medical training improved, with experienced MOsH appointed to part-time teaching posts in medical schools and universities. This growing sphere of medical work was reflected in the mainstream journals, in new spe-cialist publications, such as *Public Health* (1873) and the *Sanitary Record* (1873), and burgeoning editions of textbooks.

5 M. Pelling, *Cholera, Fever and English Medicine, 1835–65*, Oxford, Oxford University Press, 1978, 203 *et seq.*
6 On legislation in this period, see: J. Simon, *English Sanitary Institutions*, London, Cassell and Co., 1890; W. M. Frazer, *A History of English Public Health, 1834–39*, London, Baillière, Tindall and Cox, 1950, 77–146.
7 Porter, 'Stratification', 98–105.

The knowledge base that informed public health medicine was codified in 'sanitary science'. This was a synthetic subject that embraced statistics, law, engineering, chemistry, meteorology and geology, as well as medicine. In 1885, Edward Ballard (1820–97), a former MOH for Islington who was by this time a senior inspector at the Medical Department, described it as a product of 'the English Mind', being empirical and synthetic. Of course, it was not unique to England nor Britain; similar programmes were developed in continental Europe and North America.[8] Latour's description of the French sanitary science nicely captures its character – 'an accumulation of advice, precautions, recipes, opinions, statistics, remedies, regulations, anecdotes, case studies'.[9] Sanitary science was seen to be both very ancient and very modern.[10] Hippocrates' *Airs, Waters and Places* was usually cited as its foundation, and many of the textbooks, such as Edmund Parkes's influential *Manual*, first published in 1864, paid direct homage in their structure.[11] Parkes was Professor of Hygiene at the Army Medical School and a former Indian medical officer; his book reflected this background, but was a popular textbook for civil MOsH as well. All editions of the *Manual* through to the 1890s, under various editors, had successive sections on air (including meteorology, ventilation and pollution), water (plus beverages and food) and places (soil and habitations). The subject's claims to be a 'science' rested on appeals to experience, classifications and natural law, rather than on theories and experimental investigations.[12] The essence of sanitary science was to remove '. . . bad water, bad air, defective drainage, overcrowding, dirty and irregular habits' – the conditions that produced high mortality levels.[13]

The cornerstone of sanitary science was epidemiology. If patterns of disease and even individual cases could be located in geographical space, social structure and historical time, then antecedents and possibly causes could be found and preventive measures instituted.[14] The following summaries, from two local investigations published in the Report to the Medical Department for 1872, illustrate the characteristic concerns of local MOsH. For each place the reasons for the inspection, the name of the inspector and his reasons for high mortality are given:

8 A. S. Wohl, *Endangered Lives: Public Health in Victorian Britain*, London, J. M. Dent and Sons, 1983, 142.

9 B. Latour, *The Pasteurization of France*, Cambridge, MA, Harvard University Press, 1988, 20.

10 R. Rawlinson, 'Old Lessons in Sanitary Science Revived, and New Lessons Considered', *TSI*, 1880–1, 2: 127–8.

11 E. Parkes, *A Manual of Hygiene*, London, Churchill, 1864. On the origins of Parkes's *Manual*, see: D. E. Watkins, 'Explanations of Disease and the Technology of Hygiene in Parkes' *Manual*, 1864–1873', *BSHS-HSS Conference*, 5–10.

12 J. V. Pickstone, 'Ways of Knowing: Towards a Historical Sociology of Science', *BJHS*, 1993, 26: 433–58.

13 *BFM-CR*, 1867, 40: 65.

14 C. Hamlin, *A Science of Impurity: Water Analysis in Nineteenth Century England*, Bristol, Adam Hilger, 1990, 99–116, 220–4.

ABBEY HULTON, STAFFORDSHIRE. – Registrar-General's Return: high mortality, especially amongst infants from various zymotic diseases. *Dr Ballard.* Want of proper drainage. Dilapidated and overcrowded cottages, . . . filthy privies, and overloaded ash-pits.

ABINGDON, BERKSHIRE. – Registrar-General Return: fever and diarrhoea. *Dr Thorne Thorne.* Water supply mostly from surface well in porous soil, soaked with excremental and other filth. Defective sewerage. Sub-soil in part water-logged. Many nuisances from water closets and privies. No proper removal of excrement. Poor housed in dwellings unfit for habitation. Trade nuisances. Spread of infectious disease favoured by manufacture of clothing in infected houses.[15]

Each report presented a catalogue of 'defects' and 'nuisances', with the implication that these combined to produce the conditions in which diseases could arise and spread. The unwillingness of inspectors to rank the importance of various factors, or to point to critical conjunctures of conditions, was taken to mean that all had to be tackled. In one sense, the reports were political documents, intended to shame local authorities and galvanise action by cataloguing failings. The complexity of the assumed causes should certainly not be read as showing aetiological uncertainties; rather, they show the fundamental assumption that epidemic and zymotic diseases had multifactorial origins and required 'inclusive' preventive approaches.

Preventable diseases, be they miasmatic, infectious, contagious, epidemic, occupational or nutritional, were all assumed to have external exciting causes, which always operated in conjunction with many other predisposing and proximate conditions. E. A. Parkes observed that the creed of the 'School of Sanitarians' was that 'every disease . . . has its antecedents and that the problem we have to solve is to reach this antecedent and prevent the seed from bearing its fruit'.[16] MOsH often contrasted zymotic diseases with the constitutional and idiopathic afflictions dealt with by clinicians, which were nonpreventable because their origins were internal and spontaneous. This division is part of the explanation why the single largest cause of death at this time, tuberculosis (consumption or phthisis) – an inherited, constitutional condition – was not a public health disease.[17] The work of MOsH meant that they were more interested in aetiology than most other medical practitioners, and hence around 1870 they could not ignore the claims made for living germs as external, exciting causes of disease. It should not be forgotten that, as well as 'filth diseases', MOsH were usually responsible for the control of highly contagious diseases, such as smallpox. Indeed, infant vaccination against smallpox first became compulsory in 1853, during Chadwick's time at the General Board.

15 'Abstract of Inquiries Made by Medical Inspectors of the LGB during 1872', *Public Health*, 1873, I: 145.
16 *BMJ*, 1873, ii: 145. C. Hamlin, 'Predisposing Causes and Public Health in Early Nineteenth Century Medical Thought', *SHM*, 1992, 5: 43–70.
17 Another factor was that phthisis was not epidemic, causing mortality crises and political problems. In the reports of the Registrar General, it was recorded with cancer as a 'Constitutional Disease'.

Yet, dirt and filth remained the great enemies of public health; they provided both of the conditions in which disease poisons tended to arise and spread most vigorously. Murchison's ideas were the baseline; thus doctors and lay people in public health thought mainly in terms of chemical agents spread by passive diffusion in the air. With cholera and other diseases, new disease agents and types of communication were being promoted by MOsH and scientists, most of which were linked to living germ theories of disease.

CHOLERA, 1866–1880

For sanitarians, cholera had been the model miasmatic disease. Originating in India, its poison had spread several times to Europe since the 1830s, being either a gaseous poison travelling on air currents or an immaterial influence that, when settling in particular areas, induced decaying vegetable matter in the soil to elaborate poisonous 'cholera-stuff'.[18] Whatever its origins, cholera had been shown to spread and to kill in conditions of filth and overcrowding, and had proved near impossible to contain with quarantines. When epidemics threatened Britain in the 1840s and 1850s, preventive measures had focused on reducing the 'receptivity' of the country through nuisance removal, cleansing and other environmental improvements.[19] From the mid-1850s there was a movement of opinion towards cholera being spread, at least in part, via water contaminated with human wastes.[20] In July 1865, the General Memorandum advising local authorities on how to prevent cholera, issued by Simon's Medical Department, reflected this change in two new recommendations. The first was the need for 'special precautions of cleanliness and disinfection . . . with regard to infective discharges from the bodies of the sick', and the second was that all water supplies should be examined so that 'no foul water be drunk'.[21] It should not be concluded from this that Simon had fully accepted John Snow's explanation of cholera transmission; his advice merely pointed to the faecal–oral route and water-carriage as one amongst many means of communication to be targeted.[22]

Somewhat surprisingly, the epidemic saw no major state-sponsored investigation into the pathology of the disease on the model of the 1855 Committee of Scientific Enquiry, or the recent, much lauded, research of the Cattle Plague Commission. Sanderson and Thudichum, respectively, investigated cholera's communicability and chemistry, under the auspices of the newly

---

18 C. E. Rosenberg, *The Cholera Years: The United States in 1832, 1849 and 1866*, Chicago, IL, Chicago University Press, 1962.
19 M. Sigsworth, *Cholera in the East and West Ridings of Yorkshire, 1848–1893*, Unpublished PhD Thesis, CNAA, 1991.
20 Pelling, *Cholera, Fever*, 203–49.
21 J. Simon, 'Proceedings Against Cholera under the Disease Prevention Acts and Otherwise', *Ninth Annual Report of the Medical Officer of the Privy Council for 1866*, BPP, 1867, [3949], xxxvii, 1.
22 W. Luckin, 'The Final Catastrophe: Cholera in London, 1866', *MH*, 1977, 21: 32–42.

inaugurated Auxiliary Scientific Investigations sponsored by the Medical Department.[23] However, they found little of interest or use, and once the epidemic waned the investigators moved on to new topics.[24] The main interests of public health officials remained epidemiological but, as the two official retrospective reports on the epidemic show, there was growing interest in the intimate nature of 'cholera-stuff'.[25]

In his review for the Registrar-General, William Farr might have been expected to offer an epidemiological commentary, but on this, as on many other occasions, he was not backward in expressing medical opinions.[26] His report began from the presumption that the 1855 Enquiry had established the zymotic nature of cholera and, with a confidence that few MOsH shared, he stated that water was the main medium by which the disease spread.[27] He also departed from convention with his observation that zymosis was 'more striking' than ever, since Pasteur had shown that the 'zymes' had the power of reproducing themselves in successive generations, 'growing and decaying by laws like the higher forms of life'.[28] Farr was prepared to accept that 'cholera zymes' might be a fungus, Hassall's 'vibriones', Pacini's 'vibrional molecules' or the germs of Pettenkofer's soil contamination theory.[29] Yet he had not totally abandoned the idea that 'zymes' were chemicals, or that they were on the boundary of life and nonlife. In his epidemiological analysis, Farr explored three explanations of cholera's diffusion: mathematical models; air, water and contact theories; and spontaneous generation. With the latter two accounts he indulged in pathological speculation. For example, he wondered if the zyme in faecal discharges derived from 'epithelium shed from intestinal villi' or was a 'flux of the mucus membrane' of the gut; in other words, he fashioned 'cholera-stuff' as Beale's bioplasm-germs.[30] With spontaneous generation, Farr wrote of two possibilities: either that 'cholera-stuff' was derived from inorganic matter, or that benign zymes became pathogenic in certain environmental conditions. While he remained noncommittal on the exact nature of 'cholera-stuff', Farr mostly constituted it as plantlike, imaging that the 'germs of disease are as profusely expended by nature as seeds of plants'.[31] What is interesting about this statement is not only the use of the

23 J. L. Brand, *Doctors and the State: The British Medical Profession and Government Action in Public Health, 1870–1912*, Baltimore, MD, Johns Hopkins University Press, 1965, 73–5.
24 *Ninth Annual Report*, Appendices 9 and 10.
25 *BFM-CR*, 1867, 40: 1–40.
26 Pelling, *Cholera, Fever*, 81–112, and J. M. Eyler, *Victorian Social Medicine: The Ideas and Methods of William Farr*, Baltimore, MD, Johns Hopkins University Press, 1979.
27 *Report of the Cholera Epidemic in England, 1866: Supplement to the Twenty Ninth Annual Report of the Registrar-General of Births, Deaths and Marriages in England*, BPP, 1867–68, [4072], xxxvii, xi.
28 Ibid., lxvi.
29 N. Howard-Jones, 'Choleranomalies: The Unhistory of Medicine as Illustrated by Cholera', *Perspectives on Biology and Medicine*, 1972, 15: 422–33.
30 L. S. Beale, *MTG*, 1866; Cf. 'Recent Work on Cholera', *DQJMS*, 1871, 51: 178–9.
31 Farr, *Cholera*, xv.

term 'germs of disease', but its parallels with panspermic theories of sepsis and the link made to fungus theories. Farr was taken with the possible correspondence with the dry rot fungus, which was said to be a constant presence in buildings, but only grew in certain conditions. He went on to consider objections based on the supposed ubiquity of disease-germs. If cholera-stuff was well diffused, even panspermic, then why were cases of cholera unevenly distributed geographically and socially? His answers were that: (i) the activity of 'cholera-stuff' varied from day to day; (ii) its diffusion was uneven; (iii) individuals varied in their susceptibility to its effects; and (iv) the use of remedies was unequal. Thus, Farr's version of zymotic theory was sophisticated, medically sensitive, contingent contagionist and a very long way from any simple 'filth' theory. The same complexity can be found in Parkes's influential writings on cholera. Hence it is no surprise that few public health doctors were impressed by simple germ theories of diseases that rested merely on contamination and ignored contingencies in the environment and within the human body.

John Simon's report on the 1866 cholera epidemic appeared in the Annual Report of the Medical Department in 1867; however, he seems to have found the views he heard at the International Medical Congress in Weimar in 1866 more revealing than anything he learned from the epidemic itself.[32] It is worth noting that the 1866 epidemic in Britain was localised and produced fewer deaths than any previous visitation, which allowed the experience to be packaged as a great success for sanitary science and state medicine.[33] Simon was eclectic in what he reported from Weimar, but chose to emphasise: Pettenkofer's ground water theory, the mixed results of disinfection and the renewed interest in the cholera-fungus, on which the German botanist, Ernst Hallier, had recently published.[34] Simon observed that the discovery of some fungal-like agent 'would not be a surprise to pathologists', but added that such 'doctrine may be absolutely sterile of results':

Whatever may be the explanation . . . at least empirically we know that . . . the pestilence rages only where there are definite sanitary evils. This knowledge remains unchanged; and unchanged remain also our practical means of applying it. . . . Excrement-sodden earth, excrement-reeking air, excrement tainted water, these are for us the causes of cholera.[35]

This statement shows his continuing commitment to the mainstream sanitary concerns of removing the conditions in which epidemics were 'set up and propagated'. How this environmental perspective influenced his thinking is shown by the fact that, even if a cholera-fungus germ were to be found, he anticipated no changes in policy and no role for laboratory methods in

---

32 J. Simon, 'Postscript, with Particular Reference to the Cholera-Conference Recently Held at Weimar', *Ninth Annual Report*, 29–34.
33 Luckin, 'Final Catastrophe', *passim*.   34 *Lancet*, 1867, i. 266–7.   35 Simon, 'Postscript', 33.

prevention. Using microscopy to find cholera-germs in the environment would be like looking for a needle in a haystack, while examining faecal discharges was an absurdity:

Nowhere out of Laputa could there be serious thought of differentiating excremental performances into groups of diarrhoeal and healthy, or of using the highest powers of the microscope to identify the cylindro-taenium for extermination. It is excrement, indiscriminately, which must be kept from fouling us with its decay.[36]

If new facts and theories were irrelevant to preventive practice, why bother with investigations and speculation? Of course, new ideas were relevant and useful. The writings of Farr and Snow show the acceptance of water carriage over airborne transmission and, at a deeper level, the contest between those who believed in *de novo* origins and the passive diffusion of poisons, as against those who felt able to specify direct and indirect person-to-person channels of transmission.[37]

Cholera threatened Britain again in 1872. In this wave, there were very few deaths and no epidemic crisis. However, the disease remained a problem for the British government through its imperial responsibilities, especially in India, the home of the disease, where the idea that it was a 'disease of locality' continued to dominate. After the 1866 epidemic, Parkes proposed an army medical service enquiry into the aetiology of cholera.[38] He supported the faecal contamination and water-carriage theories, and was interested in how these might be linked to Hallier's new fungus theory.[39] In the summer of 1868, he recruited two promising Army Medical Service officers, D. D. Cunningham and Timothy Lewis, to pursue investigations. By way of preparation, they were sent to Germany to meet with Hallier, and visited Anton de Bary and Max von Pettenkofer. The meeting with the latter seems to have been particularly formative, as both men championed Pettenkofer's theories in India and Britain for many years. Cunningham and Lewis began work in India in 1869, and the first fruits of their labours were published in 1870.[40] They failed to find Hallier's fungus, but their experience of the disease in its homeland pointed them towards an agent that had the properties of Pettenkofer's as yet unidentified germ. They maintained this view throughout the 1870s, despite their inability to identify the agent. The results of their work and ideas for the understanding of the aetiology of cholera were paradoxical. On the one hand, they maintained the search for the germ of cholera

36 Ibid.   37 *DQJMS*, 1870, 49: 413
38 J. D. Isaacs, 'D. D. Cunningham and the Aetiology of Cholera in British India, 1869–1897', *MH*, 1998, 42: 279–305. M. Harrison, *Public Health in British India: Anglo-Indian Preventive Medicine, 1859–1914*, Cambridge, Cambridge University Press, 1994, 51–4, 99–116.
39 E. A. Parkes, *A Manual of Practical Hygiene*, London, Churchill, 1869, 480–2.
40 T. R. Lewis and D. D. Cunningham, *A Report of Microscopical and Physiological Researches into the Nature of the Agent or Agents of Cholera*, Calcutta, Office of the Superintendent of Government Printing, 1872. They acknowledged the help of Beale, Sanderson and Bastian.

of the Pettenkofer-type and became integral members of the emerging British germ-research community. On the other hand, their work supported the localist ideas that were dominant in Anglo-Indian public health, and which ran contrary to the water-carriage theory favoured by metropolitan authorities. This situation is a valuable warning against any portrayal of John Snow as a proto-germ theorist and reinforces the point that it was exactly their commitment to Pettenkofer that made Cunningham and Lewis influential germ theorists. Indeed, the majority of rank-and-file MOsH seem to have accepted water carriage for cholera, without necessarily abandoning aerial transmission.[41] At the same time, Pettenkofer's 'seasonal and topical' views were welcomed to the extent that they reinforced calls for 'inclusive' hygienic precautions, but were questioned for dismissing water carriage. In 1882, Pettenkofer was quoted as saying about cholera: 'I have never found myself in opposition to the parasitic theory; I have striven solely and always against the theory of simple contagion, which in my opinion is erroneous'.[42] As we will see in Chapter 7, when cholera first threatened in the 1880s, preventive agencies soon ceased to prioritise 'inclusive' general clean ups; instead they focused on water supplies and also considered cholera as an imported disease, to be controlled at ports by inspections that identified disease-carrying individuals.

SMALLPOX, 1865–1880

Smallpox was not on the sanitary agenda of filth diseases. However, MOsH were convinced that it was transmitted more easily in conditions of filth and that sanitary reform would indirectly lower its incidence.[43] Preventive policies were dominated by vaccinations, which was the national responsibility of the Medical Department, while locally it was the Boards of Poor Law Guardians, not MOsH and local Boards of Health, that hired public vaccinators and were responsible for ensuring compliance with the legislation.[44] Vaccination involved rubbing lymph into deep but narrow wounds made on the upper arm with a point.[45] In the 1860s, vaccinators normally used the

---

41 A. Hardy, 'Cholera, Quarantine and the English Preventive System, 1850–1895', *MH*, 1993, 37: 252–69.

42 Quoted in: F. de Chaumont, 'Pettenkofer's Views on the Parasitic Theory of the Causation of Cholera', *SRec*, 1881–2, 2: 247.

43 Most general histories of public health have followed the Chadwickian, environmental agenda and focused on diseases produced by filth and miasmatic conditions and have not foregrounded the fight against smallpox. Historians who have discussed smallpox have tended to do so in the context of the politics of compulsion in state medicine, not as a sanitary measure. See: D. Porter and R. Porter, 'The Politics of Prevention: Anti-vaccinationist and Public Health in Nineteenth Century England', *MH*, 1988, 32: 231–52.

44 R. Lambert, 'A Victorian National Health Service: State Vaccination, 1858–71', *Historical Journal*, 1962, 5: 1–18.

45 The lymph used in vaccination was produced at the National Vaccine Establishment (NVE), which had come under the control of the Medical Department in 1860. More precisely, the arm-to-

arm-to-arm method, taking lymph from pustules on the arms of previously inoculated children, but this method was beginning to give way to the use of lymph taken directly from calves with mild cowpox. The practice, empirically derived by Edward Jenner, was assumed to work by giving people a small amount of lymph containing cowpox poison (vaccinia) to produce a mild infection. It was common experience that one infection with a pox disease gave the sufferer lifetime protection from infection, but Jenner's innovation was based on the further insight that some pox diseases were so similar that they gave cross-immunity. Thus, cowpox was thought to be so closely related to smallpox (variola) that anyone who had suffered even a mild infection would be unable subsequently to develop smallpox.

The new Vaccination Act of 1867 sought to improve several aspects of the preventive system: the quality of vaccine lymph, the training of vaccinators and the effectiveness of the compulsory clauses that required all children under fourteen years to be vaccinated. MOsH strongly supported compulsory vaccinations as an effective preventive measure; its value seemed obvious, as during epidemics mortality amongst people vaccinated was at least four times lower than those unvaccinated.[46] However, vaccination was resisted locally by individuals and in certain towns by Boards of Guardians. The public feared catching the disease itself, being infected with syphilis or septic matter, and the scarring of young children. The scale and intensity of public hostility was evident in the national campaigns of the Anti-Compulsory Vaccination League, founded in 1867, and in subsequent passive resistance.[47] The high death rate in epidemics and severe pock-marking of the skin meant that smallpox had been much feared, though popular fears were waning as anti-vaccination sentiment was fuelled by the experience that epidemics had become less frequent, that more areas escaped their ravages each time and that perhaps the variola poison has lost some virulence.

Most medical texts described smallpox as a contagious disease spread by a 'virus'. The term derived from the Latin word for poison, and it was widely assumed that it was a chemical agent that acted in the blood and hence spread its effects to all tissues.[48] The aetiology of smallpox was well defined:

arm method required taking lymph from the vesicles on a child that had been vaccinated eight days earlier. This was collected on a lancet from the 'best', that is, largest, eruptions in the group. The fresh lymph was then rubbed in fresh wounds on the arms of other children, produced by scoring with a pointed instrument, often a lancet. Normally eight or ten further vaccinations could be made from a previously vaccinated child. It was believed that the lymph was altered, and perhaps weakened, by successive transmissions; hence when vesicle formation became poor, fresh lymph was sought from the NVE.

46 *BMJ*, 1872, i: 171. The typical rates were 14.9 percent mortality amongst the vaccinated and 66.2 percent in the unvaccinated.

47 R. MacLeod, 'Law, Medicine and Public Opinion: The Resistance to Compulsory Health Legislation, 1870–1907', *Public Law*, 1967, 106–28, 188–211.

48 S. Hughes, *The Virus: A History of a Concept*, New York: Science History, 1977.

transmission occurred by direct person-to-person contact, by transfer at close quarters or by contact with clothes and goods (fomites), carrying exanthemata from pustules. Unlike other zymotic diseases, there appeared to be few contingencies moderating its diffusion or effects. The specificity and power of the virus were experienced in its consistent pathogenesis: a period between infection and symptoms developing, the onset of which were signalled by the eruption of pustules in the skin, high fever and the seeming decay of the whole body. During the period of incubation it was assumed that the poison was 'elaborated' in the body, which produced internal 'disturbances' to normal structures and functions that people, literally, observed decayed and poisonous matter being thrown from the skin and in the breath. As Pelling has shown, the 'smallpox-analogy' – a standard for contagion – had been used by Budd and others to model the contagiousness of other zymotic diseases, but with only mixed success.[49] The problem was that while it was widely accepted that zymotic diseases could be contagious, none was as catching as smallpox, nor were they only spread by direct contagion. Attempts to identify and isolate the poison of smallpox and cowpox, either chemically or microscopically, had not closed around any method of preparation nor any agent, though it was a subject of new laboratory research in the late 1860s.[50]

The Sanitary Act of 1866 provided strong powers for the control of diseases at the contagious end of the spectrum, authorising local authorities to provide isolation for sufferers, either at home or in hospital, if they constituted a public 'nuisance'.[51] Hardy has suggested that a major impetus to the extension of institutional isolation was Sir James Simpson's claim in 1868 that smallpox could be 'stamped out'. With a direct acknowledgement to the lessons of the cattle plague in 1866, he proposed 'controlling the movement' of smallpox sufferers by isolating them in hospitals. He claimed that if sufferers were detained long enough, the smallpox virus would be 'poleaxed' naturally as, unable to find new bodies in which to develop and propagate, it would burn itself out.[52] Simpson was using another common metaphor for the action of zymes and living germs, namely, that they were like sparks that ignited changes in the body. In turn, the body had to be in an inflammable condition, and the way fire spread in different conditions had parallels with

49 Pelling, *Cholera, Fever*, 250–95.   50 W. B. Woodman, 'Smallpox', *LMR*, 1873, 1: 55–6.

51 E. Chadwick, 'Discussion: The Management of Cases of Small-pox and other Infectious Diseases', *TSI*, 1881–82, 3: 53–4.

52 J. Y. Simpson, 'A Proposal to Stamp Out Smallpox', *MTG*, 1868, i: 5–6, 32–3, 264, 537. For a discussion of policies to control smallpox in London, see: A. Hardy, 'Smallpox in London: Factors in the Decline of the Disease in the Nineteenth Century', *MH*, 1983, 27: 111–38. The previous objection to fever hospitals or even wards, largely articulated by anticontagionist sanitarians, was that they created a concentration of poison that was harmful to patients and staff, and could act as a foci for the dissemination of poison to the local community. See: C. Murchison, 'On the Isolation of Infectious Diseases', *MTG*, 1864, i: 210.

the varying delays, and development patterns of zymotics diseases, with their characteristic 'fevers' and 'inflammations'. Preventive measures based on people and their products were termed 'exclusive', because their advocates heretically wanted to drop some of the wider improvements that had been the mainstays of sanitary policy since the 1840s. Of course, it was easier to defend 'inclusive' policies, as in theory nothing was being left out, and it was useful to label other policies 'exclusive' to emphasise that they were not comprehensive. Very often in medicine, it was and is better not to be wrong than to risk being right.

Isolation and other 'exclusive' measures were not used extensively with smallpox until the epidemic of 1871–73, and even then vaccination remained the first line of prevention. Isolation was seen as the best response to controlling the epidemic once it was established, but public health officials hoped that this would remain a secondary line of defence. Hence, local authorities were reluctant to construct permanent isolation and fever hospitals, except in London, where the economies of scale possible through the Metropolitan Asylum Board (MAB), plus fears about the vulnerability of a port-city and migration centre to imported disease, provided the political will to invest in permanent structures in the late 1860s.

Most medical writing on vaccination in the 1860s and early 1870s concentrated on the statistics that showed its value.[53] There was surprisingly little interest in what happened when a person was vaccinated. One of the few discussions of the pathology of vaccinia was by Edward Ballard, in a long essay that won the Ladies Sanitary Association book prize in 1868. Ballard wrote mostly about the technique of inoculation and its results, with only brief speculation on the relations between smallpox and cowpox. He began on familiar ground, saying that the varioloid (pox) diseases were so closely related that they could develop in modified form in related species or take on species-specific characteristics in different bodies. If he leaned towards any theory of the nature of the virus, it was that it had 'life' and the property of 'generation', as the following account of the effects of smallpox in a cow suggests:

That when the virus, 'germinal matter', 'contagion' of smallpox is inserted into the skin of a cow, it finds there material capable, indeed, of maintaining its life and permitting its generation, but only in modified manner – so to speak in a degraded manner.[54]

Ballard argued that vaccinia-induced immunity was due to the cowpox virus using up enough of some essential pabulum (food material), so that any pox

53 For example, see: E. C. Seaton, *A Handbook of Vaccination*, London, Macmillan, 1868. There was, however, considerable interest in the history of vaccine lymph and the relationship between smallpox, cowpox and horsepox.
54 E. Ballard, *On Vaccination: Its Value and Alleged Dangers*, London, Longmans, Green and Co, 1868, 33.

virus that subsequently entered the body would not find the nutrients necessary for development. A vaccinated person would be unable, therefore, to
'take' the disease.[55] When models of immunity began to be fashioned in the
1880s, this was termed the 'exhaustion' or depletion' theory. Ballard also wrote
in a more holistic vein of vaccination making an 'impression on the constitution', and that it altered the 'proclivity of the system'. He identified three
analogies that were currently being used to explain the behaviour of the
virus: the way that yeast plants used up sugar in malt (zymosis-fermentation);
the development of parasitic entozoa; and Beale's ideas on the 'germinal
matter' of disease developing from degraded normal cells. However, Ballard
expressed no preference for any model and was wary of committing himself
to any living-virus model, but it is interesting that all of the entities he discussed had the properties of life forms. Nonetheless, the dominant chemical
zymotic model still had as much to recommend it for vaccinia; for example,
there was a dose-effect with vaccination that made the quality of lymph and
the depth and number of inoculations so critical. Moreover, the fact that
lymph could be dried and then reactivated by moisture pointed to a chemical rather than a living entity.

Experimental work by Chauveau, also in 1868, at the Lyons Veterinary
College in France had suggested that the smallpox virus was an 'organic
particle' – either a very large chemical molecule or a very small organism.[56]
Under the microscope he had found that vaccine lymph consisted of: (i) a
clear transparent fluid; (ii) leukocytes; and (iii) 'elementary granules, or minute
particles'. This led him to ask whether the virus was in the transparent lymph
or the minute particles. Microscopy could not supply the answer, though he
hoped that laboratory experiments would. He used dilution methods to
obtain particle-free lymph, which he then inoculated into susceptible animals,
finding that it did not produce disease. He concluded, by the logic of elimination rather than positive demonstration, that the 'organic particles' were
the exciting agent. This line of inquiry was taken up by Sanderson in investigations for the Medical Department in 1868.[57] He too found organic particles in vaccine lymph, referring to them as 'microzymes'. Like Chauveau,
he too was unable to demonstrate conclusively that they were the exciting
agent, though he believed that they were the most likely candidates. However,
in his 1870 Report, Simon used Sanderson's work to challenge Beale's germ-

---

55 The explanation is somewhat more complicated because it has to explain the local effects at the
 site of vaccination where vesicles were produced and how these translated into systematic protection in the blood and body as a whole. See J. J. Reynolds, *System of Medicine*, London, R. Caly
 and Sons, 1869.
56 *Lancet*, 1868, i: 626.
57 J. B. Sanderson, 'The Intimate Pathology of Contagion', *Twelfth Annual Report of the Medical Officer
 of the Privy Council for 1869*, BPP 1870, [C.208], xxxviii, 58–9, 229–56; idem., 'Further Report',
 Thirteenth Annual Report of the Medical Officer of the Privy Council for 1870, BPP 1871, [C.349],
 xxxi, 48.

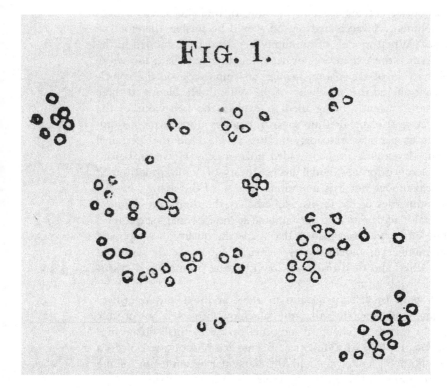

Figure 8. A drawing of the particulate matter that John Burdon Sanderson observed in vaccine lymph in his investigations for the Medical Department in 1869–70. J. B. Sanderson, 'The Intimate Pathology of Contagion', *Twelfth Annual Report of the Medical Officer of the Privy Council for 1869*, BPP, 1870, [C.208], xxxviii, 232

theory. He wrote that Sanderson had shown that the smallpox-particles were not products of the animal body, but self-multiplying organic forms of the lowest vegetable kind, in line with the ideas of Pasteur (see Figure 8). Although there was no specific agent, no causal demonstration nor any standards for establishing aetiological proofs, one reviewer still concluded that the variolae fevers 'alone, of all contagious diseases, have yielded up their germ to microscopical research'.[58]

58 *BFM-CR*, 1874, 54, 295. C. O'Rourke, 'Tyndall's Contribution to Biology and Medicine', in W. H. Brock et al., eds., *John Tyndall: Essays on a Natural Philosopher*, Dublin, Royal Dublin Society, 1981, 103–12.

Studies of both smallpox and cholera had demonstrated problems with microscopy.[59] With smallpox, all that Sanderson could show those who visited his laboratory was opaque lymph or colourless tiny globules. The illustrations that accompanied the reports of this work presented tiny circles, suggesting that the smallpox virus had no definable structure and might be merely chemical globules, implying that the limits of microscopy had been met.[60] However, in their search for the cholera-germ in India, Lewis and Cunningham had the opposite experience. They found such an abundant fauna and flora that it seemed impossible to single out any organism as a specific causative agent. Indeed, the number of microphytes present in the gut seemed to tell against the very idea that living organisms were the causes of disease; otherwise, how could the healthy body tolerate such abundant internal wildlife? Disappointed by microscopy, Sanderson turned to physical methods, such as filtration, and to chemical methods to try to learn more about the behaviour and properties of disease-poisons. Hamlin has shown that this same disenchantment with microscopy was also present in water analysis, where it was little used between the 1850s and late 1870s.[61] In this context, Tyndall's faith in light beam experiments and his assumptions about the limits of microscopy in the spontaneous generation controversy were not the odd views of an outsider physicist, but in line with evolving assumption and practices in sanitary science and experimental medicine.

Despite being the most severe recorded epidemic of the century, the smallpox outbreak in 1871–72 saw little new research on the intimate pathology of the smallpox poison, or the pathology of vaccination. In 1874, Sanderson reported on recent German work by Cohn and Weigert that associated microphytes with the disease, but was reluctant to endorse these organisms as the actual disease-agents or contagia. However, he hoped that Klein's new research on the pathology of the analogous disease of sheep-pox would confirm the 'general doctrine of the vitality of contagia'.[62] Numerous vaccinia or variola germs were announced during the early 1870s and by some well-known scientists. In 1872, Cohn described the micrococcus vaccinae, the following year Edwin Klebs (1834–1913) found the tetracoccus vaccinae, while specific micrococci were suggested by André Cornil (1837–1908), Victor Babes (1854–1926) and Klein again in 1873.[63] However, in no case was there striking visual evidence, nor did anyone report reliable inoculation experiments, which was thought to be very telling as pox diseases were so contagious.

59 See Beale's critical comments on the technical standards of work on 'fungus pathology'. *MTG,* 1870, ii: 656.
60 Sanderson, 'Intimate Pathology', 232.   61 Hamlin, *Science of Impurity,* 109–17, 218–4.
62 *Report of the Medical Officer of Privy Council and Local Government Board, New Series, No. 3, Report on Scientific Investigations,* BPP 1874, [C.1068], xxxi, 6, 30–33.
63 See listing in E. M. Crookshank, *Manual of Bacteriology,* London, H. K. Lewis, 1886, 426.

The 1871–73 epidemic reopened questions on the value of vaccination and how to control epidemics once they were established. The first response of Simon, and MOsH, was to push for more thorough and improved vaccinations. These measures, and the fact that vaccinations had not protected the nation against the disease, galvanised antivaccinationists.[64] A new factor in the epidemic was the greater resort to the isolation of sufferers. In 1871, the new London hospitals were hurriedly completed and their accommodation was supplemented with tents and other temporary shelters.[65] Other local authorities provided permanent or temporary structures for isolation and introduced more systematic methods for disinfecting the homes and possessions of sufferers. In time, isolation hospitals became physical symbols of the state's new, more 'exclusive', response to the contagious disease. They were concerned with isolating individuals who were 'nuisances' and protecting society; they were seeking to change social relations or ameliorate poor social conditions. In 1871–72, the strong popular support for contagionism was felt in the rush for revaccinations and the controversies over hospital location, especially as local residents complained about the threat to their health from transporting sufferers and their concentration in one place. With smallpox, and soon with other diseases as well, concern about people and their behaviour, rather than the environment and its pollution, became factors of growing importance in public health medicine and policy.

CONTAGION, GERMS AND SANITARY SCIENCE

Given the assumptions across medicine about the common basis of fermentation and putrefaction, it is perhaps surprising that few people linked germ speculation on zymotic diseases with that about septic diseases in surgery. This situation may point to relatively closed subcultures in British medicine, at least between surgery and public health, as well as different histories and interests across the profession. Whereas the notion of septic germs was new in surgery, speculation on the behaviour, if not the nature, of the poisons of epidemics was long-standing. Indeed, it was possible to create a modern history of notion of *contagium viva*, from Spallanzani to Henlé and Holland in the 1840s, and to the vogue for fungus pathologies in the 1850s and 1860s. Of course, Lister had eschewed theory and had contrasted his targeted, local methods with the inefficient blunderbuss approaches that sanitarians had proposed for hospitals. More important was the fact that septic and zymotic germs had quite different properties. The agents of zymotic diseases had to be powerful and specific, able to overcome the vital resistance of the healthy human body, to produce near identical pathological processes. Septic germs were saprophytes (an organism living on decaying matter) that had merely to

64 MacLeod, 'Law, Medicine', 108–25.   65 *Twelfth Annual Report*, Appendix 2.

break down dead tissue, which was seen as a general rather than a specific process and more likely to be chemical rather than organic. Thus, while surgeons were asked to imagine one type of living germ, MOsH, functionaries and lay people in public health had to imagine many types of germs and perhaps a specific organism for each zymotic disease.

The germs of surgeons and public health doctors began to be considered together in several situations at the end of the 1860s. First, in the laboratories of investigators like Sanderson and his mentors in France, any fever was ripe for their reductionist pursuit of 'the intimate pathology of contagion'. Second, anthrax, already an important disease because of several claims to have identified its germs or parasites, appeared to show zymotic and septic features, as infection led to putrefactive changes in the blood and the skin. Finally, and most importantly, in the public domain of lectures at the Royal Institution and in the letters' columns of the *Times*, John Tyndall linked the cholera-fungus, ideas on contagia and Lister's septic germs – in short, he proposed a single living-germ theory.

Tyndall's 'Dust and Disease' lecture, delivered in January 1870, has been discussed already in Chapter 3 in relation to surgery, but it has to be considered again because of its importance in public health.[66] Amongst the many reactions, MOsH objected to his simple contagionism and his absurd suggestion, to a chemically minded branch of the profession still influenced by Murchison, that cotton wool masks would protect people from catching diseases by filtering particulate matter from the air. They also took exception to his implied criticisms of existing measures, especially his observation that germ-theory would give 'a definiteness to our efforts to stamp out disease which they could not previously possess'. It was clear what balance of 'exclusive' and 'inclusive' measures that Tyndall favoured. His endorsement of germ-theory did not only aggravate doctors, an editorial in *Nature* complained that, 'In great questions affecting the health and life of nations, theories are quite out of place. They do no good, cost money, and bar scientific progress'.[67]

In the same month as Tyndall's address, the *British and Foreign Medico-Chirurgical Review* published a discussion of current theories of contagion that centred on the standing of germ theories.[68] The author opened by saying that 'considerable obscurity still surrounds the whole question of the nature, origin and prevention of contagion', but there was still plenty to discuss – though no mention was made of septic germs. The author set out three contending hypotheses on the nature of contagia: (i) Richardson's chemical or 'physical' theory; (ii) Beale's bioplasm-germs; and (iii) ideas based on Pasteur's notion of living organic ferments producing zymosis. None of these was

66 'The Dust in the Sunbeam', *MTG*, 1870, i: 125–6; J. Tyndall, 'On Dust and Haze', Ibid., 130–1.
67 'Dust and Disease', *Nature*, 1870, 1: 327.   68 *BFM-CR*, 1870, 45: 128–37.

said to be wholly convincing for all contagious diseases, so the reviewer speculated that each might explain certain classes of diseases. Richardson's chemical secretions seemed best able to account for puerperal fever, plague, smallpox and syphilis, that is, diseases where infection was by inoculation, and where local lesions led to systemic effects. The reviewer found the evidence that such 'viruses' were living organisms wanting, first, because they could survive drying and, second, because alkaloids had already been isolated. Bioplasm-germs were said to best explain diseases such as whooping cough, scarlatina, measles and typhus, which were elaborated in animal bodies and spread from person to person. The model disease for living organic ferments (also termed 'living miasmata') was said to be cholera, with the reviewer restating the cholera-fungus hypothesis. Interestingly, the action of cholera-germs was interpreted through Pettenkofer's theory of epidemic propagation in the environment. Thus, a model of the spread of cholera was built up in stages: cholera-germs were noninfective when they left the body, then underwent 'development' in the soil, gaining pathogenicity, before spreading in water or air to infect other people. The different stages and conditions of development explained the presence of milder forms of the disease and even noncontagious forms. It was once common to regard Pettenkofer as an opponent of germ theories, because of his later confrontations with Koch, but this example and the others that follow show that in Britain in the 1860s and 1870s his 'resting spore theory' was an important version of a living-germ theory of disease.[69]

Tyndall raised the stakes three months later in April, writing to the *Times* to advocate that the medical profession should adopt 'the germ theory of disease'.[70] His letter prompted the start of British spontaneous generation, and raised tensions within the profession. The first detailed response by a sanitarian to Tyndall's provocations was a paper read at the Medical Society of London in April 1870 by Jabez Hogg, an ophthalmic surgeon who was a leading microscopist and expert on water pollution.[71] Hogg also portrayed living or 'organic' germ-theory as a restatement of old style 'fungus-pathology', a term perhaps deployed in a derogatory as well as descriptive sense.[72] He also pointed to new laboratory evidence from Angus Smith, that the pathogenic features of air were due to 'emanations from human beings too closely packed together, [and] the presence of noxious gases generated by coal and

69 C. A. Cameron, 'Cholera Virus', *DQJMS*, 1869, 48: 630
70 Letters from Tyndall, *Times*, 7 April 1870, 5; 21 April 1870, 8; letters from Bastian: *Times*, 13 April 1870, 4 and 22 April 1870, 5. 'Professor Tyndall as a Pathologist', *Lancet*, i: 555–6. This whole controversy is discussed in detail in J. E. Strick, *The British Spontaneous Generation Debates of 1860–1880: Medicine, Evolution and Laboratory Science in the Victorian Context*, Unpublished PhD Thesis, Princeton University, 1997.
71 J. Hogg, 'The Organic Germ Theory of Disease', *MTG*, 1870, i: 659–61, 685–7. Hogg offered tacit support to Bastian in the spontaneous generation debates.
72 M. Pelling, *Fever, Cholera*, 157–202.

thrown off by large manufactories'.[73] Hogg's overall conclusion, following
familiar antigerm arguments, was that theories of 'fungoid bodies or organic
germs' failed to account for infectious diseases 'on analogical and experimental evidence'. Moreover, he suggested that existing multifactorial explanations could not be improved upon:

If ... we require a formula for cholera, we may take 'bad air, bad water, sewer
emanations, floating stinks, germs if you please, bad ventilation', with perhaps a dozen or
more evils ... ; but the prime occasion for its development is a mass of human beings
aggregated together, either in towns, in barracks, or the country, into a sufficiently limited
area of mud, gravel, granite, large or imposing structures, crowded courts, alleys, cellars
in St Giles, or attics in Glasgow, and the necessary conditions for cholera as well as
other zymotic diseases are provided. A vitiated atmosphere breathed and re-breathed
until it becomes lung-tainted and poisonous, to which is added bad food, bad
lodging, or some chronic disease assisting to lower vital functions, and our catalogue is
complete.[74]

In this orthodox sanitarian account of the origins of disease, the contingencies still overshadowed any contagion.

Germs were debated at medical meetings throughout 1870.[75] The controversy reached a peak in October and November following a major attack on
germ theories by Richardson at the Medical Society of London, and the
publication of Simon's Annual Report for 1869.[76] Richardson began by
admitting that 'the vital or germ-theory and his physical theory' had much
in common: they both assumed that infections were zymotic; that disease
processes had specific causes; that causative agents were particulate; and that
these agents could be transmitted person to person directly or indirectly. He
then argued that his ideas on internally produced chemical poisons, excreted
in sweat, breath and exanthemata, were better supported by clinical and epidemiological experiences. His main objection to germ theories – ferment,
fungal, bioplasm, organic, bacterial, living, parasitic or septic – was that they
rested entirely on analogy. He pointed to the fact that no one had been
able to demonstrate the causative role of any germ for any disease, even
the most contagious. He also wondered, in what became a familiar point,
why germs, given their ubiquity and powers of self-replication, were not
more damaging to health.[77] In addition, he disliked the implication of

73 J. M. Eyler, 'The Conversion of Angus Smith: The Changing Role of Chemistry and Biology in
Sanitary Science, 1850–1880', *BHM*, 1980, 54: 216–34; C. Hamlin, *Science of Impurity*, 110–17.
74 Hogg, 'Organic Germ Theory', 689.
75 The question was discussed by many at the British Association for the Advancement of Science
Meeting, at which T. H. Huxley gave his address on 'Biogenesis and Abiogenesis', *Report of the
Thirty-Ninth Meeting of the British Association for the Advancement of Science*, London, John Murray,
1870, NNN.
76 B. W. Richardson, 'The Medical Aspect of the Germ-Theory', *BMJ*, 1870, ii: 566–7.
77 Richardson's view was summed up as follows: that 'the hypothetical germs, being omnipresent,
reproductive, and indestructible by conditions which are fatal to higher organisms ... would sup-

germ pathologies that diseases must be entities – 'manifestly a retrograde step for science'.

The Annual Report of the Medical Department for 1869, which appeared in the same month, started new controversies. Simon praised Sanderson for having found that the active particles of contagia were particulate 'living, self-multiplying organic forms'.[78] As we know, Sanderson held complex views on contagia and was claimed as an ally by all sides. In the early 1870s, all that he would say was that the likely causes of zymotic diseases were the 'germs' of bacteria, in the sense of being their seeds, and that these were 'particulate'. Despite the spin that Simon put on his work, Sanderson would not actually say that disease-germs were living organisms. Nonetheless, Beale was incensed at what he saw as state endorsement of 'fungus pathology' and the neglect of his bioplasm ideas. He maintained that Sanderson's work was empirically and theoretically flawed, and cited Lewis's failure to find any specific cholera fungus in India against the new researches.[79] Sanderson responded to his many critics in a reply to Richardson's Medical Society lecture. He was typically ambivalent, saying at the outset that he agreed with Richardson's main points! In fact, he imagined several resolutions to the chemical versus living contagium issue: that bacteria (or their germs) were sources of chemical-poisons, or that bacteria carried chemical poisons (what some called 'the raft theory'), or that bacteria were the actual disease-causing agents.[80] Sanderson was also seen as equivocal on spontaneous generation, though he maintained that he was against the doctrine.[81] This issue was a critical one in public health medicine because of its relevance to the *de novo* origins of epidemics and the priorities to be given to 'inclusive' and 'exclusive' policies. Chemical theories of zymosis were associated with two propositions: that zymotic diseases could arise *de novo*, and the anticontagionist view that 'inclusive' preventive strategies offered the best hope for disease prevention. Living-germ theories, on the other hand, were associated with ancestral theories of disease, contagion and 'exclusive' measures. These associations were not necessary ones. It was possible to believe in living germs, the *de*

---

plant all others, and that the life of the universe would come to consist of germs alone.', *Lancet*, 1870, ii: 643–4.

78 *Twelfth Annual Report*, 5–8

79 Beale wrote to Sanderson saying that, when Simon moved from accepted zymotic diseases to supposing that tubercle and cancer might be included, 'Some wicked little microzymes must have been pirouetting amongst the particles of the living matter of the cells in the cortical portion of his cerebral convolutions'. 16 November 1870. Sanderson Papers. Add 179/1 22–23. Copies of Burdon Sanderson's replies, if any, are not available. However, in the *Medical Times and Gazette* a colleague of Sanderson, George Buchanan, defended him by saying that he was only reporting the views of others and that he had yet to make up his own mind. *MTG*, 1870, ii: 628–9, 687, 658.

80 J. B. Sanderson, 'Further Report', 763.

81 Also see: G. W Child, 'On Protoplasm and the Germ Theories', *British Association for the Advancement of Science, Report of the 40th Meeting in Liverpool*, London, John Murray, 1871, 129.

novo origins of epidemics, anticontagionism and support 'inclusive' measures, as did Bastian and Pettenkofer, though for different reasons. Similarly, the chemical models could support ancestral theories, contagion and 'exclusive' measures, as with the (chemical) virus of smallpox and Richardson's glandular theory. Indeed, Bastian claimed that the sporadic outbreaks of zymotic diseases was amongst the best evidence for spontaneous generation, and the best reason for avoiding 'any narrow or "exclusive"theories'.[82] Theory and practice were seen to be inextricably linked, though the associations were political rather than logical. The spontaneous generation controversy was of direct relevance to disease control for the following reasons. First, if fermentation was shown to be due to the action of living organisms, then so probably was zymosis. Next, if disease poisons (and zymotic agents) were living organisms, and if cell theory was correct – that *Omnis cellula e celluli* (only cells begat cells) – then the *de novo* origin of disease was impossible. Over the 1870s, the debate on spontaneous generation turned more and more to laboratory work; however, the field of public health medicine remained a resource for speculation over the *de novo* origin of diseases, and by implication the spontaneous generation of life.

Edmund Parkes introduced reflections on the nature of contagia into his annual report to the Army Medical Department in 1872 and mentioned alternatives to chemical accounts of zymosis for the first time in the next edition of his influential *Manual* in 1873.[83] The alternatives he gave were bioplasm-germs, fungal pathologies and the new ideas that made the causes of infections 'minute animal organisms, previously known as Bacteria, Zoogloea, Microzymes, Vibrios, Monads, & c'.[84] The attractions of the new ideas to Parkes were evident when he wrote on cholera in the same year, expressing his dissatisfaction with the explanations favouring miasmas and 'local conditions', against the definiteness of the approaches focused on poisons carried by humans and spread by water, air and food.[85] For cholera, Parkes now leaned towards 'exclusive' policies of isolating sufferers, disinfecting their wastes and depriving germs of the specific 'nutritive conditions' that allowed them to bear fruit. The arguments were not just about policy differences between groups within public health medicine; this whole area was still influenced by political differences. 'Exclusive' measures were opposed by liberals, who objected to the state interfering in personal affairs and introducing policies that damaged the economy. Popular opinion was also wary of medical power, as was shown in the support mobilised by the groups in the 1870s

82 H. C. Bastian, 'Epidemic and Specific Contagious Diseases: Considerations as to their Nature and Mode of Origin', *BMJ*, 1871, ii: 400–9.
83 D. E. Watkins, *The English Revolution in Social Medicine, 1889–1911*, Unpublished PhD Thesis, University of London, 1984, 18–22.
84 E. Parkes, *Manual of Hygiene*, fourth edition, Churchill, London, 1873, 475.
85 E. Parkes, 'Address in Medicine', *Lancet*, 1873, i: 180.

campaigning to repeal the Contagious Disease Acts.[86] Also, sanitarians suspected that 'exclusive' measures were being promoted by chemical manufacturers, irrespective of their value, simply to boost the demand for disinfectants and other products.

Simon's famous essay on the evils of 'filth' in his Annual Report for 1874 also pondered the 'inclusive' versus 'exclusive' dilemma.[87] He called for specific controls, such as isolation and quarantines, to be applied to 'cases of dangerous infected disease' so that sufferers could not 'scatter abroad the seeds of their infection'. However, he continued to stress 'inclusive' measures against the evils of 'filth' – the medium in which all germs, both those whose 'sole birthplace' was the living body and those with 'a birthplace exterior to man', were able to 'continue their existence' or develop disease-causing properties. He added new questions about the effectiveness of chemical disinfectants against living organisms in the environment, in comparison to their successful application against weaker septic germs in the narrow confines of wounds. He was certain that in public health, the best methods were the natural disinfectants of cleanliness, ventilation and drainage.[88] In 1874, Richardson yet again put the case for chemical theories, still painting a picture of disease-germs as panspermic, all-powerful and necessarily fatal. By linking these properties with spontaneous generation, he invented what he hoped was an untenable position for his opponents:

> Could we conceive of disease 'germs' to have an existence, and were we obliged to admit their ceaseless spontaneous origin, all attempts to check contagion would be paralysed, and spontaneity would be able to conquer anything. The theory may, however, be discarded as an obstruction to science, and the dictates of hygiene may be obeyed with the conviction that obedience will be rewarded.[89]

Thus, spontaneous generation was not only an affront to scientific naturalism, it was an anathema to ordered, moral and optimistic sanitary policies.

In his *Handbook of Hygiene* in 1873, George Wilson, one of Stevenson's paradigmatic sanitarians, supported 'inclusive' policies, though he added that 'In order to be able to apply such measures judiciously, some knowledge of the mode of propagation of the several epidemic diseases is essential'.[90] The disease-by-disease approach that he recommended was one consequence of

86 J. Walkowitz, *Prostitution and Victorian Society: Women, Class and the State*, Cambridge, Cambridge University Press, 1980.

87 J. Simon, 'Filth Diseases and Their Prevention', *Report of the Medical Officer of Privy Council and Local Government Board, New Series, No. 2: Supplementary Report on Inquiries in 1874*, BPP, 1874, [C.1066]. xxxi, 33.

88 J. Simon, 'Memorandum on Disinfection', *Ninth Annual Report*, 236–9. Cf., J. Dougall, *The Science of Disinfection*, Glasgow, Macclehose, 1875.

89 *BMR*, 1874, 3: 64–5.

90 G. Wilson, *A Handbook of Hygiene*, London, Churchill, 1873, 280. The same point is made in Pettenkofer-like terms in: W. Squire, 'On the Development and Propagation of Epidemic Diseases', *PH*, 1873, 1: 161.

the growing medical influence in sanitary affairs. Wilson stated that there should be different priorities and practices for each disease. The main task with cholera and typhoid fever was to disinfect discharges from the intestines, and stop their spread in polluted water supplies. With scarlet fever, where he used Richardson's glandular theory, Wilson recommended isolating patients and disinfecting all bodily emanations, especially sweat and scales of skin. Many historians have placed the change in public health policy and practice, from measures centred on 'environment' to 'people', much later in the 1880s and 1890s, and have seen it as indicative of the change from state medicine to preventive medicine. The range of opinion and policies that I have discussed, from Tyndall, through Parkes and Wilson, to Richardson, shows that person-centred approaches were debated and used much earlier. They were always the priority in the control of smallpox outbreaks. Their extension to attempts to disinfect and control the excretions of cholera and typhoid fever sufferers in part followed new water-carriage ideas, but they were also shaped by the manner in which disease prevention more generally focused on specific nuisances and their removal. Thus, calls for notification and isolation were in part about removing people who were 'nuisances'.[91] It is also worth noting that antiseptic dressings were understood by Listerians to seal in the effluvia of wounds to prevent hospital epidemics, another example of person-centred prevention.

Parkes's narrative on different types of germ-diseases in the 1873 edition of his *Manual* was developed in the chapter on disinfection, indicating how the nature of germs was of practical interest. Indeed, the objectives that MOsH had for disinfection changed in the 1870s, becoming more limited and concentrating on neutralising or destroying disease-poisons or contagia. Previously, disinfection had many purposes: deodorisation, altering the environment so that poisons did not arise and even hurrying the providential process of decay.[92] One manufacturer produced a new disinfectant called 'Sporokton', the name being a compound of 'spore' and 'roke' – a mist. Parkes warned that if contagia were independent living germs, then disinfection would be more difficult as organisms had vitality, and would be harder to counter than mere chemicals or feeble bioplasm.[93] If disease-agents were living, ancestral and contagious, directly or indirectly, then there were new problems for epidemiological studies. Zymotic diseases ought to be less capricious and more predictable than previously thought, following the slower patterns of biological development rather than the rapid reactions of chemistry.

91 A. Carpenter, *On the Right of the State to Obtain Early Information of the Appearance of Epidemic and Infectious Disease*, London, P. S. King, 1876.
92 H. Letheby, 'On the Right Use of Disinfectants', *PH*, 1873, 1: 193–5. Disinfectants were said to work in one or more of the following ways: enabling a substrate to resist decay; creating new compounds in the substrate that resist decay; accelerating providential decay or destroying the special agent of disinfection.
93 *MTG*, 1879, ii: 409.

However, it seems that rank-and-file MOsH, and the wider public health community, remained committed to chemistry and *de novo* origins, as was only too evident in the vexed debates about the prevention and control of typhoid fever in the 1870s.

TYPHOID FEVER, DE NOVO ORIGINS AND PREVENTIVE POLICIES, 1870–1880

Lloyd Stevenson suggested that typhoid fever was 'the exemplary disease' for modelling the pathology of fevers in the mid-Victorian era.[94] The strategic medical role ascribed to this disease has been extended by McTavish, who sees it as paradigmatic of changes in late Victorian therapeutics. I want to continue this line of argument and suggest that typhoid fever was an exemplar in debates on the prevention of zymotic disease in public health in the 1870s.

The clinical differentiation between typhoid and typhus fevers, based on William Jenner's studies in the late 1840s, was widely accepted and used in Britain, though it was not until 1869 that the Registrar-General recorded deaths separately.[95] The national incidence of typhus fever declined steeply after 1869, while that of typhoid fever waxed and waned on a slower downward trend. However, it was local epidemics that attracted the most attention, for their apparent randomness and mortality.[96] The Medical Department made more investigations of typhoid fever than any other disease in the 1870s. Public awareness had been raised in 1861 when it killed Prince Albert, and in 1871 it was again newsworthy when the Prince of Wales had a near-fatal infection. In public health more generally, Wohl suggests that typhoid fever served as 'a barometer of inadequate water supplies and sewerage', a view recently endorsed by Luckin and Hardy.[97] It was also the model for contingent contagionism; hence, typhoid fever was amongst the first diseases to be

94 L. G. Stevenson, 'Exemplary Disease: The Typhoid Pattern', *JHM*, 1982, 37: 159–81; J. R. McTavish, 'Antipyretic Treatment and Typhoid Fever', *JHM*, 1987, 42: 486–500.

95 L. G. Wilson, 'Fevers', in W. F. Bynum and R. Porter, eds., *Companion Encyclopaedia of the History of Medicine*, London, Routledge, 1993, 401–6. The diseases were first differentiated by their symptoms and pathology. Typhoid fever caused a steady rise in temperature, extreme lethargy, a rash and eventually abdominal pains and diarrhoea. While regarded primarily as a blood disease, it was recognised at postmortem by the inflamed Peyer's patches on the intestinal wall. Case mortalities varied considerably, with deaths usually due to a haemorrhage or peritonitis arising from the rupture of the intestine. That sufferers required such a long convalescence confirmed that its effects were systemic, as well as local in the digestive system.

96 In 1870, typhoid or enteric fever had the fifth highest mortality of the eighteen zymotic diseases. Those with higher mortality rates in rank order were (mortality per million population in brackets): scarlet fever (1461); diarrhoea (1136); whooping cough (534); typhoid fever (398); measles (339).

97 Wohl, *Endangered Lives*, 127, 173; W. Luckin, *Pollution and Control*, Bristol, Adam Hilger, 1983, 118–38; A. Hardy, *The Epidemic Streets: The Rise of Preventive Medicine in London, 1850–1910*, Oxford, Oxford University Press, 1993, 151–72.

assessed in terms of the new aetiological and pathological germ models developed after 1870. However, the central issue throughout the decade was how often, if at all, did local epidemics arise *de novo*, and what the answer to this question meant for preventive policy. The intimate nature and properties of any 'typhoid-stuff' was secondary in public health medicine, yet the claims of laboratory scientists throughout the 1870s to have found the typhoid fever germ, together with their denial of the possibility of its spontaneous generation, raised important issues for preventive policy.

From the 1840s, typhoid fever had been linked by sanitarians to 'sanitary defects' and was the archetypal 'pythogenic' disease.[98] However, as early as 1861, William Budd had proposed that the disease was caused by a specific poison that passed from person to person, usually via drinking water, in a manner similar to Snow's water-carriage theory for cholera.[99] Neither authority was 'exclusive': Murchison allowed for contagion in some circumstances, while Budd acknowledged the role of poor sanitation in propagating and spreading the specific agent. However, there was an important difference: Murchison proposed that the disease usually arose *de novo* and that contagion was secondary, whereas Budd supposed that every case had its ancestry in an earlier one, though the lineage might be lengthy and circuitous.[100] Most sanitarians took both models to point to the same methods of prevention: remove filth and promote cleanliness to reduce the chances of the disease-poisons arising, developing and spreading.[101] However, in the 1870s the two approaches became associated with different priorities and different political philosophies. Pythogenic theory was linked with 'liberalism', as sanitarians and older MOsH required that priority be given to 'inclusive' measures that removed the conditions in which the disease-poisons originated, so that individuals could be free to live in a safe environment and to avoid quarantine and similar measures that infringed on personal freedoms. On the other side, modernising MOsH tried to make a necessary connection between living-germ theories; ancestral origins; controlling personal infection; 'exclusive' methods and legislative powers for notification, isolation and the control of movements. As previously with cholera, agreement on contingent contagionism did not prevent wide divisions of opinion on priorities.

In the early 1870s, the implicit endorsement of Budd's ideas on typhoid fever by authorities such as Simon and Parkes, and their linkage to 'exclusive' approaches, worried many established MOsH. John Fox, MOH for Cockermouth, wrote in January 1874 that until the exact nature and means

98 C. Murchison, *Continued Fevers of Great Britain*, London, Parker, Son and Bourne, 1862.
99 C.-E. A. Winslow, *The Conquest of Epidemic Disease: A Chapter in the History of Ideas*, Princeton, NJ, Princeton University Press, 1943, 286–90.
100 See: *BMJ*, 1870, i: 308, 426. Clifford Allbutt's view, that typhoid fever had a specific poison, was challenged by Thorne Thorne, who favoured its spontaneous origin. Cf. *MTG*, 1870, i: 205.
101 J. M. Fox, 'Typhoid Fever and Sanitary Administration', *PH*, 1874, 2: 7–9, 20–3, 8.

of spread of the *materies contagii* was known, any changes in sanitary work ought to be suspended 'on the ground of logic and public safety'.[102] Furthermore, he worried that 'if the view became popular that only typhoid or choleraic discharges were sources of imminent danger . . . a powerful motive to action would be taken out of our hands'. His point was that filth theories gave MOsH greater political leverage to argue for general sanitary improvements, whereas germ theories would be used to support cheaper and narrower methods.[103] He surmised that 'exclusive' measures would inevitably be opposed or flouted, so that they would achieve nothing. One influential supporter of Budd was William Corfield, Professor of Hygiene at University College Hospital and a colleague of Bastian. He drew the opposite conclusion to Fox, arguing that controlling personal infection was the most effective strategy. In June 1874, he spoke at the Epidemiological Society against the spontaneous development of the typhoid fever poison, saying that such ideas were 'erroneous' and 'mischievous', because they 'discouraged persons from attempting to stamp out the disease by destroying the poison at the earliest possible moment after its exit from the body'.[104] Most of those who spoke in the discussion disagreed, and supported Fox's view that exclusivity would produce only partial benefits and offered a cheap, inferior alternative to the 'economist' factions on local councils. There also was much speculation in the discussion of Corfield's paper about the 'germs' of the typhoid fever, with confusion coming from the fact that many doctors were using the term metaphorically while others were actually talking about living organisms. One of the most telling responses to Corfield was by Alfred Carpenter, MOH for Croydon, who had recently completed a report on an epidemic in the town. He suggested that 'The germs which can produce typhoid fever, existing everywhere, are only waiting for the condition required for development, for them to grow into the typhoid state'. This occult germ-theory can be read as a synthesis of Dobell's work in the early 1860s, the panspermism of Lister and Tyndall, and Pettenkofer's theories, though Carpenter's preferred the dry-rot fungus analogy. Although he spoke as a germ theorist, he said that his experience and ideas led him to support 'inclusive' policies rather than 'exclusive' ones.

The publication of William Budd's book, *Typhoid Fever*, in 1874 prompted John Tyndall to write to the *Times* once again to promote the germ-theory of disease and attack spontaneous generation.[105] Many doctors were again irritated that a physicist and polemicist should interfere in their affairs, not least with his advice to treat the digestive systems of sufferers with

102 Ibid., 21.   103 W. Procter, 'Our Epidemics', *PH*, 1874, 2: 97–100, 131–4.

104 W. H. Corfield, 'On the Alleged Spontaneous Development of the Poison of Enteric Fever', *PH*, 1874, 2: 155–8.

105 J. Tyndall, *Times*, 9 November 1874, 7e. His intervention provoked a considerable debate. See 10 November 1874, 7d; 11 November 1874, 5f; 12 November 1974, 7d and 12a. A letter from Lionel Beale was published on 16 November 1874.

antiseptics.[106] There were complaints that he had misrepresented both Budd and Simon, as correspondents said that neither would have abandoned cleanliness, drainage and ventilation for the singular attack on the 'seeds' of typhoid fever recommended by Tyndall.[107] Tyndall claimed that his decision to bring Budd's work to the public's attention at this time was due to the discovery of the specific typhoid fever germ:

... the crowning fact, already published in the medical journals and to which my attention was recently drawn by my eminent friend Mr Simon, that Dr Klein has recently discovered the very organism which lies at the root of all the mischief, and to which medical and sanitary skill will henceforth be directed.[108]

Later in the year, Simon also celebrated Klein's work, when it was published officially, saying that the 'microphyte' he had identified offered 'for the first time the contagion of enteric fever as something recognisable to the eye'.[109] In January 1875, the *Practitioner* published an account of Klein's work and reproduced versions of his drawings, showing how the claim was based on histology-based microscopy (see Figure 9).[110]

Simon constituted Klein's' typhoid fever germs as 'parasitic fungi' and speculated that this would lead the profession 'to direct our utmost energies to the task of preventing the deadly entrance of these deadly fungus germs into the organism'. Although the finding was described as 'sensational', what became known as the Tyndall Typhoid Controversy centred more on Tyndall's propaganda than on Klein's typhoid fever germ.[111] Tyndall had gained more notoriety in 1874 with his address to the Belfast Meeting of the BAAS, in which he had advocated a materialist philosophy. With germs, Tyndall faced the problem that the genre and rules of 'germ discovery' had yet to be invented. In the spontaneous generation debate in 1870–3, he had tried many times to designate certain experiments 'crucial', but with little success.[112] With disease theories, he faced the problem that accepted aetiological ideas were multifactorial and the idea that the microscopic, structureless objects found by Klein were powerful, and specific and were alone responsible for typhoid fever, was hard to accept. Germ 'discoveries' became 'events' of a sort after Koch's work on the anthrax bacillus was published at the end of 1876, but mostly it took years for particular aetiological and pathological claims

106 However, see: E. J. Syson, 'The Antiseptic Treatment of Zymotic Diseases, *PH*, 1877, 8: 301–3.
107 A. Carpenter, *Times*, 13 November 1874.
108 Klein's first publication on this had appeared in Germany in September. *Centralblatt fur die Medizin Wissenschaft*, 1874, 12: 692, 706.
109 *Report of the Medical Officer of the Privy Council and LGB, New Series, No 6: Report on Scientific Investigations*, BPP, 1875, [C.1371], xl, p. 5. Also see: *Practitioner*, 1875, 24: 472–3, and *PH*, 1876, 4: 463–4.
110 T. L. Brunton, 'Dr Klein and the Pathology of Small-pox and Typhoid Fever', *Practitioner*, 1875, 24: 10.
111 T. L. Brunton, 'Another Aspect of the Tyndall Typhoid Controversy', *Practitioner*, 1875, 24: 62–7. Matters had not been helped by reactions to Tyndall's Belfast Address in 1874, in which he advanced a materialist philosophy.   112 Strick, *British Spontaneous Generation*, Ch. 6.

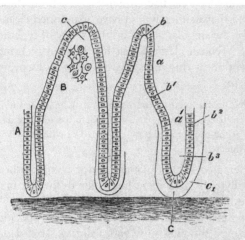

FIG. 1.—Diagram to show the positions of the round organisms and micrococci in relation to the villi and Lieberkühnian follicles of the intestinal mucous membrane. A, Lieberkühniah crypt or follicle; B, a villus, in one part of which is shown the adenoid tissue of which the substance of the villus is composed; c, a lymph space surrounding a Lieberkühnian follicle; $a\,a'$, first position of the organisms and micrococci at the surface of the intestine and mouths of the Lieberkühnian follicles; $b\,b'\,b^2\,b^3$, more advanced position of these bodies in the epithelium of the villi, under the epithelium of the villi, in the epithelium and in the lumen of the Lieberkühnian follicles; $c\,c'$, still more advanced position in the tissue of the villi and the lymph spaces surrounding the follicles.

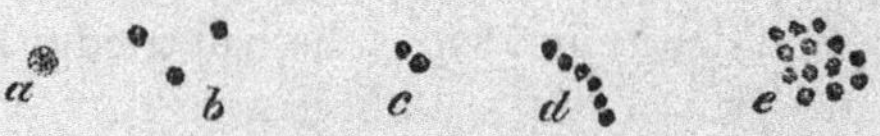

FIG. 2.—Micrococci under a low power at a. Under a high power: isolated at b, in twos, forming a dumb-bell at c, forming a necklace at d, and a zoogloea at e.

Figure 9. The illustrations from the *Practitioner* that accompanied the discussion of Klein's claim to have identified the micrococcus of typhoid fever. These diagrams are simplified versions of the coloured drawings of sections of the wall of the intestine from the Report of the Medical Department which showed the micrococci in situ at the points labelled a, b and c. From *Practitioner*, 24, 1875: 10

to gain widespread acceptance. With anthrax, Koch had the good fortune to work with relatively large organisms, with definite forms, that were relatively easy to find in the blood, and which he was able to fashion as parasitic diseases, one area of medicine where the overriding importance of one factor – large worms and flukes – was hard to deny. Koch had exhibited his anthrax germs to Cohn and his colleagues in a 'theatre of proof' –

experimental demonstrations backed up by microscopy and detailed drawings. Cohn spread the word of his performance, and Koch reported his techniques and findings in such detail that he was able to create a 'virtual theatre of proof' in the minds of his readers. Against this, Klein's typhoid germs had been presented in the tradition of histological research, two-dimensional drawings of sections of the intestine with the actual germs represented as mere dots.

Reactions to the Tyndall Typhoid Controversy rumbled on into 1875, with MOsH pondering the conundrum that, while pathological investigators were suggesting that contagia were living organisms and of ancestral origin, epidemiologists and the majority of workers in public health still believed that they were combating a chemical poison with *de novo* origins. When drawn into the issue in 1875, William Jenner stated that the question would be settled in the field rather than the laboratory, which many MOsH took as an invitation to submit evidence of their experiences to the medical press and meetings.[113] The majority of letters maintained that the disease could 'begin anew at any time in a person in a low condition inhaling some fermenting (zymotic) nuisance', usually referred to as the 'typhoid-poison'.[114] A review of twenty-seven small epidemics by C. B. Fox, MOH for Essex, led him to admit a personal struggle between 'theory' and 'experience': 'my mind . . . is prejudiced in favour of the more philosophical view that enteric fever never arises spontaneously, yet my judgement points to the opposite conclusion'.[115] Opinion amongst MOsH was divided, though in more complex ways than Farr's suggestion that rural MOsH tended towards contagionism, because they found it easier to find antecedent cases, whereas urban MOsH reported many more isolated cases and *de novo* origins.[116]

Jenner's assumption about the secondary position of the laboratory seemed to be vindicated in the spring of 1876, when Charles Creighton showed that Klein's micrococci of typhoid fever were merely 'some albuminous matter' and an artefact of the methods used.[117] A report in the *BMJ* referred to this as a 'sudden and fatal shock' to living-germ theory and that without Creighton's intervention 'organisms would have been saddled with all the bodily evils known to us'.[118] Klein never replied, tacitly conceding his error.

---

113 W. Jenner, *BMJ*, 1875, i: 233–6; *BMJ*, 1875, i: 486; *SRec*, 1876, 4: 81–2, 115–16, 151.

114 Note again how the soil (the 'person in a low condition') is cited before the seed (the 'fermenting nuisance'). *BMJ*, 1875, i: 639, 772; Ibid., ii: 720; 1876, Ibid., i: 444, 659.

115 C. B. Fox, 'Is Enteric Fever Ever Spontaneously Generated', *BMJ*, 1876, i: 374–7.

116 *BMJ*, 1875, i: 486, 639; *SRev*, 1875, 2: 254; Ibid., 1876, 4: 81–2, 115–16, 151. Also see: G. Wilson, *BMJ*, 1881, ii: 510, and R. B. Low, 'The Origin of Enteric Fever in Isolated Rural Districts', *BMJ*, 1880, i: 733–6. Budd's conviction of the contagiousness of typhoid fever was believed to have come form his experiences of the disease in villages.

117 C. Creighton, 'Note on Certain Unusual Coagulation Appearances Found in Mucus and other Abdominal Fluids', *PRSL*, 1876–7, 25: 140–4. At the same meeting, Bastian read a paper on the chemical theory of fermentation.

118 *BMJ*, 1876, ii: 499. These criticisms were never publicly answered by Klein.

It was later suggested that Creighton's finding had seriously damaged laboratory medicine in Britain in the mid-1870s, which Klein had also harmed in his evidence to the Royal Commission on Vivisection in 1875, in which he appeared to be indifferent to animal cruelty.[119] As discussed with surgery, there was a stalemate in the debate on germ theories at the Pathological Society in April 1875 that had been a setback for germ theorists. There were further problems in 1876, especially when Sanderson, to Simon's embarrassment, wrote that septic ferments were 'unformed' and hence not living organisms.[120] Like many others, Sanderson had assumed that some disease-germs were the spores or seeds of bacteria, but he now suggested that such seeds might be 'molecular aggregates' and not living beings. He reiterated the point in an address to the Society of Medical Officers of Health in January 1877 entitled '*Contagium Vivum*'.[121] This paper annoyed Tyndall, who attacked the 'grave' position that Sanderson had taken and he regretted the ammunition that this gave to Bastian and supporters of the *de novo* origin of disease.[122] An editorial in the *Lancet*, a journal not known for its enthusiasm for living-germ theories, wondered what the profession was to do if the 'army of germ theorists is divided'.[123] An indication of the weakness of living-germ theories was that in 1876 the spontaneous generation debate flared up again, and in medicine the issues were little different to those in the early 1870s. The new debate was reviewed by John MacDonald, in a Glasgow MD thesis in 1878, for which Sanderson was an external examiner. Sanderson made a number of comments in the margins, but intriguingly made no remarks about being listed with Bastian, Cohn and Huitzinga as an advocate of spontaneous generation on the first page.[124] MacDonald was not a strong student, but his confusion is indicative of the uncertainties and ambiguities in germ ideas and work at this time, a decade after the cattle plague, the cholera crisis and the announcement of Lister's great principle.

119 '[They gave] strong encouragement to . . . scepticism, and in this country, for a time, probably gave a check, if not to the progress on investigation . . . yet to the publication of its results'. *BMJ*, 1881, ii: 877. Ironically, Creighton's paper had been read to the Royal Society by T. H. Huxley. On the long-run consequences of Klein's evidence to the Royal Commission, including the extent to which he was a model for uncaring doctors in late Victorian fiction, see: C. Lansbury, *The Old Brown Dog: Women, Workers and Vivisection in Edwardian England*, Madison, WI, University of Wisconsin Press, 1985, 130–8, 155.

120 *Report of the Medical Officer of the Privy Council and LGB, New Series, No 8: Report on Scientific Investigations*, BPP, 1876, [C.1608], xxxviii, 455.

121 J. B. Sanderson, 'Contagium Vivum', *PH*, 1877, 8: 59–63.

122 UCL Archives, Sanderson Papers, Add 179/3 5. Also see: Tyndall's reply to Corfield's last lecture, 'The Laws of Health', *PH*, 1877, 8, 322. Also see: J. Tyndall, 'Further Research on the Deportment and Vital Resistance of Putrefactive and Infective Organisms', *PRSL*, 1878, 26: 228–38; *idem.*, 'Notes on Dr Burdon Sanderson's Latest Views on Fermentation and Germs', *PRSL*, 1878, 26: 353–6. J. B. Sanderson, 'Remarks on the Attributes of the Germinal Particles of Bacteria, in Reply to Professor Tyndall', Ibid., 416–26.

123 *Lancet*, 1877, i: 691–4, 692.

124 J. McDonald, *A Few Remarks on the Germ Theory and its Relation to the Germ Theory of Disease*, MD Thesis, University of Glasgow, 1878–79.

The second round of the spontaneous generation debate was relatively short-lived and will be discussed in more detail in the next chapter. One reason for its short life was that the technical standards for the laboratory study of germs had improved, and while it was still impossible to prove the negative proposition that spontaneous generation never occurred, it became easier to show the life history or ancestry of microorganisms. In Britain, the work of members of the microscopical societies brought a new order to the microworld, and in medicine the work of four people, all based in Liverpool, was critical: William H. Dallinger, John Drysdale, Frances Vacher and P. M. Braidwood.[125] Between 1873 and 1875, Dallinger and Drysdale published a series of studies on the 'Life History of Monads', which demonstrated life cycles and spores for many bacteria and botanised germs in general. In 1875, Braidwood and Vacher, who was MOH for Birkenhead, began publishing the results of BMA-funded investigations, 'On the Life History of Contagion.[126] This typically British work on the natural history of microorganisms predated Koch's displays of the life cycle of the anthrax bacillus, and was widely cited before and after Koch's work on anthrax became known.

Koch first demonstrated his methods and findings on anthrax in Cohn's laboratory in April 1876. In August, Cohn visited London and spoke with Tyndall about the work. Koch's seminal paper was published in Germany in October, and was first brought to the attention of British audiences by Tyndall in a talk in Glasgow and in an article in the *Fortnightly Review*. Tyndall stated confidently that the bacillary cause of anthrax 'has been place beyond on all doubt'.[127] He went on to suggest that Koch had gone beyond previous studies of germs and disease, which had merely demonstrated constant associations, and devised new techniques to manipulate the anthrax bacillus to be able to build up both aetiological and pathological demonstrations of its behaviour. Given the size of anthrax germs and their powers of multiplication, it was quite easy to see how they might produce structural alterations to the body (blocking capillaries, lowering vitality and breaking up tissues), though many doctors supposed that their systemic effects were due to chemical poisons, excreted wastes or their use of the body's oxygen.

Koch's ideas, techniques and findings did not initially attract much attention in Britain, certainly not in the medical press. Anthrax was not a

125 Adam, *Spontaneous Generation*, 82–6.
126 W. H. Dallinger and J. Drysdale, 'Researches on the Life History of Cercomonad: A Lesson in Biogenesis', *MMJ*, 1973, 10: 53–58; *idem.*, 'Further Researches into the Life History of Monads', *MMJ*, 1873, 10: 245–49; 1874, 11: 7–10, 69–72, 97–113; 1874, 12: 261–69; 1875, 13: 185–97. P. M. Braidwood and F. Vacher, 'First Contribution to the Life History of Contagion', *BMJ*, 1875, ii (Suppl.) 18–22; 1877, ii: 301.
127 J. Tyndall, 'Fermentation and its Bearing on the Phenomenon of Disease', *Fortnightly Review*, 1876, 20: 567. Tyndall stated categorically that the bacillary cause of anthrax 'has been placed beyond on all doubt by [recent] research'.

public health disease, it was not scheduled in veterinary legislation, and its occupational form – Woolsorters' disease – was a very local problem. Also, as Klein discovered, having Tyndall as your promotions' manager hardly helped. Thus, it would be wrong to imagine a domino effect whereby once the first germ aetiology was constructed for anthrax, this opened the way for the application of an 'anthrax analogy', and it was only a matter of time before other diseases fell into place. Rather, the question was not when diseases would fall into line, but which diseases would turn out to be due to living germs and which would remain with a chemical or other explanation. Also, in one sense Koch's work and techniques made the search for disease-germs that much harder, as he set such high standards in technique and aetiological proof. The anthrax analogy required investigators to show life histories, parasitism and the pathological effects of bacteria; indeed, Koch himself could only rarely make germs behave quite so cooperatively again. Finally, Koch pathologised bacteria, which in the minds of many doctors, especially, as we shall see in the next chapter, those around Lister, made other types of microorganisms harmless.

Koch, like the Liverpool group, had advanced the cause of microscopy, though the possibility remained that some disease-germs would be ultramicroscopic, or that instruments were unreliable. In 1876, Lister convinced a German visitor to Edinburgh that the 'supposed bacteria' they had found under an antiseptic dressing 'were only a microscopical illusion'.[128] Indeed, for those who believed that disease-germs were pleomorphic and that their effects came from their poisons, function mattered more than form. Sanderson stated in December 1877, in lectures on 'The Infective Processes of Disease', that 'in deciding the question of the presence or absence of living matter capable of germinating, the microscope has no voice'.[129] In what was a major address, in part correcting the 'misunderstandings' he had recently fostered and also introducing Koch's anthrax work to a metropolitan medical audience, it is revealing that he only bothered to provide illustrations of the life history of the anthrax bacillus in the printed version of the talk (see Figure 10).

The year 1877 was much better for germ theorists. They took heart from the absence of challenges to Koch's work on anthrax and from Pasteur's willingness to confront Bastian over spontaneous generation. Sanderson had fallen back into line and, as we will see, Lister's work continued to be celebrated overseas. However, the pivotal moment that signalled the improved prospects for germ theorists came not from events in continental Europe or the work of the Simon, Sanderson, Tyndall circle, but from an address by a Manchester physician at the BMA's Annual Meeting in the summer. William

128 *EMJ*, 1876, 22: 467.
129 J. B. Sanderson, 'The Infective Processes of Disease', *BMJ*, 1877, ii: 879–81, 913–15; Ibid., 1878, i: 1–2, 45–7, 119–20, 179–83, 914.

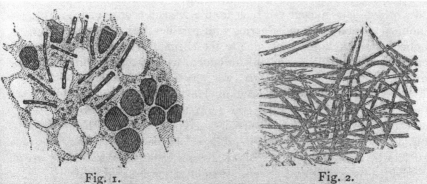

Fig. 1. Fig. 2.

ig. 1.—Bacilli, as seen in a fresh preparation of an animal affected with splenic fever. The blood-corpuscles and bacilli are deeply stained by an aniline solution, which has been added for the purpose.

ig. 2.—Felt-work of long unjointed filaments, into which the rods grow when transferred to humor aqueus, and kept at a temperature of 32 deg. C.

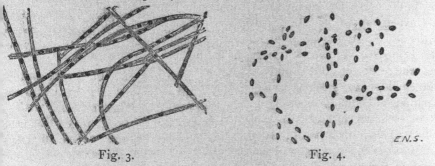

Fig. 3. Fig. 4.

ig. 3.—The same filaments twelve to twenty-four hours later. The formation of "spores" in their interior has already commenced.

ig. 4.—The spores in their complete stage. Some are free, but the most are still held together by the scarcely distinguished remainder of the filaments. The infecting power of these spores has been recently tested in the course of experiments now in progress.

Figure 10. The drawing of the anthrax bacillus that accompanied the published version of Sanderson's final lecture on the infective processes of disease. These appeared in the British Medical Journal on 9 January 1878, and were the first public display of this crucial work in a major medical journal. *BMJ,* 1878, i: 181. (Reproduced by courtesy of the Director and University Librarian, the John Rylands University Library of Manchester)

Roberts, who had been active on Tyndall's side in the spontaneous generation debate in the early 1870s, developed what was in essence a clinician's version of the bacterial theory of disease, which linked laboratory findings with experience and practice in surgery, public health and the

clinic.[130] I discuss this address in detail in the next chapter, so here I shall
simply note that his whole argument was built from a refutation of spontaneous generation, an accommodation of germs with parasites, and with the
idea that zymotic disease syndromes were due to the chemical poisons produced by disease-germs.[131] Charles Cameron's introductory address in Dublin
that year, also on the 'Pathology of Contagia', was very similar, also beginning with an attack on spontaneous generation. He completely ignored
chemical theories and discussed the same two germ theories as Roberts:
Beale's 'disease grafts' and 'the more generally accepted opinion that
each contagious disease is caused by . . . a living thing'.[132] However, he ended
in a traditional vein by saying that 'all contagious diseases were filth diseases
and could be subdued or eradicated by the most rigid national and private
cleanliness'.

In respect of typhoid fever, Koch's aetiology of anthrax, with its dormant
spores in the soil, gave new credence to Pettenkofer-type notions of 'stuff'
from the gut of sufferers developing pathogenicity in the environment, and of
'resting spores' in the soil.[133] The attempts to accommodate laboratory findings
with the field experience of the disease led to some ingenious suggestions.
For example, the dissemination of germs or spores was attributed to human carriers, one idea being that vagrants, wandering in the night and fouling out-
buildings, were the source of isolated outbreaks in rural areas.[134] Pettenkofer's
ideas were also employed to explain *de novo* origins, without reliance on spontaneous generations or chemical theories. In 1879, Bruce Low, MOH for the
rural district of Helmsley in Yorkshire, explained *de novo* outbreaks in his
district as follows, 'This is not at all a question of the development of a living
organism out of matter independently of antecedent life, but merely the production, by means of a process of evolution, of that which gives an already
existing organism that property by which it become infective'.[135] Alfred
Carpenter repackaged Pettenkofer's ideas in terms of x, y, z variables, where x
was the human body, y the waste products of human metabolism, and z the

130 W. Roberts, 'The Doctrine of *Contagium vivum* and its Applications to Medicine', *BMJ*, 1877, ii:
   168–73.
131 See the similarities with E. J. Syson, MOH for Huntingdon, who wrote of the 'gradations' of
   'Germ Theory', from the 'fineness of scarlet or typhoid fever to the coarseness of trichinosis'.
   PH, 1877, 8: 302; Cf. J. Lane Notter, 'The Chemical Theory of Contagion, Compared with the
   Corpuscular Theory', *BMJ*, 1877, ii: 301.
132 C. A. Cameron, 'The Pathology of Contagia', *PH*, 1877, 7: 284.
133 W. Cayley, 'Croonian Lectures on Some Points on the Pathology and Treatment of Typhoid
   Fever', *BMJ*, 1880, i: 391–3, 671, and ii: 1881, 507. Cayley's list of possible poisonous agents
   included: a fungus, microzyme, protoplasm (*contagium vivum*) or a derivative of albumen – the
   microzyme was the most commonly assumed. Cf. Robert King of the Middlesex Hospital, who,
   in 1879, said that by giving up the idea that the typhoid poison was a living entity removed
   the objection of its de novo origin. *MTG*, 1879, ii: 119. Dr. Davidson, Chester County Asylum,
   stated that the 'supposed specific germ . . . only exists in the cineritious matter of the brains of
   a few theorists'. *BMJ*, 1880, i: 982.
134 *BMJ*, 1876, i: 659.   135 *BMJ*, 1880, ii: 736.

germ or 'matter from without'.[136] In other words, y represented the different pabula and wastes ('filth') where different germs (z) could develop and become pathogenic before spreading to humans (x). He concluded that there were two duties of sanitary authorities:'first, to remove [and alter] the pabulum "y", upon which "z" is able to increase and multiply . . . [and] second, to prevent the importation of"z", or if it be in our midst alter its nature that it cannot fructify [bear fruit]'. Carpenter was quite happy to play with analogies and said little on the materiality of any of his factors. His approach typified the way living germs were integrated into multifactorial aetiologies – the presence of the 'seeds' was never enough on its own to produce disease. A suitable 'soil' was needed in two senses: environmental conditions in which living germs could develop and spread, and humans who were vulnerable to infection. Either way, he used living-germ theories to support the priority of 'inclusive' sanitarianism over narrow, 'exclusive' measures.

Despite the lower profile of Bastian after his appointment as Physician at University College Hospital, London, and the accommodation offered by Carpenter and others, the controversy over the *de novo* origin of the disease continued. Many MOsH remained worried about the consequences of accepting living-germ theories because of their linkage to 'exclusive' sanitary policies. Dr. Whitgreave, MOH for a rural sanitary district in Nottinghamshire, feared that if the ideas of Tyndall and the germists were correct, 'there would be little necessity to continue efforts to remove nuisances from the neighbourhood of human habitations'.[137] Thomas Walker, a surgeon from Peterborough, observed that the recent drainage and water supply improvements in the town had come about because the doctors in the town had been 'Unanimous in believing and teaching that typhoid fever was to be prevented, not by isolating patients and burning their beds and clothing, etc., but in getting rid of impure water and sewage-polluted atmosphere'.[138] Others warned that saying typhoid fever was contagious would cause the public to panic at any outbreak, lead to cases being hidden and generally make control measures more difficult.[139]

These concerns were made in response to views such as those of Dr. Hudson of Redruth, who had recommended the ideas of Tyndall to his local board of health in 1877:

Adopt the germ view, and you have something definite to guide you in your sanitary precautions. Adopt the pythogenic view, and you have scepticism and silence, if not avowed, opposition from the public who know that the biggest stinks in a parish

136 A. Carpenter, 'On the First Principles of Sanitary Work', *BMJ*, 1879, ii, 643–8; 1880, i: 79; *idem.*, 'The Dual Requirements Which Are Necessary for the Production of Enteric Fever, and a Consideration of the Fallacies Which Are Based upon a Narrow View of the Germ Theory', *BMJ*, 1879, ii: 336–7 *et seq.* Cf. Winslow, *Conquest*, 326.
137 *BMJ*, 1875, i: 486.   138 T. J. Walker, 'Typhoid fever', *BMJ*, 1879: i: 584.
139 *BMJ*, 1881, i: 392.

have not their invariable complement of fever-cases. . . . Destroy the specific germs before they mix with the filth; look on filth as the agent for the dissemination of the poison, not the poison itself, and you are more likely to be rewarded by success.[140]

Brudenell Carter, a medical journalist and ophthalmic surgeon, who supported germ theories of contagion but not sepsis, welcomed the fact that germ aetiologies made life easier for MOsH by giving them more circumscribed tasks.[141] He said that MOsH should, in an ideal world, be 'inclusive', and aim to improve all of the places in which typhoid fever germs or poisons might have arisen; however, in practice, they mostly reacted to control outbreaks as and when they occurred, with their limited powers and resources. In these circumstances, their first task was to identify the homes affected and manage sufferers to prevent the further spread of the disease. This work usually involved some help with treatment, advice on isolation in the home, trying to contain the disease within the family and neighbourhood by attention to discharges, and disinfecting the house and its contents.[142] Alexander Collie, a medical officer at Homerton Infectious Fever Hospital, London, accused those who ignored personal measures as showing 'a masterly inactivity' that was 'practically dangerous to life in as much as it diverts attention from the real sources of danger: viz., the sick person and the sick person's diseased excreta'.[143] The number of MOsH who saw advantages in focusing on the home, family and person-centred work grew. They saw it as the area where MOsH could make a difference, and was closest to their clinical training and other work, remembering that most MOsH were part-time. MOsH only rarely had the influence and support to effect the wide-ranging improvements that the classic sanitarian programme demanded. They tried to turn epidemics to their advantage, but local crises were mostly over too quickly to enable support to be assembled for improvements. Indeed, when sewage systems, water supplies and urban improvement programmes were built, they were more the province of engineers and town clerks, and, as Hamlin has shown, economics and amenity often mattered more than health.[144]

In 1879, William Thomson, MOH for Peterborough and a supporter of the 'ancestral theory', conducted a survey of opinion amongst MOsH of the

140 *BMJ*, 1877, i: 741.
141 'If it could be proved to be true that the zymotic diseases constantly originated anew – that they arose out of certain combinations of favourable conditions, then the work of sanitary reformers, although by no means hopeless, was almost inconceivably more difficult and more arduous.' R. Brudenell-Carter, 'On the Present Possibilities of Sanitary Legislation', *SRec*, 1877, 7: 239.
142 Until the 1890s a mere ten percent of typhoid fever deaths were in fever or isolation hospitals.
143 A. Collie, 'The Etiology of Enteric Fever', *BMJ*, 1879: i, 341.
144 C. Hamlin, 'Muddling in Bumbledon: Local Governments and Large Sanitary Improvements: The Cases of Four British Towns, 1855–1885, *Victorian Studies*, 1988, 32: 55–83.

extent of contagion in typhoid fever outbreaks.[145] He reported that seventy respondents, out of the eighty self-selected MOsH who replied, supported contagion, and that most used isolation and disinfection to prevent the spread of the disease.[146] Contagion was seen to occur in two main ways: directly from person to person via bodily excreta (Farr) and exhalations (Richardson), and indirectly when the poison-germ was carried in water, food, dust and air currents, especially in sewer gas or soil contaminated with faecal matter.[147] The enduring influence of contingent contagionism was evident in the qualifications that were offered, for example, that communicability was affected by the cleanliness of towns, the ventilation of homes and family affinity to the disease.[148] Those maintaining belief in *de novo* origins were a declining minority. On the other hand, contagion was not exclusively associated with living-germ aetiologies, though if MOsH imagined that sufferers were 'a hot-bed swarming with living organisms', then to switch from public to 'private sanitation' became easier.[149]

A new balance of opinion towards contagion and a living-germ theory for typhoid fever was clear in a discussion of the disease at the Public Medicine Section at the BMA in August 1881.[150] However, the nature of any living germ was barely touched upon, being considered 'a question of theoretical rather than practical interest'.[151] Henry Cayley outlined four types of communication: (i) direct person-to-person; (ii) by fresh stools; (iii) from decomposed stools via water and food; and (iv) from decomposed stools by air. While suggesting that the differences were narrow, he said that they were important politically, as MOsH wanted to avoid unnecessary restrictions and worries for the public. These points highlight a neglected aspect of the work of MOsH, the management of public opinion as well as public health. At times of epidemic crisis the task was particularly difficult, as they tried to steer a middle course between panics about contagion and indifference to infection. The public were known to panic with infections such as smallpox, while with other diseases they would be indifferent to warnings. Indeed, many mothers routinely exposed their children to catching diseases, such as measles, in the hope that children would take the disease and acquire immunities. In the control of public opinion, contingent contagionism was a valuable resource, allowing MOsH to reassure the public that the spread of disease was patterned and the efforts of individuals and families could make a difference. When Edward Seaton issued new advice on 'Measures to be taken

---

145 In 1879, the ancestral theory was given the official blessing of the two leading inspectors with the Medical Department, Edward Ballard and George Buchanan.
146 W. Thomson, 'Typhoid Fever: Contagious, Infectious and Communicable', *BMJ*, 1879, i: 343–5.
147 W. Cayley, 'Croonian Lectures', 392.   148 *SRec*, 1882–83, 5: 121.
149 A. G. Davey, 'The Prevention of Enteric Fever', *BMJ*, 1881, ii: 509; C. Cameron, 'Micro-Organisms and Disease', *SRec*, 1881–2, 4: 157.
150 S. F. Murphy, 'The Etiology of Enteric Fever', *BMJ*, 1880, ii: 736.
151 Cayley, 'Croonian Lectures', 391.

when threatened by epidemics' in the Annual Report of the Medical Officer the three main priorities were to focus on the poor as sources and spreaders of infection, remove filth and disinfect filth.[152]

The reports from Klebs in 1880 and Eberth in 1881 that the specific bacillus of typhoid fever had been 'discovered' barely registered in public health medicine in Britain.[153] They were typical of many discovery claims emanating from Continental laboratories. They were reported in the medical press without any comment on their veracity, seemingly as possible additional factors in the multifactorial aetiology of the disease. The new germs were said by germ theorists 'strongly to corroborate' that the development of typhoid fever depended on microorganisms, but it was stressed that there had been no demonstration that the bacilli were the specific cause.[154] Indeed, in reviews of the status of the link between microorganisms and disease in the following years, typhoid fever remained a disease where there was 'meagre evidence' for specific causation by bacteria.[155]

The issue of *de novo* versus the ancestral origin of epidemics was also debated with other zymotic diseases in the 1870s, especially with diphtheria, where the death rate for children was rising.[156] The belief amongst medical practitioners was that diphtheria was a relatively new disease to Britain, having been introduced from France in the 1850s. Experience suggested that it had moved from the countryside to towns, perhaps changing type, becoming most serious in London, where the mortality rate was sixty percent higher than the national average. Diphtheria was separated from scarlet fever in mortality returns from 1861; however, diagnosis was so uncertain that the official returns were understood to be unreliable. Diphtheria began with a sore throat and raised temperature, but developed into blood poisoning and possible complications with the heart, kidneys and nervous system. Its most characteristic feature was the growth of a membrane in the throat that could cause rapid death by asphyxiation. Doctors found it difficult to distinguish early and mild cases from sore throats and croup. Such uncertainties complicated attempts to explain the aetiology of the disease, especially the way in which clusters of mild cases of sore throat developed into local epidemics of diphtheria. If the disease itself was variable, so too might be its causes.

The aetiology of diphtheria was the subject of four enquiries by the Medical Department before 1880. Each pointed to different sets of causes:

---

152 *Supplement to the Eighth Annual Report of the LGB, Containing the Report of the Medical Officer for 1878*, BPP, [C.2452], xxix, 1, Appendix 6.
153 E. Klebs, *Archiv fur experimental Pathologie und Pharmkologie*, 1880, 12, 231; 1881, 13: 232–3, 381. *BMJ*, 1880, ii: 629.
154 'The Bacillus of Typhoid Fever', *BMJ*, 1881, ii: 877–8. C. Eberth, *Virchow's Archiv*, 1880, 81: 58; 1881, 83. Cf. *MTG*, 1882, ii: 385. There is one piece of contrary evidence. The *London Medical Record* in July 1883 said that the first claims of a bacterial etiology in 1881 were first received with 'incredulity'.
155 J. Dreschfeld, 'Micro-organisms in their Relations to Disease', *BMJ*, 1883, ii: 1055.
156 *BMJ*, 1876, i: 131; ii: 804; 1878, ii: 882; 1879, i: 8; 1879, ii: 623; 1881, i: 281.

low-lying places, communicability, soil wetness, filth, sewer gas, the water supply, the seasons and preexisting sore throats. The outcome of these investigations was summed up in 1878 as showing that 'there is no affection the aetiology of which much less is known'.[157] During the 1870s the possibility that diphtheria was caused by a specific contagion was also widely debated, though no clear candidate emerged as the specific cause. The colour, nature and growth of the characteristic membrane in the throat made fungi the most favoured agents; some doctors even thought that the disease was akin to potato blight.[158] Buhl (1867), Oertel (1871) and Klebs (1875) published accounts suggesting that micrococci were specific causes, though there was little interest amongst doctors in using microscopy to identify agents and the absence of bacterial forms became a problem. Yet, this did not stop Pettenkofer-like speculation that the germs of diphtheria altered their virulence with the seasons, outside of the body and in throats.[159]

In May 1877, Sir Thomas Watson published an article in the first volume of the periodical *Nineteenth Century*, entitled 'The Abolition of Zymotic Diseases.'[160] Watson was an elite physician, in his eighty-sixth year, whose *Principles and Practice of Physic* was a leading textbook from the 1840s to the 1870s. Watson's optimism was based on his conviction that all zymotic diseases were caused by living contagia, or, to quote his words, 'more popularly they are called its germs, or, in plain and more accurate English, its "seeds"'. He argued that the way to abolish zymotic diseases was to stop contagia from being spread by the adoption of four measures: notification, isolation, disinfection and preventing importation. His starting point was that medical experience had shown zymotic diseases to be specific and contagious, and that, 'according to the verdict of exact scientific experiment, there is no such thing as spontaneous generation'. Watson identified the *de novo* origin of disease, as endorsed by Murchison and his chemical theories, as the principal obstacle that exclusivists like himself had to overcome. He made extensive use of the smallpox analogy, but mainly relied on epidemiological evidence to show that zymotic diseases were contagious and never arose *de novo*. At no point did he refer to any evidence of laboratory studies of the intimate nature of the 'seeds' of disease. The final element in his argument was to take James Simpson's suggestion of extending the lessons of the control of the cattle plague to smallpox a stage further and apply 'exclusive', personcentred measures to all zymotic diseases; in

157 *BMJ*, 1878, ii: 882; *BMJ*, 1879, ii: 623; *BMJ*, 1880, ii: 747.
158 *BMJ*, 1879, i: 8 and 189; *BMJ*, 1881, i: 281 and 356.
159 Dr. Fussell wrote in 1876 how virulence varied between the homes of the rich and the poor, and in 1881 Dr. Airy reported to the LGB that the 'morbidific agent' was more prevalent in the autumn. *BMJ*, 1867, ii: 826; 1881, i: 281.
160 T. Watson, 'The Abolition of Zymotic Diseases' *Nineteenth Century*, 1877, 1: 380–96. The essay was expanded and published as a book in 1879. Idem, *The Abolition of Zymotic Diseases*, London, Kegan Paul, 1879.

other words, notification, isolation, disinfection and preventing importation. He rejected objections that notification led to stigmatisation and isolation infringed on liberties; instead he chose to portray infected people as dangerous, if not akin to murderers, and a burden on ratepayers. Watson was, of course, typical of the many doctors, MOsH and lay people who had accepted living-germ accounts of zymotic disease, in the absence of accepting any specific organism as the cause of any important human disease.[161] What is difficult for us to grasp, especially with our bacteriological notion of germs as real, living organisms, is that this did not matter in the 1870s. Living germs and their properties were most valuable as a resource for analogical reasoning and deployment in professional and political debates in public health.

While not directly decisive for any disease, the work of laboratory scientists crucially changed the terms of debate on zymotic disease. This was as much for what was not produced as what was. The chemical explanation of fermentation, the key analogue for zymosis, was overturned in chemistry and replaced by a vital process, thereby robbing Murchison's pythogenic theory of its chemical foundation.[162] Richardson's glandular theory, despite his protestations, remained 'theory', as no chemist was able to identify reliably any poisonous bodily secretions and his attempts to paint germs as all-powerful parasites were eroded by the new revelations of the diversity of the microworld. The repeated attacks by scientists on Bastian took their toll on the doctrine of spontaneous generation and, by implication, the *de novo* origin of epidemic diseases. However, he never felt personally defeated, and his relative absence from germ debates after 1878 owed more to his career than any refutation of his position. At the same time, the exploration of the nature and properties of microorganisms became a major research programme in a number of disciplines; and while precise, medically relevant results were few, by 1880, living-germ theories were the most plausible explanation of zymotic disease on the grounds of analogy and experiment. Many older sanitarians were bemused by the new science of germs, but had been drawn into using its language, if not its aetiological and pathological models. The comments of Robert Rawlinson, speaking at the Royal Sanitary Institute in 1880, no doubt summed up the views of many sanitarians when he said, 'I have used the word "germ" as applicable to disease without in the least being enabled to explain satisfactorily what is meant by it'.[163]

161 William Corfield's classes in hygiene at University College in the summer of 1882 were firmly based on living-germ aetiologies, though he still spoke of 'material particles that act like ferments' and full consent to all 'doctrines' was still withheld. WIHM, Western Manuscripts, MS 269. William Halliburton's Lecture Notes.

162 Lyon Playfair acknowledged in 1875 'that long ago he was a strong advocate of the chemical theory of contagion' but that modern research had 'given little support to this view. The very specific character of contagion – its power of reproduction – was an argument in favour of germ theory'. *BMJ*, 1875, ii: 265.

163 Rawlinson, 'Old Lessons', 128.

The growing use and influence of germs by MOsH public health was not only a product of the elaboration and use of new theories of disease. More sophisticated epidemiological investigations had made infectious diseases less capricious, and there was greater confidence that key variables could be identified. In the day-to-day work of local public health bodies there was a greater division of labour, leaving MOsH to concentrate on more 'medical' matters. MOsH were attracted to 'exclusive' measures as they were more targeted and precise, and, to the extent that living germ theories were part of the same package, they bought into it. MOsH were also to speak with greater authority on person-centred matters that were clearly medical and could be associated with the improving ideologies of science and technology. Both of these features were used to enhance the authority and independence of MOsH in their local communities, with their employers and with other medical practitioners. Indeed, as will be shown in Chapter 7, it was this identity of medical modernisers that leading MOsH increasingly adopted and exploited in the 1880s and 1890s.

5

'Deeper Than the Surface of the Wound': Surgeons, Antisepsis and Asepsis, 1876–1900

In his inaugural lecture at King's College Hospital, London, in 1877, Joseph Lister offered his first direct support for living-germ theories of disease to a medical audience in Britain since 1871.[1] His talk was based on his own experiments and concentrated on the point that lactic fermentation was produced by living organisms. The significance of this phenomenon for doctors rested on analogies too familiar to require spelling out. Lister also introduced important techniques and ideas, most notably serial dilution to isolate single microorganisms and his commitment to fixed bacterial species. That said, his experimental style and the issues he raised were closer to early 1870s spontaneous generation work than the new bacteriological and microbiological work emerging in Germany and France. He made no reference to the experimental work with animals that Robert Koch had recently used with anthrax, a disease that Pasteur was also studying. Indeed, when Lister gave a similar talk to the Pathological Society at the end of the year, Koch's work was mentioned only for showing that bacteria could have 'germs', in the sense of spores, not for its new aetiological construction of anthrax as a disease caused by specific bacterial parasites.[2] It is revealing that, ten years after announcing his founding principle, Lister was still trying to convince his metropolitan peers of the reality of germs rather than exploring their role in septic and other diseases. Yet within five years it was being observed that the importance of germs in disease was being overstated, and that in surgery everyone was an antiseptic practitioner. This chapter supports the view of many contemporaries that there was a decisive shift towards surgeons accepting living-germ theories of sepsis and in using antiseptic methods. However, I argue that the theories of sepsis current at the end of the 1870s were distinct from those first articulated by Lister, and that what was practised as antisepsis was a much broader enterprise than old-style Listerism.

The chapter begins with a discussion of what I take to be the catalyst of this transition, William Roberts's Address in Medicine to the BMA in August

1 J. Lister, 'On the Nature of Fermentation', *QJMS*, 1878, 18: 177–94.
2 J. Lister, 'On Lactic Fermentation and its Bearing on Pathology', *TPSL*, 1877, 29: 425–67.

1877.[3] This talk, rather than Lister's lectures, became a reference point for surgeons' thinking on germs and antisepsis. Sanderson articulated similar ideas to those of Roberts in a lecture series over the Christmas period at the end of 1877. They both proposed a crucial modification into antiseptic theory, namely, that 'the principles which underlie the success of the antiseptic treatment are deeper than the surface of the wound'.[4] In other words, they argued that instead of just focusing on combating the 'seeds' of sepsis coming from outside, surgeons had also to consider the human soil in which they might 'germinate' and produce disease. Next I consider the laboratory research on germs and sepsis that informed this revision. There had been many investigations of this question in Britain and elsewhere, but little attention had been paid to these as Listerians emphasised clinical assessments of their practice and finding better ways to kill germs. Ironically, one reason why surgeons became so much more receptive to germ ideas was that, cumulatively, reports from laboratories posed problems for Listerian versions. Lister's opponents welcomed reports that the atmosphere was not full of panspermic germs, that germs were often found in antiseptic dressings, that carbolic acid had limitations as an antiseptic, and that the healthy body had a vital resistance to septic germs. Listerians tried to answer these points with their own findings, but they also rolled with the punches and began to change their practice and the meaning of antiseptic surgery. They made it more inclusive and claimed that it represented an *end* rather than a *means*. In the 1880s they had to contend with organised opposition from the so-called Cleanliness School, who claimed to be able to achieve the end of antisepsis by non-Listerians means. The elaboration of germ theories also produced differences within the Listerian camp, most notably when Lister and his 'bulldog' – William Watson Cheyne – clashed with Alexander Ogston over the role of micrococci in wounds and deep abscesses.[5] This controversy was short-lived and actually helped Listerians become more eclectic in their practice and more explicit about their theories. In the early 1880s it seemed likely that Cheyne and Ogston would become the country's first bacteriologists, but both abandoned germ research for clinical careers and left no followers, leaving surgical bacteriology in Britain to be a largely German import. Given this condition, it was unsurprising that the next challenge to Listerians, aseptic surgery, also came largely from Germany, though there was a distinct British school led by Charles Barrett Lockwood. On this topic I suggest that the powerful position that Listerians occupied in British surgery enabled them once again to

3 W. Roberts, 'The Doctrine of *Contagium vivum* and its Applications to Medicine', *BMJ*, 1877, ii: 168–73.
4 J. B. Sanderson, 'The Infective Processes of Disease', *BMJ*, 1877, ii: 879–81, 913–5; 1878, i: 1–2, 45–7, 119–20, 179–83.
5 C. Lawrence and R. Dixey, 'Practising on Principle: Joseph Lister and the Germ Theories of Disease', in C. Lawrence, ed., *Medical Theory, Surgical Practice*, London, Routledge, 1993, 186–95.

absorb opposition and turn it to their advantage as they accrued the credit for all new methods in surgery and, in fact, for creating a revolution in surgery.

That surgeons and other medical practitioners still needed to be persuaded of the reality of germs and their role in disease in 1877 cannot be doubted. The success of Bastian at the Pathological Society debate in April 1875 and the indifference to germ theories at the Metropolitan Medical Society at the end of that year had been setbacks to germ theorists. These events led John Tyndall to begin new experiments to try to refute spontaneous generation and to enrol Pasteur in his attempts to discredit Bastian.[6] The cause of germ theories and scientific medicine generally was not helped by the introduction of the Cruelty to Animals Act in 1876, which put a brake on the use of animals in investigations of the causes and processes of disease.[7] Klein's 'error' with the typhoid fever micrococci revealed in the spring of 1876 was another blow. Matters worsened during the winter of 1876–77 in the dispute between Tyndall and Sanderson over *contagium viva*.[8] However, the tide had begun to turn at the end of 1876. The second round of the spontaneous generation controversy waned quite quickly, aided by Bastian's effective abandonment of experimental work after his appointment as Physician to University College Hospital in 1878. Support for chemical theories of sepsis and zymosis had also been weakened. However, the key events came in the second half of 1877, following the favourable reception given to talks by William Roberts (see Figure 11) and John Burdon Sanderson, both of whom developed clinically related accounts of the latest germ science and technology.

In 1877, Roberts was a Physician at Manchester Royal Infirmary, whose main interests were in digestive diseases. He had published a number of important papers based on his experimental work on spontaneous generation in the mid-1870s and had stood out against the doctrine.[9] Sanderson

6 J. E. Strick, *The British Spontaneous Generation Debates of 1860–1880: Medicine, Evolution and Laboratory Science in the Victorian Context*, Unpublished PhD Thesis, Princeton University, 1997.

7 R. D. French, *Antivivisection and Medical Science in Victorian Society*, Princeton, NJ, Princeton University Press, 1975.

8 J. B. Sanderson, 'Contagium Vivum', *PH*, 1877, 7: 59–63; J. Tyndall, 'Notes on Dr Burdon Sanderson's Views on Ferments and Germs', *PRSL*, 1877, 26: 353–6, 354. Tyndall quotes Sanderson as saying that ferments 'occupy the borderland between living and non-living things' and might be regarded as 'molecular aggregates'. For Sanderson's reply, see: Ibid., 416–26. *Lancet*, i: 1877, 691–3, 692. Also see correspondence between Tyndall and Sanderson, 20 May 1877 and 21 May 1877. UCL, Sanderson Papers, Add 179/3, 1–5. This whole episode was seized upon by Bastian to suggest that Sanderson was supporting spontaneous generation.

9 Roberts was qualified in both surgery and medicine, and his interests in physiology took him to Paris and Berlin. He worked at the Manchester Royal Infirmary from 1854 to 1883, and taught

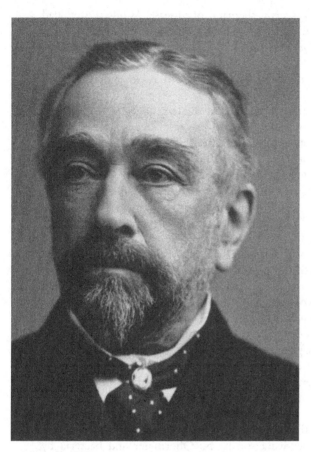

Figure 11. William Roberts (Reproduced by courtesy of the Wellcome Institute Library, London)

was, by this time, Professor of Physiology at University College, London, with interests moving away from zymotic diseases and towards heart diseases. Roberts's address in the summer of 1877 was initially entitled 'On the doctrine of contagium vivum and its applications in medicine', but was subsequently published with a significant new title, *On Spontaneous Generation and the Doctrine of Contagium Vivum*.[10] The address provided evidence and ideas that were subsequently used by all sides in the debates about the merits of

at Owens College. After working on spontaneous generation in the 1870s, he became well known for his studies of digestive ferments and the dietary treatment of disease. See: D. J. Leech, *The Life and Works of Sir William Roberts*, Manchesker, no date.

10 W. Roberts, *On Spontaneous Generation and the Doctrine of Contagium Vivum*, Manchester, Cornish, 1877.

antiseptic surgery and living-germ theories of disease. While Lister had attacked spontaneous generation by implication, Roberts was dismissive. He offered counterevidence from his own experiments and used the heat-resistance of bacterial spores to develop a naturalistic explanation of purported instances of the phenomenon in the laboratory and *de novo* outbreaks of disease. He spoke of the two germ theories: Beale's bioplasm theory (which he associated with the 'graft theory' of his Manchester colleague, James Ross) and the living-germ theory of Pasteur. As his first title suggests, Roberts was attracted by the notion that all zymotic infections, contagious, infectious and septic, were due to *contagium viva*. He was also attracted to analogies with parasitic diseases. Throughout his talk he used the word 'germ' sparingly, pre-ferring to speak of 'minute organisms', 'bacteria' and 'saprophytes'. Indeed, he believed that the adoption of the distinction between bacteria and germs, in the sense of the spores of bacteria, would remove a lot of confusion. The term 'germ-theory' remained in professional and popular use, though more and more it was understood as the 'bacterial theory of the disease', with these agents seen to be saprophytic or parasitic organisms. Roberts was not the only one trying to link germ-theory with parasitism; Thomas MacLagan explored the idea in his volume *The Germ Theory* in 1876, as did John Drysdale in his *The Germ Theories of Infectious Diseases* in 1878.[11]

In the last part of his paper Roberts illustrated the role of *contagium viva* in disease by reference to septicaemia, relapsing fever and anthrax. His evidence on septicaemia relied on Sanderson's work on septic poisons and on the clinical success of Listerism. Roberts made no mention of the direct microscopical observations of the pathogenic bacteria, implicitly endorsing Tyndall's and Sanderson's views on the limitations of microscopy. However, with relapsing fever and anthrax, he relied almost wholly on direct micro-scopic identification of, respectively, spirilla by Obermeier and bacteria by 'Davaine, Bollinger, Tiegel, Klebs, and, most of all, Koch'.[12] Roberts showed drawings of the 'dots', 'rods', 'oval bodies' and 'threads' observed by Koch and briefly outlined his methods of artificial cultivation and inoculation. For further evidence of the role of specific contagia in diseases such as vaccinia, smallpox, sheep-pox, diphtheria, erysipelas and glanders, Roberts referred his audience, not to Koch and continental work, but to the reports of Peter Braidwood and Frances Vacher.[13] Roberts concluded his address with

11 T. J. Maclagan, *The Germ Theory Applied to the Explanation of the Phenomenon of Disease*, London, 1876; J. J. Drysdale, *The Germ Theories of Infectious Diseases*, Liverpool, Baillière, Tindall and Cox, 1878. Drysdale was known in the 1870s for his work with Dallinger on the life history of micro-organisms. In the 1840s, he had been editor of the *British Journal of Homoeopathy* and published the *Hahneman Materia Medica* in 1852.

12 Sanderson observed that, despite all of the efforts made, the germs of only two diseases had been identified: relapsing fever and anthrax. *BMJ*, 1875, i: 199.

13 Peter Braidwood and Frances Vacher published a series of literature reviews on what they called the 'Life History of Contagion'. Their work was supported over a number of years by grants for

speculation on bacterial variability and parasitism, seeking a Darwinian explanation of the difference between septic and infectious diseases in a unified germ-theory. He suggested that some species of contagia were subject to 'variation or sporting', while others were more stable.[14] He speculated that sepsis was due to simple, little evolved organisms that could only develop in dead tissue, and that these organisms were successful because they could grow in any organism after death; that is, they were *saprophytes*. Against this, specific infections were due to more complex and powerful organisms, which through variation had become specific parasites and were evolved only to develop in the living tissues of a particular species or groups of organisms; that is, they were *pathophytes*.

In his discussion of septicaemia, Roberts made an observation on aetiology that was seized upon time and time again by surgeons:

[C]ontact of the septic germs with the dead tissues never fails to produce successful septic inoculation. But it is quite otherwise with the same tissues when alive and forming part of our bodies. You cannot successfully inoculate the healthy tissues with septic bacteria. . . . The healthy living tissues are an unsuitable soil for them; they cannot grow in it; or, to put it another way, ordinary septic bacteria are not parasitic on the living tissues. . . . for we find no traces of them in the healthy blood and healthy tissues'.[15]

He went on, in what became the most quoted part of his lecture, to comment on the controversy over Lister's ideas and methods:

We should probably differ less about the antiseptic treatment if we took a broader view of its principle. We are apt to confound the principle of the treatment with Lister's method of carrying out. The essence of the principle, it appears to me, is not exactly to protect the wound from the septic organism, but *to defend the patient against the septic poison*. Defined in this way, I believe that every successful method of treating wounds will be found to conform to the antiseptic principle and that herein lies the secret of the favourable results of modes of treatment which at first sight appear to be in contradiction of the antiseptic principle'. [Italics in original]

Thus, it could be argued that the open method 'worked' by allowing the rapid escape of the septic poison or that it simply dried out, that cleanliness 'worked' by removing the poison, that washing with water 'worked' as it diluted the concentration of poisons and that rest and older antiphlogistic

scientific investigations from the BMA. Vacher was MOH for Birkenhead. See: P. M. Braidwood and F. Vacher, 'First Contribution to the Life History of Contagion', *BMJ*, 1875, ii (Suppl.): 18–25; *idem.*, 'Third Contribution to the Life History of Contagion, *BMJ*, 1882, i: 41–3, 77–9, 107–13, 143–6, 181–4, 219–22, 257–68.

14 Roberts felt that some of these variations would revert to their original type, while others, on finding a new parasitic niche, would keep their new form. Cf. W. F. Bynum, 'Darwin and the Doctors: Evolution, Diathesis and Germs in Nineteenth Century Britain', *Gesnerus*, 1983, 40: 43–53.

15 Roberts, 'Doctrine', 171.

methods 'worked' by strengthening the patient's constitution.[16] It is significant that it was a physician rather than a surgeon who first broadened what
counted as 'antiseptic', and to argue directly that sepsis was a product of the
interaction between internal and external forces.

Sanderson's Christmas lectures reflected his recent visit to Germany and
his recent differences with Tyndall.[17] Like Roberts, he also gave a detailed
account of Koch's anthrax work and, for the first time in a medical journal,
reproduced drawings of the anthrax bacillus and its spores. However, he spoke
at greatest length on septicaemia, acknowledging what everyone concerned
had long known, namely, that every antiseptic operation could be regarded
as analogous to 'one of Professor Tyndall's or M. Pasteur's experiments on
spontaneous generation'.[18] Sanderson maintained that septic infection was
produced by poisons produced by bacteria, and that such organisms could
not develop and produce their poisons in healthy tissues. He also spoke of
'two pathological theories': 'the theory of *contagium vivum* and the germ-
theory'.[19] What he termed the 'germ-theory' related to inflammations and
surgical injuries, while *contagium vivum* involved 'the intervention of living
organisms – microphytes . . . in the communication of specific diseases from
diseased to healthy individuals'. He said pointedly that the two theories were
often 'wrongly conflated', but he did not say who had done this or with
what consequences.

SEPSIS AND GERM RESEARCHES, 1871–1879

Although renowned as a laboratory researcher, Sanderson observed in his
Christmas lecture series that the best evidence for the germ-theory was still
the effectiveness of Listerism. Judging Listerism by its results rather than its
rationale had become a common ploy amongst its supporters. It was one way
of avoiding the surgeon's no-go area of theory and the anomalies emerging
from clinical and laboratory research. The disputes over the statistical results
of different practices were protracted, and the Listerian cause was not helped
by the variety and changes in the methods used. However, Listerians also
faced worrying laboratory findings, including reports of germs being found
in healthy tissues, studies that showed that germs in the air were less numer-

---

16 James Spence, an Edinburgh colleague of Lister and doubter of his methods, told an audience in
   December 1877 that 'there was no surgeon now who did not treat on "an antiseptic plan".' He
   believed that a wound treated by the open method was as antiseptic as those treated in a special
   manner, since the putrefactive discharges were allowed free exit. *EMJ*, 1877–78, 23: 550–4, 550.
17 Sanderson, 'Infective Processes', *passim*.
18 Ibid., 180. An editorial in the *BMJ* in 1876 had observed that 'Professor Tyndall's experiments
   are of immense force in confirming the value and importance of the such precautions as are
   involved in Professor Lister's antiseptic practice'. *BMJ*, 1976, i: 138. Sanderson made the reverse
   point, that Lister had introduced laboratory 'exactitude and cleanliness' into patient care. See: *PH*,
   1877, 7: 61.
19 Sanderson, 'Infective Processes', 179.

ous and malign than panspermism required, accounts of germs being found in antiseptic wound dressings and that germs were 'tenacious of life' and actually able to survive in carbolic acid solutions. Many of these problems had been around since the early 1870s, and a number had actually emerged from Sanderson's researches for the Medical Department. As long as Listerism was represented as an innovation in practice rather than theory, such issues were disregarded, but in the late 1870s they were given new significance by the changing terms of the debate on germs in sepsis.

Sanderson had been publishing on the physiology and pathology of sepsis since the early 1870s, when his work had supported Lister's claims that healthy tissues were germless and that septic mischief always came from without.[20] However, the idea of germ-free healthy tissues was challenged in 1875 by Tiegel and Billroth in Germany, and by Walter Moxon (b. 1836) and James F. Goodhart (1845–1910) of Guy's Hospital, London.[21] This led Sanderson to take up the problem again and to develop new ideas.[22] The position he had adopted by the end of 1877 was that blood and muscle might briefly harbour septic bacteria, but that they were unable to survive due to the 'antibiotic' properties of blood – be that its alkalinity, oxygen level or by the 'struggle for existence between the blood-corpuscles and the bacteria'.[23] John Chiene, of the Edinburgh Royal Infirmary, and John Cossar Ewart, of University College, London, published a paper in April 1878 that confirmed the germlessness of healthy tissues but accepted that there were exceptions, for example, in diseased organs (e.g. bladders in cystitis) and in the digestive system, which was beginning to be pictured as a dangerous germ-ridden sewer running through the body.[24] Their suggestion was that the liver and mucous membranes normally acted as, respectively, internal and external barriers to the entry of germs, and that any germs that made it through these portals were killed by the vital resistance of the blood. Chiene and Ewart were clear about what was at stake, saying that 'If the wound is liable to contamination from within, Lister's system of treatment is comparatively useless'.

Another earlier and troubling finding that had reemerged in the late 1870s was that ordinary air was not loaded with septic germs. As early as 1871, the year in which Lister introduced the spray, Sanderson had speculated that if

20 J. B. Sanderson, 'Preparation Showing the Results of Certain Experimental Inquiries Relating to the Nature of the Infective Agent in Pyaemia', *TPSL*, 1872, 23: 303–8. Cf., Anon, 'Traumatic Fever and Purulent Infection', *BFM-CR*, 1873, 53:43–60.

21 W. Moxon and J. F. Goodhart, 'Observations on the Presence of Bacteria in the Blood and Infective Products of Septic Fever and the "Cultivation" of Septicaemia', *Guy's Hospital Reports*, 1875, 20: 229–60. Moxon and Goodhart reviewed the work of Billroth and Tiegel.

22 J. B. Sanderson, 'The Occurrence of Organic Forms in Connection with Contagious and Infective Diseases', *BMJ*, 1875, i: 69–71, 199–200, 403–5.

23 *BMJ*, 1878, i: 120.

24 J. Chiene and J. C. Ewart, 'Do Bacteria or their Living Germs Exist in the Organs of Healthy Animals?', *Journal of Anatomy and Physiology*, 1878, 12: 448–53.

germs were tiny living organisms, they would be easily killed by drying in air currents. Thus, he suggested that they would have to be conveyed to wounds by moisture, or introduced directly into wounds from germ-carrying objects.[25] It was this querying of the role of airborne germs that led Lister to undertake his own experimental investigations and publications on fermentative and putrefactive agents.[26] One of the weaknesses of Listerism as a practice was its seeming vulnerability to the entry of a single germ, though Listerians had tried to use this to their advantage, arguing that the potency of the threat reinforced the need for ritual attention to detail. However, critics continued to ask what good was a wound treatment that was so easily undone. Continuing experience of success by some surgeons with the open treatment and the healing of untreated wounds in wild and domestic animals was further ammunition against panspermism. Attempts to find germs in the air and to determine the levels of 'aerial sewage' largely failed. And even if they had succeeded, investigators would have faced the same problems of interpretation as water analysts had with their findings.[27] When Sanderson returned to this question in 1878, he was quite clear that germs did not just fall into wounds from the air, being far too few and fragile; rather, they mainly came from other diseased sources and had to be 'introduced' into the body.[28]

Most alarming of all to Listerians were reports of germs in antiseptic dressings themselves, which supported other evidence on the limitations of carbolic acid as an antiseptic.[29] Indeed, the reports of germs in carbolic acid dressings prompted Cheyne, then Lister's house surgeon, to begin research on wound pathology in 1876. After three years' work, he came up with two answers to this troubling phenomenon. The first and most predictable was that it was due to poor technique, for example, carbolic acid solutions being made up wrongly or applied unevenly. His second and more surprising conclusion was that there was nothing to worry about, as any germs surviving in properly dressed antiseptic wounds were harmless micrococci. His views were set out in detail in a

25 J. B. Sanderson, 'Further Report on the Intimate Pathology of Contagion', *Thirteenth Report of the Medical Officer of the Privy Council for 1870*, BPP, 1871, [C349], xxxi, 48. Also see: J. B. Sanderson, 'The Origin of Bacteria', *QJMS*, 1871, 11: 323.

26 J. Lister, 'A Contribution to the Germ Theory of Putrefaction and other Fermentative Changes, and the Natural History of Torulae and Bacteria', *TRSE*, 1875, 27: 313–44. Sanderson's work was noted by Ferdinand Cohn in 1872. See: F. Cohn, 'Bacteria and their Relations to Putrefaction and Contagion'; *QJMS*, 1872, 12: 208.

27 C. Hamlin, *A Science of Impurity: Water Analysis in Nineteenth Century Britain*, Bristol, Adam Hilger, 1990.

28 Sanderson said in 1877 that the 'Dangers from infection . . . are of *pathological* not *meteorological*, origin', 'Infective Processes', 180. His notion that bacteria were not the direct cause of septic infection was widely quoted. This left bacteria to be either the carriers of infection or the producers of septic poisons. See the ideas of the Manchester surgeon: S. M. Bradley, *Lancet*, 1876, i: 768–9.

29 Bastian had argued this as early as 1871. H. C. Bastian, 'Epidemic and Specific Contagious Diseases: Considerations as to Their Nature and Mode of Origin, *BMJ*, 1871, ii: 400–9.

WOODCUT 18.

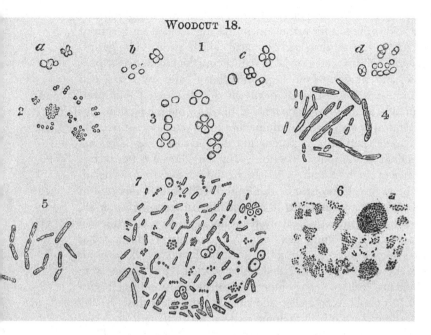

Figure 12. The drawings from Cheyne's paper on micrococci and bacteria in antiseptic wounds published in May 1879. (1a–d) Drawings were copied from Lister's 1875 paper, 'The Germ Theory of Putrefaction', and show micrococci as seen under the microscope. (2) Micrococci from an antiseptically treated wound growing in cucumber infusions, which demonstrated that micrococci were not necessarily killed by carbolic acid. (3) Micrococci growing in cucumber infusions containing carbolic acid, making the same point as above. (4 and 5) 'Forms of bacteria injected into animals, causing death'. (6) A drawing of 'the discharge from a wound treated antiseptically'. It is important to note the absence of rod-shaped bacteria. (7) The organisms that ordinarily grew on cucumber infusions that were not treated antiseptically. The point being made here is the number of bacterial forms compared to drawing 3. W. W. Cheyne. 'On the Relation of Organisms to Antiseptic Dressings', *TPSL*, 30: 1879: 569. (Reproduced by courtesy of the Director and University Librarian, The John Rylands University Library of Manchester)

paper read to the Pathological Society in May 1879 (see Figure 12).[30] He argued that a distinction had to be made between bacteria and micrococci: the former were pathogenic and were killed by carbolic acid; the latter were nonpathogenic, and hence it did not matter that they survived in antiseptic

30 W. W. Cheyne, 'On the Relation of Organisms to Antiseptic Dressings', *TPSL*, 1879, 30: 557–82, 569. Pleomorphism was used to explain the presence of germs in healthy tissue with the proposition that they only became pathogenic in altered conditions. An editorial in the *Medical Times and Gazette* accepted Cheyne's ideas, but worried that if micrococci could find their way into

solutions. He was engaged in a nice piece of circular reasoning, using vulnerability to carbolic acid as the test for pathogenicity, having decided a priori from
the experience of Listerism that carbolic acid killed pathogenic germs.
Nonetheless, Cheyne's points were crucial in reinforcing the link between 'bacteria' and disease, and showing how important 'form', and even size, had
become in germ research. Interestingly, Cheyne cited Koch's 1878 publications
on the role of different forms of micrococci in traumatic wound infections, but
only for their technical innovations in staining and microscopy. He missed the
point that they contradicted his conclusions and showed that parasitic micrococci caused specific types of septic infections. Why did Cheyne fail to recognise the significance of Koch's findings? Perhaps he did not read them in detail,
though he was the eventual translator of the English edition that appeared in
1880. Perhaps Koch's results seemed to have little clinical relevance; after all,
his experiments were on mice and involved producing infection artificially
by inoculating septic material into the body. The experiments showed that
different animals had differing susceptibilities to particular micrococci, a point
that could have encouraged Cheyne's belief that not all septic germs were
pathogenic to humans. Perhaps it was simply that micrococci were not 'bacteria', and seemed too small, structureless and nonparasitic? Of course, Koch's
findings had no essential meaning; different readers, with different cognitive
assumptions and different interests, constructed different meanings. Thus,
a major investigation of pyaemia by four of Britain's leading pathologists
in 1878–79 also mentioned Koch's technical innovations and work but saw no
significance at all for their study, which was mainly on the morbid anatomy
of the disease.[31]

Assumptions about micrococci were also influenced by the idea that they
were merely the spores or degenerate forms of bacteria and not organisms
in their own right.[32] Improved magnification and staining techniques showed
that micrococci had little or no 'structure'. They were presented as mere 'dots'
and 'circles', seemingly too small and physiologically feeble to be pathogenic
in such a large creature as humans. They were, as Klein had found with
typhoid fever, easily mistaken for other things. As pleomorphism went out of
favour, 'form' mattered more and more in germ research. Indeed, the demonstration of the life cycle of the anthrax bacillus, which was parasite-like in its
elaborate change of forms, set new standards for microorganisms to qualify
as serious contenders for the status of disease-germs.[33] One of the most

Mr. Lister's carefully dressed wounds, what organisms might find their way into those dressed by
less scrupulous surgeons? *MTG*, 1879, i: 565.
31 Koch's monograph on septic infection was translated by Cheyne and published in Britain in early
1881. R. Koch, *Investigations into the Etiology of Traumatic Infective Diseases*, (trans. by W. W. Cheyne),
London: New Sydenham Society, 1880.
32 L. G. Wilson, 'The Early Recognition of Streptococci as Causes of Disease', *MH*, 1987, 31: 403–13.
33 J. C. Ewart, 'The Life History of the Bacillus Anthracis', *QJMS*, 1878, 18: 161. Also see: J. C. Ewart,
'The Life History of Bacterium termo and Micrococcus, with Further Observations on Bacillus',
PSRL, 1878, 27: 474–85.

persuasive features of Koch's work was how the size, complex life-forms and reproductive powers of the anthrax bacillus were readily correlated with the clinical symptoms and the aetiology of the disease.

VITAL RESISTANCE: SEED AND SOIL, 1877–1879

Many surgeons continued to ignore the new work on germ theories, but this seems increasingly to have been a rhetorical gesture as part of their stance as practical men and unreconstituted empiricists.[34] More significantly, surgeons of all persuasions began to use the newly accessible knowledge of bacteria and their likely actions to explain and legitimate a variety of practices. The 'germ controversy' was said to be a diversion 'from the far more important point of how to remove from the tissues the materials of putrefaction, without which we may be sure that germs (if germs there be) would prove innocuous'.[35] Living-germ theories were no longer presented by their supporters as an alternative to the chemical theory; they were part of it – bacteria were the manufacturers of septic poisons. However, what surgeons used most was the notion from Roberts and Sanderson that germs did not always produce disease. Whether this was due to the type of bacteria, or the absence of a suitable *nidus,* or some other factor, the conclusions were the same: Lister's simple contamination model of sepsis was inadequate. Lister remarked in 1879 that 'Some years ago, he had pointed out that healthy tissues had a power of resisting the development of minute organisms, but that enfeebled tissues had no longer this power'. However, few surgeons seem to have heard him, as the notion that germs did not always interfere with health was said in a *BMJ* editorial in response to Cheyne's work to be a 'startling conviction'.[36]

The use of newer germ theories against Lister was pivotal in perhaps the last set-piece attack on his system by an elite metropolitan surgeon, William Scovell Savory (1826–95), at the Annual Meeting of the BMA in August 1879.[37] Savory first visited familiar ground by objecting to the exclusivity of Listerians and their rejection of other methods. He surprised many in his audience by accepting that the antiseptic system was based on 'a sound theory', but went on to say that it was 'imperfect in practice'.[38] His main

---

34 A review of antiseptic surgery in the Birmingham Medical Review in 1878, said that it was unnecessary for surgeons to believe in germs, as Listerism could be judged by its results – or, as the reviewer put it, 'A tree can always be known by its fruit.' *BMR,* 1878, 7: 225–36.
35 *BMJ,* 1878, ii: 224.   36 *BMJ,* 1878, ii: 172; 1879, ii: 782.
37 W. Savory, 'Address in Surgery', *BMJ,* 1879, ii: 210–17. Godlee describes this as 'the swan-song of the already dwindling race' of opponents of Listerism. R. J. Godlee, *Lord Lister,* Oxford: Clarendon Press, 1924, 323. Norman Moore stated that Savory's 1879 declaration against Listerism 'will always be interesting as the last public expression by a prominent surgeon of opposition to the now universally accepted methods of modern surgery'. W. MacCormac, *Centenary Festival of the Royal College of Surgeons of England and Short Biographical Accounts of Each Master and President,* London, Ballantyne Hanson, 1900, 204.
38 Editorial, 'Mr Savory's Address in Surgery', *MTG,* 1879, ii: 187. Opposition to Lister seems not to have harmed Savory's practice, as in the early 1880s he was estimated to earn £2,000 per

point was that Listerians gave too much attention to the 'external' cause of sepsis and not enough to the 'internal' conditions, that is, how the general health of tissues determined whether any septic material was absorbed into the body and the degree of mischief produced.[39] Thus, he said,

Allowing the principle to be sound, the antiseptic system only attacks the question from one side; but on the other hand, if a wound be maintained in a perfectly healthy condition, and all discharges be allowed to escape freely, the danger of absorption of putrid elements is minimised'.[40]

Roberts's address was evoked to support his claim that less exclusive methods now took 'most cognisance of all the facts before us'.[41] In the same year, Sampson Gamgee noted how Lister feared the 'ubiquity and the potency of Pasteur's germs', while Savory had been comfortable with vibrios because of his confidence in other means of combating them.[42] To support his anti-Listerian views, Gamgee drew upon the authority of none other than Lister himself. He claimed that in the autumn of 1878, during a visit to Birmingham, Lister had made a 'very large concession', namely, 'that the healthy tissues have the power of preventing the development of bacteria in their vicinity'.[43] Lister's talk to the Midland Medical Society was on 'Healing Wounds without Antiseptic Treatment', but disappointingly there is no published version.[44] Gamgee asked, if wounds can be healed in strong healthy bodies without antiseptics, why pursue the 'hit and miss' methods of trying to kill bacteria in the air and the wound, rather than the certain path of helping the whole body resist sepsis? Gamgee championed rest as an alternative to what he termed 'carbolism', claiming that not moving affected parts of the body allowed vital energies to be channelled into healing.[45] He saw the constant changes of dressings in Listerian methods as interrupting rest and nature's ways of healing, and felt that such methods were best confined to the management of a wound already filled with dead tissue and pus. Disingenuously, he suggested that perhaps in this latter and limited area of surgery, 'a special triumph will be reserved for Professor Lister's treatment'.[46]

annum, making him probably the highest paid surgeon in London. He became surgeon to the Queen, and was made Baronet in 1890.

39 BMJ, 1879, ii: 906, 1000–2. Savory favoured scrupulous cleanliness and detailed variations on this theme for different types of tissues, wounds and patients, but he insisted that on its own these would never be enough. In addition, there had to be pure air, hence ventilation and the avoidance of overcrowding, plus the patient had to rest and have their general health maintained.

40 'Mr Savory's Address', 187. Some of the leading opponents to Listerism, for example, Callender and Savory, were opponents of reform of the Royal College of Surgeons that would have opened up membership to rank-and-file doctors and undermined existing hierarchies.

41 BMJ, 1879, ii 216. For replies to Savory, cast in terms of germ-theory, see: Ibid., 446–8.

42 S. Gamgee, 'On Wound Treatment', Lancet, 1879, ii: 342–8, 456–8.

43 Ibid., 457; also see: S. Gamgee, 'On Wound Treatment', Lancet, 1878, ii: 869–71, 871.

44 BMR, 1879, 8: 106. Lister spoke on 30 October 1878.

45 T. H. Bartleet, 'The Treatment of Wounds', BMR, 1878, 7, 166–78.

46 Lancet, 1879, ii: 457.

In the 1880s, Savory was the first champion of the what became known as the Cleanliness School of surgeons, a group opposed to Listerians' methods who claimed to be able to achieve the same end of sepsis-free surgery by other means. The other leading members were Lawson Tait, Timothy Holmes, Sampson Gamgee and Thomas Bryant.[47] Gamgee even suggested that there were 'two camps' in British surgery and that they were 'more widely asunder' than ever.[48] However, the Listerians adoption of the seed and soil model brought the two sides closer together. By 1879, both camps accepted that germs caused sepsis, but they differed over the circumstances and what to do to prevent it. For example, Tait agreed that 'the germ-theory was substantiated' for putrefactive changes but emphasised that there was no evidence that germs could produce putrefaction in the healthy human body – a point that Lister could make.[49] Tait maintained an absolute distinction between dead and living tissues, and wrote that 'he cared not a fig for germs' as his surgical methods removed 'any nest for germs to breed in'.[50] He rejected the germ-killing preoccupation of old-style Listerism as inefficient and damaging to the body. He preferred to ensure that there was no soil on which germs could grow, to reduce their numbers by absolute cleanliness and to work with nature rather than use artificial methods.

The month after Savory's attack, Lister was lionised by Europe's medical and surgical elite at the International Medical Congress in Amsterdam.[51] However, Lister chose not to revel in the accolades, but instead dwelt on the opposition that he faced at home on several fronts: spontaneous generation, pleomorphism, germs in antiseptic dressings and vital resistance. The following brief report of the address nicely sums up the issues that were troubling him:

47 A. Greenwood, 'Lawson Tait and Opposition to Germ Theory: Defining Science in Surgical Practice', *JHM*, 1998, 53: 99–131. Tait joined Holmes and Savory in speaking against the method and theory of Listerism at the Royal Medical and Chirurgical Society in December 1880. See *BMJ*, 1880, ii: 976. Tait's standing with his fellow surgeons was not high. *MTG*, 1881, ii: 659.
48 Gamgee, 'Wound Treatment', 342. Cf. L. Granshaw, '"Upon this Principle I Have Based a Practice": The Development of Antisepsis in Britain, 1867–90', in J. V. Pickstone, ed., *Medical Innovation in Historical Perspective*, London, Macmillan, 1992, 40.
49 *MTG*, 1880, i: 246.
50 Tait's distinction between dead and living tissue was dismissed on clinical grounds by William Stokes, who observed that 'those who hold this view ignore the elementary fact that there never was a wound, and especially one in which vessels are tied and twisted [i.e. an operative wound], in which dead and living tissue were not at once brought into contact'. *BMJ*, 1882, ii: 258. Also see: *Lancet*, 1876, i: 768–9, and *BMJ*, 1887, ii: 169.
51 A correspondent to the *Lancet* in 1878, who called himself Flaneur (i.e. Idler), noted how Listerism had been 'eagerly adopted by the scientific Germans, and a little grudgingly by the semi-scientific Scotch', while it had 'never been in any degree appreciated by the plodding and practical English surgeon'. However, Flaneur's conclusion was that this had been no disadvantage as the English surgeons had for a long time been 'practising a partially antiseptic system, thanks to his cleanly English habits'. *Lancet*, 1878, i: 36. This repeated the old observation that it was only 'dirty' continental hospitals that saw benefits from Listerism.

[Lister] briefly set forth the scientific basis on which the theory rests, describing the simple means by which urine freshly passed and protected from the admission of septic germs may be indefinitely preserved without undergoing change; he referred to his experiments on the specificity of the bacterium concerned with lactic fermentation, by way of part answer to those who object that certain bacteria not known to be specific may be found beneath antiseptic dressings; and on this subject, more particularly to Mr Watson Cheyne's recent researches on the bacteria of wounds; to those who allege favourable results without antiseptic precautions as a reason for putting them aside, he replied by giving reasons for believing that living animal tissues in sound states do oppose the pullulation [germination] of specific or septic bacteria. . . .[52]

On the latter point Lister separated this type of vital resistance from the constitutional measures favoured by other surgeons.[53] He admitted that those who complained that he neglected the condition of the patient were correct, as 'questions of diathesis were not so much neglected by the antiseptic surgeon; they were rather removed out of the way'. He was making two points. First, if there were no germs, then the vitality or the state of tissues was irrelevant; but second, it was the condition of the local tissues immediately surrounding the wound that mattered, not the general health of the patient. With clinical audiences, Lister maintained that he did all he could for the patient and never neglected constitutional measures, though his clinical work was directed at the local management of the wound and the surrounding tissues.[54] Thus, when it came to explaining septic infection, Listerians were no longer happy to be seen as simple contaminationists; they wanted to be 'contingent contaminationists', having reshaped their theory in terms of the metaphor of seed and soil.[55]

ANTISEPTIC THEORY, 1879–1881

In 1879 Jonathan Hutchison claimed that 'all surgeons were in these days antiseptic'.[56] What he meant by this was not that all surgeons had become strict 'spray and gauze' Listerians, but rather that all surgeons now aimed to achieve the end of antisepsis, albeit by different means.[57] The Listerians' appropriation of the 'antiseptic' had always given them an advantage, as no opponent would want to advocate its opposite – 'septic surgery'. All surgeons might be said to have become Listerians in two senses: first, wound management had become a more important part of surgeons' work and was no longer delegated to dressers; and second, it seems that most surgeons

52 *BMJ*, 1879, ii: 454.
53 See the summary of the principles of antiseptic treatment by Cheyne in *BMJ*, 1879, ii: 860.
54 *BMJ*, 1879, ii: 782.
55 S. M. Bradley, 'The Prevention of Blood Poisoning', *BMJ*, 1879, ii: 446.
56 *Lancet*, 1879, ii: 922.
57 H. Pennington, 'Osteotomy as an Indicator of Antiseptic Surgical Practice', *MH*, 1994, 38: 178–88.

used some adaptation of Listerian methods, to some degree, in some cases.[58] Thus, Listerism was no longer understood as a fixed menu to be rigidly followed; it was now available á la carte and in cut-price versions.[59]

This shift in the meaning of antiseptic surgery was evident at a meeting of the Metropolitan Counties Branch Meeting of the BMA in December 1879 that featured Lister's first domestic response to Savory's summer offensive and the renewed criticisms of Timothy Holmes.[60] The meeting was dominated by claims and counterclaims over the success of different methods, and whether statistics were the best way to judge the effectiveness of surgical procedures. Lister set out his own results, but he went on to the surprise of many to introduce a new 'principle'. This was the ability of living tissues to replace or absorb dead matter in a way that 'I had never before supposed possible'.[61] He noted that many surgeons recognised that separated pieces of liver and bone could be absorbed or 'organised' by adjacent living tissue. He now linked this process to the observation that carbolised catgut, the standard ligature used by Listerians, was also 'organised'. The important 'principle' was that the absorption of ligatures was the result of an active biological process, not a chemical or physical one, where they were merely dissolved. Lister regretted that he had not brought this to the attention of his colleagues earlier with sufficient force and he now recommended, in a leap of logic that few would have followed, that Mr. Holmes should try carbolised catgut ligatures and then 'he might see something in the germ-theory'.[62] So what had the absorption of a catgut ligature to do with germ-theory? First, it showed the importance of biological over chemical processes in wound healing; second, it showed that carbolised materials did not inhibit normal physiological processes; and third, it highlighted the distinction between living and dead tissues – the latter could not 'organise'. In responding to his critics, Lister had been led to construct an account of events in wounds that went beyond the contamination and poisoning model that had become the trademark of Listerism. However, not just the theory changed, its ideology also shifted. The central aim remained keeping germs out of wounds, but Listerism was now portrayed as an adjunct to natural healing. While it was still important to keep germs at bay, this was not to be done at all costs. This was because surgeons had to rely to some extent on the 'vital resistance' of healthy tissues and had to be careful that their antiseptic methods did not damage this in any way.

58 W. Thomson, 'Blood Poisoning and Antiseptics', *BMJ*, 1879, ii: 446–8, 851. T. H. Bartleet, 'Inaugural Address', *BMR*, 1881, 10: 223.

59 G. T. Beatson, 'Some Remarks on the Exciting Causes of Expense in the Antiseptic Treatment of Surgical Cases, *GMJ*, 1879, 11: 440–51.

60 'The Debate on Antiseptic Surgery', *Lancet*, 1879, ii: 850–4.

61 Ibid., 854.

62 Timothy Holmes remained one of the few elite surgeons who was willing to express his doubts about the living-germ theory in public. See *BMJ*, 1880, i: 34.

William MacCormac (1836–1901), from the Listerian stronghold of St. Thomas's, London, organised the publication of the proceedings of the Metropolitan Branch meeting, with additional material on Listerian theory and practice, in a volume entitled *Antiseptic Surgery*. This was the first British book by a Listerian devoted wholly to the subject.[63] The reports of the meeting in the medical press said that most surgeons who attended had showed little interest in germ-theory, but the published proceedings tell a different story.[64] For example, John Wood (1825–91), a colleague of Lister at King's College, used what he now termed 'the bacterian theory' against old-style Listerism:

1. How is it that, if bacteria have a power so terrible in their effects, in 999 cases out of 1000 they are unable to exercise it? 2. How is it that a patient may die of pyaemia or septicaemia, self-poisoned, without an external wound at all, the source of infection being a deep-seated abscess, far secluded from contact with the air? 3. How is it that bacteria may exist in abscesses originating inwardly, and yet no blood poisoning ensues? 4. How is it that wounds of the face heal so quickly and so well, and yet bacteria are found in number in the fur of the tongue and mucus on the surface of those cavities?[65]

By highlighting deep-seated septic abscesses, Wood was picking on one of the weak points in old and new Listerian theory: how did bacteria from the air reach deep into the body to create a septic abscess? Wood's answer was that bacteria were only one factor amongst many in the production of sepsis, and that surgeons needed to know much more about the interactions between bacteria and all of the other factors. What was at stake for Listerians was not germ-theory or antiseptic surgery as such, but their versions of them.

An attempt to answer Wood's first and fourth points was made by MacCormac in the chapter he contributed to the book that was entitled *Antiseptic Theory*.[66] He made reference to Koch's work on traumatic wound infections and specific micrococci, and used it to support the contention that there were several different kinds of bacteria – 'some potent for evil, others harmless, acting variously in different animals, and in different forms of disease'.[67] This construction of variable germs and different hosts allowed him to explain how normal wound healing had ever occurred before Listerism. This question had been neglected since the early 1870s as the 'open treatment' went out of favour, a decline that was not unconnected with the

63 W. MacCormac, *Antiseptic Surgery*, London, Smith Elder, 1880. For reviews see: *BMJ*, 1880, ii: 976–7; *Lancet*, 1880, ii: 15–16.
64 *Lancet*, 1879, ii: 853, 922. The followup editorial surprised no one when it reported: 'Very little was said by the surgeons who took part in the debate regarding germ theory, but they at once proceeded to consider the real problem at issue, as to whether Mr Lister's system of dressing affords patients a better chance of recovery than other methods of treatment.' 882.
65 MacCormac, *Antiseptic*, 76.
66 A review in the *Medical Times and Gazette* says that this chapter was 'very vague and unsatisfactory'. *MTG*, 1880, ii: 21.
67 MacCormac, *Antiseptic*, 106.

hospitalism crisis and the Listerian promotion of panspermism. So how did a Listerian now account for simple, natural healing by first intention'? MacCormac argued that this occurred when tissues were brought together so promptly that there was no opportunity for germs to enter, or because the surfaces had retained their 'vitality' and could resist any germs that might be around. He went on to add that in other types of wound healing, the degree of septic activity depended on 'the relative quantity, and probably quality of the organic particles in the atmosphere', on these particles finding 'a suitable soil', on the vitality of the parts affected and or the speed at which granulation tissue or scabs were formed.[68] He wrote of a range of 'antiseptic actions': artificial ones such as carbolic acid dressings and drainage, or natural ones such as scabs (described as 'an antiseptic plug'), the diluting effects of wound exudates and, of course, vital resistance.[69] However, while admitting that 'all modern surgical practice is antiseptic in a degree', he added that 'the aim of the ordinary plans of treatment [non-Listerian methods] is to combat the consequences of putrefaction', whereas the aim of Listerism was 'completely to arrest its development'. In the years that followed, the term Listerism fell into disuse, with all surgeons increasingly using the term 'antiseptic surgery', a broad church rather than an exclusive sect.

Wood was surprised at all of this, saying that what Listerians now spoke of as the body's 'power to reduce putrefaction depended on what in the old language was called the vital power of the blood'. He went on to say, echoing Gamgee, that perhaps traditional Listerism had at last found its true place in surgery as an ancillary method for patients with unhealthy tissues, for example, sufferers from diabetes and people with weak constitutions. Erichsen commented scathingly that the new rationale and advice from Listerians went against the whole thrust of prior principles and methods, which had been to make 'everything local and nothing constitutional'.[70] He also recognised the changes in ideology. Previously, Listerians had played on the threat posed by just one potent germ and used this to insist on strict obedience to specific techniques. Now they were more relaxed, relying on new allies, such as natural antiseptic actions and vital resistance. Previously, surgeons had been made to feel personally responsible for any septic complications, now the moral burden had been eased by admitting uncontrollable variables, such as highly virulent germs and patients with lowered vitality.

Lister himself answered Wood's second and third questions on deep-seated abscesses at the BMA in August 1880, in yet another confrontation with his

---

68 Lister himself was beginning to qualify his position. In August 1880 he stated that, 'it was only necessary that one bacterium should be present in order that, *as soon as life left the inflamed or injured part*, it should develop itself, and produce a septic abscess'. [emphasis added] *BMJ*, 1880, ii: 340.

69 Also see: 'Experimental Inquiry into the Value of the Antiseptic Spray', *MTG*, 1881, i: 276–7, 302–3.

70 *BMJ*, 1880, ii: 343.

critics. Old ground was revisited, with the bulk of comments around statistics and their meanings.[71] Lister tried to explain how deep-seated abscesses could occur without external contamination by bacteria. He began by referring to his own earlier ideas that inflammation, tension and nervous activity, as well as germs and their poisons, could produce suppuration and hence abscesses.[72] Thus, a deep-seated abscess need not be septic and, if not, would pose no threat of blood-poisoning – which neatly disposed on Wood's third query. Lister implied that any bacteria found in deep-seated abscesses had probably been introduced by the surgeon during drainage or excision – the familiar tactic of impugning critics for their poor technique. He went on to repeat the claim that antisepsis should not be solely identified with the 'spray and gauze' and acknowledged that drainage, ventilation, cooling and even the selection of cases were all ways of avoiding and halting sepsis. He summed this up by saying that 'every good surgeon was, whether consciously or unconsciously, an antiseptic surgeon'.[73] Erichsen's frustration with the changing meanings of Listerism boiled over as he complained that the word antiseptic had 'simply lost all significance'.[74] While Listerians were not unhappy about the widening of the term, they began to try to claim back a special position for their methods. They argued that in fact antisepsis had been a misnomer for their methods and that they had always aimed to achieve what they now called 'asepsis', that is, 'the total exclusion of septic agencies, which differed *toto coelo* from antiseptic treatment'.

Granshaw has suggested that there was a 'compromise' between Listerians and non-Listerians in the early 1880s as their methods and theories were amalgamated.[75] However, as argued above, it would be wrong to suggest that differences were settled or a truce declared. All sides became less exclusive and a wider variety of practices were termed 'antiseptic', but old divisions remained and new ones emerged. For example, surgeons continued to debate the value of wet (carbolic acid) and dry (sterilised cotton wool) dressings, the value of the spray and whether the partial adoption of Listerian methods could ever be effective. With theories, there was agreement that 'bacteria' were the essential cause of sepsis, but the use of the seed and soil analogy for sepsis allowed more complex theories about the action of germs to be developed by surgeons.[76] Also, any compromise was between unequal parties,

71 The debate followed a paper by John C. McVail on 'Ten Years' Surgery in the Kilmarnock Infirmary', where dry dressings rather than carbolic acid 'wet dressings' had been used. *Lancet*, 1880, ii: 340–4.
72 Lawrence and Dixey, 'Practising on Principle', 164–71.
73 *BMJ*, 1880: ii: 340. At the Metropolitan Counties Meeting of the BMA in December 1979, Jonathan Hutchison had remarked that 'all surgeons were these days antiseptic', but disparagingly referred to Listerian methods as merely 'spray and gauze'. *Lancet*, 1879, ii: 922.
74 *BMJ*, 1880, ii: 342.
75 Granshaw, 'On this Principle', 40–6.
76 Holmes wrote a long footnote in Sanderson's chapter on 'Inflammation', in T. Holmes and J. W. Hulke, *System of Surgery*, London, Longmans, Green, 1883, 41–3.

as Listerians now set the terms of the debates. They were helped by the wider medical uses of germ theories, and the fact that they had appropriated many of their opponents' practices. Finally, Listerians enjoyed the support of modernisers in medicine and science, not least in the growing international community of medical scientists, and gained particularly from their association with Pasteur, Koch and their followers.

In Britain, the new terms of engagement were evident in the debate in the early 1880s over the value of antiseptic precautions in elective operative surgery, particularly in ovariotomies. The removal of the ovaries had been one of the most controversial operations of the middle quarters of the century because of its high mortality.[77] During the 1860s and 1870s mortality fell, which surgeons attributed to improved techniques from specialisation, better selection and management of patients and a reduction of septic complications. Both Listerian and non-Listerian ovariotomists claimed similar rates of success. In the early Listerian world of panspermic germs, opening the abdomen to expose diseased organs seemed tantamount to murder. In this context, it was the spray that liberated Listerism from a mere wound treatment to become a surgical system applicable to operations and surgical treatments. Yet, the spray was the feature of the Listerian armatarium that was most often forsaken.[78] For example, Spencer Wells initially resisted its use due to fears of carbolic acid poisoning and its depressive effects on the body's physiology, and only took it up in 1877.[79] Surgeons who did not use the spray claimed to avoid sepsis by taking care not to damage tissue – by quickly removing diseased tissue in which bacteria might develop, by maintaining absolute cleanliness and by relying on the vital power of abdominal tissues, all of which would have seemed very non-Listerian before 1880.

The issue raised by successful non-Listerian ovariotomies was whether the great icon of Listerism – the spray – was really necessary.[80] In no lesser forum than the International Medical Congress (IMC) in 1881, Lister himself offered a commentary on what he said had become 'the touchstone of the efficacy of antiseptic treatment'.[81] In fact, Lister gave two addresses to the Congress, as befitting his status as the British equal of Pasteur and Koch and his continuing willingness to separate theory and practice. He spoke to the Pathology Section on microorganisms and inflammation, and three days later to the Surgical Section on the treatment of wounds.[82] Lister's intervention on wounds came in reply to criticisms by Savory and Gamgee of his 'meddle-

77 O. Moscucci, *The Science of Woman: Gynaecology and Gender in England, 1800–1929*, Cambridge, Cambridge University Press, 1990, 134–64.
78 Two well-known Listerians, John Chiene and S. Messenger Bradley, were using the spray only in selected cases in 1877. *BMR*, 1878, 7: 225–36.
79 *MTG*, 1878, ii: 64–5.
80 'Editorial', *Lancet*, 1881, ii: 423–5; 'Experimental Inquiry', 277.
81 J. Lister, 'An Address on the Treatment of Wounds', Lancet, 1881, ii: 863–6, 901–3.
82 J. Lister, 'On the Relation of Micro-Organisms to Inflammation', *Lancet*, 1881, ii: 695–8.

some surgery'.[83] His response surprised many. He began by admitting that 'the brilliant success' of ovariotomy had not been wholly due to strict Listerism. Indeed, he claimed that when Keith had first proposed antiseptic ovariotomies, he had 'strongly dissuaded him from his purpose'. Why? He had doubts about the effectiveness of the spray over such a large wound, and he felt that carbolic acid might be an irritant and upset the balance between the effusion of the wound and the absorption of the serum. Lister explained that his caution had come from his belief that prior tissue damage in the abdomen was unlikely and that the peritoneum anyway had a 'high vital power'. He also attributed his reevaluation of the spray to his own experimental work that showed that 'the serum of blood is not at all so favourable a soil for the growth of micro-organisms as I had previously imagined'.[84] Thus, at the meeting that elevated him to international fame as a surgeon and medical scientist, Lister's response to his domestic critics carried the admission that, in one of the most invasive operations then practised, the spray – the main symbol of his practice – was perhaps least needed.[85]

THE BEGINNING AND THE END OF SURGICAL BACTERIOLOGY, 1881–1889

It might be expected that Listerism and the debates that it generated in Britain would lead to surgeons being well represented in the first generation of bacteriologists.[86] As was shown earlier, Lister apart, surgeons were slow starters as germ researchers even before vivisection was controlled. This was because so few of them believed in germs and because those who did were more interested in learning how best to kill them rather than in studying their form and function. However, in the early 1880s, two British, actually Scottish, surgeons emerged as leading international researchers on germs: Lister's assistant Cheyne and Alexander Ogston, Surgeon at Aberdeen Royal Infirmary (see Figure 13).[87] Their research work and preeminence as medical

83 The main Address in Surgery was delivered by John Erichsen, who concentrated on operative technique, though when he did comment on wound treatments he once again bemoaned the neglect of constitutional measures in favour of local factors. *BMJ*, 1881, ii: 213, 305.
84 *Lancet*, 1881, ii: 863.
85 Lister suggested that, while it was probably safe to abandon the spray in operations where surgeons had an unbroken skin to start with, and where the operation was well away from any source of putrefaction, in other circumstances it was essential. There was another discussion of ovariotomies in 1881 led by Spencer Wells at which Thornton, Keith and Tait spoke. The latter noted that 'surgeons had still not fully appreciated the extent to which the peritoneal cavity can be interfered with without a disproportionate danger'. *Lancet*, 1881, ii: 304.
86 G. H. Brieger, 'American Surgery and the Germ Theory of Disease', *BHM*, 1866, 40: 135–45.
87 Edgar M. Crookshank, who took over as Lister's bacteriologist from Cheyne in the mid-1880s, was also a surgeon. He made a career in bacteriology for ten years, publishing important bacteriological textbooks and manuals. However, in the 1890s he adopted heterodox views on vaccination, and moved into politics and eventually big game hunting. W. Bulloch, *The History of Bacteriology*, London, Oxford University Press, 1938, 360.

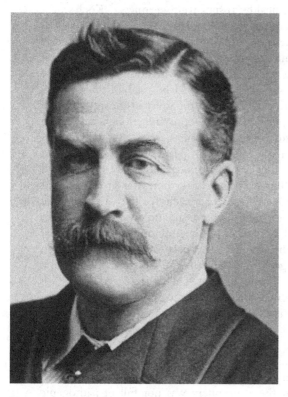

Figure 13. Alexander Ogston (Reproduced by courtesy of the Wellcome Institute Library, London)

scientists was relatively short-lived, and neither established a research school. By 1890 both had abandoned bacteriological research for clinical careers, by which time British bacteriology was becoming dominated by physicians, public health doctors and pathologists. Nonetheless, Cheyne and Ogston played a crucial role in developing and disseminating the new ideas and techniques of bacteriology to surgeons at a crucial moment, and were instrumental in securing the place of Listerian ideas at the heart of British surgical culture.

Lister and his followers were quite relaxed about the more complex bacterial theories of disease being fashioned in the early 1880s. Indeed, changes in theory and practice demonstrated that their work was informed by new knowledge and not based on dogma. However, there were two points that Listerians were unwilling to concede: first, that the origins of sepsis were always external and, second, that healthy tissues were germless.[88] Koch's pioneering work on traumatic infections, published in Cheyne's translation in 1880, had been equivocal on these questions. On the one hand, his experimental protocol of inoculating mice with septic material had relied on 'external' contamination of the body, albeit by artificial methods. On the other hand, his results showed that septic infections could be established in seemingly healthy tissues.[89] What later became seen as the great originality of these studies, the demonstration that specific types of septic infections were due to distinct species of microorganisms (in this case micrococci), was not seen as significant in Britain until after 1882. This was in part because Koch worked on animals rather than humans, and in part because antiseptic theory faced more troubling findings from other sources.[90] First, there was growing laboratory and field evidence of the 'extraordinary tenacity of life' of pathogenic bacteria. If they could survive all manner of chemicals and even boiling, might they not readily survive the 'vital' properties of human blood, cells and tissues? Second, Pasteur's new work on the attenuation of bacteria was used to reopen the possibility that innocuous germs, already on the body, might become pathogenic in certain conditions. This complicated what the 'germlessness' of tissues actually meant and reopened the issue of the spontaneous origin of pathogenicity, though not of life itself. Third, and slow to catch on, was Koch's own admission that he had found it very difficult to observe micrococci in the body, and had only succeeded by developing microscopic techniques and new stains.[91] Thus, tissues and surfaces that had appeared germless under old techniques might now be seen to be riddled with microorganisms. Last, it was increasingly accepted that the atmosphere was not full of pathogenic germs regularly raining down on the body. Rather, septic germs were concentrated in and on diseased people, and were part of the ordinary fauna and flora of human skin. Many of these findings came from researchers in Germany, and it was Ogston who introduced their substance, and the style of the work that had produced them, into British debates on antiseptic surgery.[92] Although a convinced Listerian practitioner, it fell to Ogston to challenge Listerian assumptions about micrococci and the germlessness of living tissue.

Ogston had first revealed his interest in germ theories in April 1879, in a

88 The most recent troubling findings were: V. Horsley and F. W. Mott, 'On the Existence of Bacteria or their Antecedents in Healthy Tissues', *Journal of Physiology*, 1880–82, 3: 188, 296.

89 The experiments were unequivocal on this as they showed specific micrococci active in different species, which was contrary to the views of Sanderson and Roberts, who had regarded septic germs as active in all species in the common conditions of dead tissue.

90 'Experimental Inquiry', 276.

91 J. C. Ewart's talk on 'Bacteria' to the Aberdeen Branch of the BMA in February 1880 was amongst the first in Britain to be based on types of organisms rather than diseases.

92 G. Smith, 'Ogston the Bacteriologist', in A. MacDonald and G. Smith, eds., *The Staphylococci*, Aberdeen, Aberdeen University Press 1981, 9–21. Also see: Wilson, 'The Early Recognition', 403–13.

talk to the Aberdeen Branch of the BMA, in which he summarised the latest German and French work. He supported the notion of a single bacterial-infection germ-theory and that there were distinct species of disease-germs, all of which could be linked to specific septic and contagious diseases. Significantly, he did not mention the emerging distinction between the role of bacteria in dead and living tissues.[93] In that same year, Ogston began an investigation into the role of micrococci in abscesses, using methods that he had learned firsthand from Koch in Germany. The results were reported in Germany in 1880, with subsequent publications in Britain in successive years.[94] Ogston's main finding was that micrococci were the cause of all abscesses, including those deep in the body. Lister took exception to this, first, because it contradicted his own beliefs and the recent finding of Cheyne that micrococci were nonpathogenic and, second, because it was impossible for a septic germ to survive in blood serum or healthy tissues to reach the site of a deep-seated abscess. Lister maintained his view that deep-seated abscesses were due to mechanical, chemical or nervous causes, and that the presence of micrococci in abscesses examined by Ogston was 'a mere accident' and 'of entirely insignificant importance' – everyone knew that bacteria produced disease, not micrococci. Ogston's work was, of course, welcomed by Lister's opponents; for example, John Duncan, Surgeon to the Royal Infirmary Edinburgh, mused in 1883 on 'the fate of Listerism had our knowledge been formerly as it is now'.[95] He asked,

How would these methods have been received had we known that under antiseptic dressings organisms may flourish while the wound follows what has been called an aseptic course; . . . that all suppurations of an acute character . . . are attended by microbia although unexposed to the air; . . . that contamination of a wound through the atmosphere is comparatively unimportant, while the means taken to prevent it are inefficient?'

John Lowe, a provincial surgeon from Norfolk and self-confessed 'full believer' in the germ-theory, stated that the exchanges between Ogston, Cheyne and Lister had vindicated his reluctance to adopt Listerism.[96]

Ogston's ideas were practically and ideologically troubling for Listerians, and they were attacked by Lister himself at no lesser forum than the 1881 International Medical Congress.[97] This represented a change in tactics for Lister, who until this time tried to keep germ theorists together as a united group. For example, at the BMA in 1880 Lister had publicised Koch's work

93 A. Ogston, 'Bacteria and Disease', *BMJ*, 1879, i: 592.
94 A. Ogston, 'Über Abscesse', *Arch. f. Klin. Chir.* 1880, 225: 588–600; *idem.*, 'Micro–organisms in Surgical Diseases, *BMJ*, 1881, i: 369–75; *idem.*, 'Micrococcus poisoning', *Journal of Anatomy and Physiology*, 1882, 16: 526–67, 1883, 17: 24–58.
95 J. Duncan, 'Germs and the Spray', *EMJ*, 1883, 28: 778.
96 J. Lowe, 'The Germ Theory of Disease', *BMJ*, 1883, ii: 53–5.
97 *BMJ*, ii: 1881, 697.

on anthrax; Pasteur's on chicken cholera; the attenuation of bacilli by Pasteur, Toussaint and Greenfield; and associated all of these developments with his own work and ideas.[98] During the IMC in 1881, demonstrations of Koch's methods were made in Lister's department at King's College, and he was only too pleased to be associated with Pasteur and Koch as one of the founders of the new science of germs.[99] However, between 1881 and 1883, and unlike the schools of Pasteur and Koch, Listerians made a firm distinction between two germ theories, those of putrefaction and infection. They said that the former, upon which Listerism had always been based, referred only to the action of saprophytic microorganisms on dead tissues, while the latter applied to specific, parasitic microorganisms causing disease in living tissues.[100] In his volume on *Antiseptic Surgery*, published in 1882 but written a year earlier, Cheyne complained that it was 'from mixing up these two theories that the confusion, and much of the difficulty in accepting the principles of antiseptic surgery, have arisen'. Of course, Listerians had been at the forefront of 'mixing up' things, and had been slow to adopt the distinction offered by Roberts and Sanderson. Reviewers of Cheyne's *Antiseptic Surgery* made no mention of the two theories, which was just as well because by 1883 Cheyne was giving them up.[101] Indeed, he did well not to be hoist on his own petard as the distinction was, of course, central to the Cleanliness School and to antivivisectionists. Perhaps he escaped because *Antiseptic Surgery* looked back rather than forward. It began by setting the scientific groundwork with accounts of fermentation and putrefaction, followed by practical details of Listerism and three chapters attacking spontaneous generation.[102] The other chapters set out the impressive statistics of antiseptic surgery and repeated the new line that Lister's practice had always been about 'asepsis' rather than 'antisepsis'.[103] There was no reference to the work of Koch and Ogston on micrococci, nor was there much on the form and actions of the germs causing sepsis.

98 J. Lister, 'On the Relation of Micro-Organisms to Disease', *QJMS*, 1881, 21: 330–42. The version printed in the *QJMS* contained additional paragraphs on Pasteur's work on the attenuation of chicken-cholera and Greenfield's 'Brown Lectures' on anthrax.

99 *MTG*, 1881, ii: 227.

100 W. W. Cheyne, *Antiseptic Surgery: Its Principles, Practice, History and Results*, London, Smith, Elder, 1882, 287. Cheyne wrote, 'We have seen that antiseptic surgery is simply a struggle with the causes of putrefaction. I have not mentioned the germ theory of infective disease at all. That has no essential bearing on the *principles* of antiseptic surgery. All that is required of antiseptic surgery is to prevent the occurrence of all kinds of fermentation. The germ theory of infective disease is, I say, an independent view, and not part of those principles at all.'

101 See reviews of Cheyne's *Antiseptic Surgery*: *BMJ*, 1881, i: 740; *Lancet*, 1882, ii: 143–4. The volume was written in 1881, when it won a Prize Essay for the best account of Listerism. For comments on the neglect of Listerism in British surgical textbooks, see: *Lancet*, 1880, ii: 15; *BMJ*, 1882, ii: 740.

102 The review in the *Medical Times and Gazette* noted how important it was for Cheyne to make this refutation. *MTG*, 1882, i: 480.

103 Cheyne, *Antiseptic*, 265–89. This was a strange point to make for a method that had always been regarded as a wound treatment as well as a surgical system.

At the very moment *Antiseptic Surgery* was published, Cheyne took on the role of gatekeeper for the diffusion into Britain of the burgeoning bacterial research of Continental laboratories, especially those of Koch and his followers.[104] Several events combined to create his new situation. Awareness in Britain, largely from the IMC in the previous year, that the strength of its medical research was behind that of other countries led in March 1882 to the creation of the Association for the Advancement of Medicine by Research (AAMR), which aimed to promote 'exact researches in physiology, pathology and therapeutics'.[105] This initiative was backed by political and religious leaders, along with leading clinicians and scientists, with Lister already a figurehead for the cause. Amongst its main targets were antivivisectionists and the government for failing to fund research and support research careers. Worries about the decline of British science were heightened again when Charles Darwin, a supporter of the AMMR, died the following month.[106] Three days after Darwin's death there was another crucial moment: John Tyndall announced in the *Times* that Koch had identified a *Tubercle bacillus* that was the essential cause of consumption, the single largest killer in Europe. He went on to state boldly that Koch had shown the disease to be contagious and hence as preventable by means of disinfection and isolation. Tyndall also predicted that in time a protective vaccine would be produced by the methods that Pasteur had used against anthrax at Pouilly-le-Fort the previous summer.[107]

Also in April 1882, Sanderson was giving yet another lecture series on inflammation and infection. He reflected on the changed position of germs, saying that:

[Now] the tendency exists to believe germs explain everything, so that whereas formerly one had to vindicate the very existence of such things as parts of pathological processes, it has now become one's business to protest with all needful vehemence against the attribution to them of functions which they do not possess.[108]

He too quietly abandoned the distinction between septic and infective diseases, saying that inflammations and their exudates anywhere in the body were favourable soil in which micrococci could develop. And once this process had started, micrococci could become 'infective' in the sense of being capable of spreading sepsis to any part of the body, living or dead. But according to Sanderson what happened was a contingent matter, 'although the seed is indispensable . . . whether that seed becomes morbidific or not depends not

04 L. Kern, *Deutsche Bakteriologie im Spiegel englischer medizinischer Zeitschriften, 1875–1885*, Zurich, Juris Druck and Verlag, 1972.

05 *Lancet* 1882: i: 542–3. The Association for the Advancement of Medicine by Research was supported by the surplus from the 1881 International Medical Congress.

06 A. Desmond and J. Moore, *Darwin*, London, Michael Joseph, 1991, 644–77.

07 *Times*, 22 April 1882, 10.

08 J. B. Sanderson, 'Lumleian Lectures on Inflammation', *Lancet*, 1882, i: 553–6, 554.

on the seed but on the soil'. The significance of all of this for surgeons was explained in July by Solomon Charles Smith, Surgeon to the Halifax Infirmary. He told the Yorkshire Branch of the BMA that recent developments meant that it was now necessary 'to add to the bare and naked germ theory the hypothesis that there is a varying resisting power in living tissue, and that germs do not always find it a fit nidus for their development and multiplication'.[109] Smith's explained that his confidence in germ-theory had been

strengthened by the recent discovery of the bacterial origin of tubercle; for here we have an instance in which the contagion habitually passes over the strong to attack . . . a feeble member of the flock and . . . is usually impotent against those portions [of the lung] whose functional activity is greatest and is prone to affect those . . . which have been inflamed.[110]

The *Tubercle bacillus* was also interpreted to have implications for surgeons operating on tubercular joints, one of Cheyne's special interests. They had long faced septic complications in severely diseased joints, but now they were either operating to remove infective material or using rest, tonics and pressure to help the body resist an infective process. Lister too was thinking in terms of seed and soil, as in 1884 he suggested that drugs might be used to alter the chemistry of the blood sufficiently 'to kill off or to prevent the development of any special bacteria'.[111]

Within three weeks of Tyndall's announcement, the *Tubercle bacillus* was being displayed at King's College by Cheyne and Goltdammer, Koch's private assistant.[112] Along with the *Tubercle bacillus*, the 'bacilli' of leprosy, septicaemia, erysipelas and anthrax were shown. Similar demonstrations, with up to sixty 'see-for-yourself' microscopes, toured national and local medical societies over the summer.[113] Another surgical 'bacterium' soon on show was the gonococcus, first identified by Neisser in 1879.[114] However, germ theorists did not have it all their own way; surgeons continued to use other theories, as with syphilis, where the 'virus' might still be a 'specific cell' (Beale-type bioplasm),

109 *Lancet*, 1882, ii: 309–11. Smith had begun by observing that research on the relationship between microorganisms and disease was now advancing on two separate lines, 'the microscopic line of inquiry as to the nature of the germs of disease' and 'the nature of those conditions which make man's body a fit nidus for the hatching of those germs, and the development of the diseases to which they are related'.

110 S. C. Smith, 'Modern Study of Micro-Organisms and its Influence of Medical Thought', *Lancet* 1882, i: 309. Also see: Holmes *System of Surgery*, third edition, 42.

111 *MP*, 1884, i: 336.   112 'Bacilli in Tuberculosis', *Lancet* 1882: i: 797.

113 *BMJ*, 1882: i: 735, 787, 1213, 1221.

114 Germ-theory was used to unsex the pathology of gonorrhoea. Previously, many surgeons had assumed that the poison arose spontaneously in the body and that women's bodies provided the better conditions for this process to develop. Also, because the poison had been elaborated in women, they were seen to be less susceptible to its effects than men, who could thus contract the disease from a perfectly healthy woman. C. R. Drysdale, *Syphilis and its Nature with a Chapter on Gonorrhoea*, London, Baillière, Tindall and Cox, 1872, 1–4, 24–5.

a 'cryptogamic vegetation' (fungoid origin à la Klebs) or a specific ferment that 'multiplied in the system'.[115] Many doctors were given the opportunity to come and see disease bacteria for themselves. However, uncertainties about the *Tubercle bacillus* remained and in the summer the AAMR sent Cheyne to Toulouse to investigate Toussaint's claim to have found the 'tubercle micrococcus', and then on to Berlin to learn about Koch's methods and confirm his results. Cheyne returned a full convert to the *Tubercle bacillus* and to the Koch school of bacteriology, which implied acceptance of a specific, parasitic, bacterial model of pathogenesis. But more important was that he returned the leading British exponent of Kochian bacterial practices.[116] As well as the specific innovations, Cheyne promoted what became Koch's postulates – the experimental steps required to confirm a bacterial aetiology. These requirements, first set out by Loeffler, not Koch, in 1883 were that: (1) A specific microorganism must be shown to be constantly present in diseased tissue; (2) the specific organism must be grown and isolated in pure culture; (3) and the pure culture must produce the disease when inoculated into a healthy animal. In time a fourth postulate was added, that the pathogenic microorganism had to be recovered from the infected animal and produced again in pure culture. The confidence that germs had moved from 'theory' to 'fact' was not universal, despite visually and aetiologically impressive demonstrations, and the sense that every septic and zymotic disease was now a candidate for germ causation.[117] When Edward Lund, Surgeon to the Manchester Royal Infirmary and a Listerian of over ten years standing, spoke on the 'Antiseptic Question' in July 1883, he began by saying that he would suppress as far as possible certain well-known terms which to some people '. . are painfully provocative – carbolic acid, septic germs, the germ theory, bacteria and the like'.[118]

With the new techniques acquired in Germany, Cheyne continued to investigate micrococci. In his next major publication on sepsis in September 1884, he admitted that he had earlier 'missed the discovery . . .

15 J. E. Erichsen, *The Science and Art of Surgery*, London, Longmans Green, 1877, 843. Local treatment was little used as the poison penetrated deep into the body so rapidly; hence the basis of mercury treatment was to promote constitutional improvements that might lead to the elimination of the poison.

16 W. W. Cheyne, 'Report to the AAMR on the Relation of Micro-Organisms to Tuberculosis, *Practitioner*, 1883, 30: 240–320. In 1886, Cheyne was the editor of an immensely important collection of papers. Cheyne also published one of the first bacteriological manuals in Britain, though it was aimed at MOsH rather than surgeons. W. W. Cheyne, W. H. Corfield and C. E. Cassell, *Public Health Laboratory Work*, London, Williams Clowes and Sons, 1884. In 1886, Cheyne published an important collection of translations of key German and French articles. W. W. Cheyne, *Recent Essays by Various Authors on Bacteria in Relation to Disease*, London: New Sydenham Society, 1886.

17 In the previous year, in a debate in Birmingham, Langley Brown had challenged Lawson Tait, saying that he should stop talking about 'germ theory' as it was now 'germ law'. *BMR*, 1881, 10: 79–93, 90

18 E. Lund, *The Antiseptic Question*, Manchester, Cornish, 1872, 7.

that micrococci are present in all acute abscesses' and were their cause.[119] He blamed his 'error', not on his Listerian preconceptions, but on his failure to use Koch's techniques, and he still queried Ogston's view that micrococci were the sole cause of septic inflammations. Cheyne set out his revised position in a new volume, *The Antiseptic Treatment of Wounds*, in 1885.[120] The preface referred readers to *Antiseptic Surgery* for 'the scientific basis of antisepsis', though he added that readers would find nothing there on the character of germs – the time had not then been ripe for such detail. His abandonment of the two germ theories was clear in his statement that wound infection was 'almost entirely due to the growth of minute vegetable organisms in the discharges of wounds *or in the living tissues of the body*' (emphasis added).[121] The short chapter on 'Bacteria and Disease' was structured around the four types of 'bacteria' defined by form (bacteria, bacilli, micrococci and spirilla), not types of septic diseases or their pathologies. The final irony was that he illustrated the relationship between bacteria and specific septic diseases with examples from his 1880 translation of Koch's *Traumatic Infective Diseases* – a text he had barely used in his volume on *Antiseptic Surgery* that had appeared in 1882.[122] The best gloss that Cheyne was able to put on the change was that antiseptic surgery had been 'enlarged' to include the causes to fermentation as well as putrefaction.[123]

Cheyne continued to be one of Britain's leading 'bacteriologists' and published one of the earliest practical manuals in 1884; however, this was specifically aimed at public health applications and not surgery.[124] More significant for the wider diffusion of germ theories was the collection of German papers he edited, *Bacteria in Relation to Disease*, for the New Sydenham Society in 1886. This contained seminal works by the Koch school on bacterial technique and aetiological claims for both septic and infectious diseases. In 1886, he and a new assistant, Edgar M. Crookshank, offered an extramural course in bacteriology at King's College, the first time the subject was formally taught in a British medical school. Together, as we will see later, they championed Koch's postulates and the 'discoveries' of his school, often against the claims against British followers of Pasteur and of the group that formed around Edward Klein. Cheyne also translated the 1886 edition of Flügge's *Micro-organisms*, which was regarded as one of the best accounts of the new science, though this did not appear until 1890.[125] Before then, Cheyne

119 *BMJ*, 1884, ii: 553, 645; *MP*, 1884, i: 325.
120 W. W. Cheyne, *The Antiseptic Treatment of Wounds*, London: Smith, Elder, 1885, v.
121 Ibid., 10.   122 *BMJ*, 1884, ii: 553, 645.
123 W. W. Cheyne, 'Antiseptic Surgery', in C. Heath, ed., *Dictionary of Surgery*, Vol. 1, London, Smith, Elder, 1886, 71.
124 Cheyne, *Public Health*. Later versions of this volume, written by Kenwood, were the text for MOsH through the 1880s and 1890s.
125 C. Flügge, *Micro-organisms: With Special Reference to the Etiology of Infective Disease*, (Translation of the second edition of *Fermente und Mikroparasiten*), London, New Sydenham Society, 1890.

reviewed the state of knowledge on suppuration and wound management in February 1888 in a series of lectures at the Royal College of Surgeons.[126] Three things stand out in these lectures. First, only three of the ninety references cited were by British authors, and all of these were early 1880s publications of Ogston, Lister and himself. Little or no significant research on the bacteriology of septic diseases had been pursued in Britain during the 1880s. Second, he used the seed and soil metaphor extensively. He said that in septic diseases there were 'two forces' at work, 'on the one side the bacteria and on the other the body'. He added that the discovery of bacteria had not settled the question of the aetiology of sepsis because so many other factors were involved. Finally, he noted 'a certain antagonism . . . between bacteriologists working in laboratories and clinical observers', the former emphasising the 'seeds' of disease and the latter the 'soil'. He tried to reconcile these views by pointing to the weaknesses of both positions. The germs of sepsis had been shown not to be all-powerful, their virulence varied and where and how many entered the body mattered. On the other side, it was correct to say that the aetiology of sepsis was complex, but a particularly virulent germ, or large numbers entering at a vulnerable point, could override all other variables.[127]

Exactly who the 'bacteriologists working in laboratories' that Cheyne refers to is puzzling. Both he and Ogston had given up germ research to follow clinical and teaching careers.[128] The only British germ researchers from the 1870s to remain active throughout the 1880s were Sanderson and Klein, though Sanderson did so part-time after he moved to Oxford as Professor of Physiology in 1880.[129] Defined by publications, Britain's leading bacteriologists in the late 1880s were Klein, Crookshank, German Sims Woodhead, A. W. Hare, W. R. Grove and John Tyndall, of whom only Sanderson had worked directly on sepsis.[130] Lister himself continued his own private research, but this focused on finding alternative antiseptic agents to carbolic acid, because its effects on healthy tissue had become a major issue. In 1884, Lister extolled the virtues of 'corrosive sublimate' (mercuric chloride) and in 1887 those of 'double salt' (cyanide of zinc and mercury).[131] The Annual Report of the

126 W. W. Cheyne, 'Lectures on Suppuration and Septic Diseases', *BMJ*, 1888, i: 404, 452, 524–30. W. W. Cheyne, *Suppuration and Septic Diseases*, Edinburgh, Young J. Pentland, 1889.

127 Cheyne, *Suppuration*, v.

128 I. A. Porter, 'Sir Alexander Ogston (1844–1929)', in G. P. Milne, ed., *A Bicentennial History, 1789–1989*, Aberdeen Medico-Chirurgical Society, 1989, 179–89.

129 J. B. Sanderson, 'The Progress of Discovery Relating to the Origin and Nature of Infectious Diseases, *BMJ*, 1891, ii: 983–7, 1033–7, 1083–7, 1135–59.

130 E. Klein, *Micro-Organisms and Disease*, London, John Murray, 1884; E. M. Crookshank, *Manual of Bacteriology*, London, H. K. Lewis, 1886; G. S. Woodhead and A. W. Hare, *Pathological Mycology*, Edinburgh, Young J. Pentland, 1885; W. B. Grove, *A Synopsis of the Bacteria and Yeast Fungi and Allied Species*, London, Chatto and Windus, 1884.

131 J. Lister, 'Corrosive Sublimate as a Surgical Dressing', *TMSL*, 1885, 8: 2–19; idem., 'On a New Antiseptic Dressing', *TMSL*, 1890, 13: 32–50.

Medical Department showed an increasing number of investigations of disinfection, by Sanderson and Klein amongst others, but most of these addressed the question in public health and not surgery.[132]

The only area of active research on sepsis after 1880 in Britain was on ptomaines or the chemical poisons of germs.[133] This seems to have a consequence of three factors. First, the whole logic of the germ-theory of putrefaction and the systemic effects of infective bacteria had long pointed to a role for chemical poisons. Sanderson had worked on this in the 1870s, and in 1881 Victor Horsley produced a review of the subject for the Medical Department. Second, there was the relative strength of physiology in Britain, especially under Foster at Cambridge and Sanderson at University College, London and Oxford. Finally, this was an area of research that required only limited use of vivisection, as poisons could be isolated from culture plates and the tissues of infected humans and animals. However, the seminal work of the 1880s was produced in Germany; Ludwig Breiger's three-volume *Über Ptomaine* was published in 1886.[134] The subsequent work of Behring, Kitasato and Roux was followed closely in Britain, and in the late 1880s and early 1890s Britain had a burgeoning group of researchers working on both toxins and antitoxins (what Sanderson then called 'alxines'). In 1892, Woodhead identified such work as a particular strength of British bacteriology and identified a dozen researchers.[135] The most prominent figure was Sidney Martin, who worked on the toxins of tetanus, anthrax and diphtheria, and who in 1892 boldly suggested that there ought to be a fifth Koch postulate: the identification of the chemical toxin of each disease.[136] The manner in which this work developed in the context of the new bacterial therapies and preventive products will be discussed in more detail in the next two chapters.

There were a number of attempts in the late 1880s to produce an account of bacteriology directly relevant to surgeons. One influential example was in A. A. Bowlby's *Surgical Pathology*, first published in 1887, which was said to

132 *Supplement to the Fourteenth Annual Report of the LGB, containing the Report of the Medical Officer for 1884*, BPP, 1884–85, [C. 4516], xxxiii, 227, Appendix B.

133 The term was coined in 1878 by the Italian chemist Francesco Selmi (1817–1881), for alkaloid bodies found in putrefying matter.

134 N. Morgan, 'Pure Science and Applied Medicine, Bacteriology and Biochemistry in England after 1880', Paper given at the BSHS-HSS Conference on *Science in Modern Medicine*, Manchester, 1985.

135 G. S. Woodhead, 'Address in Bacteriology', *Lancet*, 1892, i: 238. He identified: Sanderson, Sidney Martin, William Halliburton, Lauder Brunton, John McFadyean, R. W. Philip, Edward Hankin, Armand Ruffer, Edgar Crookshank, Herroun, William Hunter and George Cartwright Wood. Woodhead was speaking in the aftermath of the introduction of Koch's failed tuberculin remedy for consumption. Philip, Crookshank, Herroun and Hunter worked for only a brief period on bacterial chemistry in relation to tuberculin. Woodhead could have cited the following in addition: Allen McFadyen, Leonard Wooldridge, Rubert Boyce and Vaughan Harley.

136 S. Martin, 'Chemical Pathology of Diphtheria Compared with Anthrax, Infective Endocarditis and Tetanus', *BMJ*, 1892, i: 641, 696, 737.

be representative of the 'English School'.[137] In the familiar style of pathological texts, Bowlby's started with degenerations but broke new ground by
placing a chapter on microorganisms before the discussion of inflammations,
implying that microorganisms were the prime source of inflammation. This
juxtaposition also showed how pathology now routinely considered the
pathogenesis of disease, not just its results. In his Bradshawe Lecture on 'Bacteriology and its Relations to Surgery' in 1888, Henry Power began with an
account of the different types of organisms as defined by shape: micrococci
(single round organisms), staphylococci (groups of round organisms forming
a grape shape), streptococci (chains of round organisms) and bacilli (thin, rod-
shaped organisms), and discussed the diseases that each caused.[138] This was
one of the first examples of the abandonment of such terms 'as septic germs',
'septic bacteria' and 'pyogenic bacteria', and the adoption of the language of
staphylococci, streptococci and 'cocco-bacteria', and later 'staphs and streps'.
However, the bacteriological sections incorporated into revised editions of
surgical textbooks in the late 1880s were often decidedly dated. The fifth
edition of Holmes' *Treatise on Surgery* in 1888 still referred to 'organised irritants' and was still quite chemically minded.[139] The 1889 edition of Walsham's
Surgery still referred to 'ferments' and only in the fifth edition in 1895 was
there a significant modern bacteriological input from A. A. Kanthack and
C. R. Drysdale.[140] However, this was nothing compared to the importance
accorded the topic in new volumes. For example, Frederick Treves's *System
of Surgery*, first published in 1895, opened with a chapter by Woodhead on
'Surgical Bacteriology', followed by two chapters by Cheyne on 'Inflammation' and 'Suppuration'.[141] The iconic significance of bacteriology for surgery
was signalled by the volume's frontispieces, expensive colour plates of all of
the important known bacteria.

SURGERY, GERMS AND NEW LISTERISM, 1882–1890

Through the 1880s the Cleanliness School continued to challenge the authority and methods of Listerians. It was, however, an unequal struggle. Lister and

137 A. A. Bowlby, *Surgical Pathology and Morbid Anatomy*, London, Churchill, 1887. The structure of
Bowlby's volume was significant in that it begins with processes and places the morbid anatomy
of particular organs last. After two initial chapters on atrophy and degeneration, the next seven
chapters are on microorganisms, inflammation and septic diseases, in that order.

138 H. Power, 'Bacteriology in its Relations to Surgery', *Lancet*, 1886, ii: 1111–6. Power warned of
the technical difficulties of bacteriological work. Other accounts in surgical textbooks took their
lead from Cohn's classification.

139 T. Holmes, *A Treatise on Surgery: Its Principles and Practice*, fifth edition, edited by T. Pickering
Pick, London, Smith and Elder, 1888, 10. The 1888 edition of Erichsen's textbook dealt with
the topic by reference to ferments and organised irritants, though it did give details of micrococci, bacilli and spirilla.

140 W. J. Walsham, *Surgery: Its Theory and Practice*, second edition, London, Churchill, 1889; fifth
edition, 1895.

141 F. Treves, *A System of Surgery*, London, Cassell and Co., 1895–6.

his supporters increasingly dominated the institutions and ideology of British surgery, and from the early 1880s the authors of surgical textbooks began to signal the end of hostilities by declaring themselves Listerians. The first edition of Keetley's *Index of Surgery* in 1881 had tried to be impartial between Lister and his critics, but in the next edition three years later the author regretted this 'mistake' and recommended that surgeons 'regard every surgical operation and dressing as a chemico-biological experiment demanding nicety, and extreme care'.[142] The adoption of laboratory theories was perhaps that much easier if surgeons were being persuaded, and even flattered, by the idea that their clinical practice was analogous to laboratory work. In the 1884 edition of his *The Science and Art of Surgery*, even Erichsen admitted that Lister's principles were 'intact and unchangeable' – and by 1888, in an edition revised by Beck, the preface opined that Lister's practice was based 'on facts now beyond dispute'.[143] Lister continued to tell surgeons that they could separate practice and theory, but this was unnecessary as he was now winning on both fronts.[144] As germ-theory was converted into a series of demonstrable bacterial aetiologies, the adoption of anti-bacterial measures became difficult to resist.[145] In addition, the spread of Listerism and antiseptic practice had coincided historically with safer and more successful surgery. The question that Listerians asked was how these two trends were related; their answer was, of course, that germ science had led to antiseptic technologies and to the surgical and social benefits. However, progress was a mixed blessing. In 1888, MacCormac suggested that hospital hygiene had improved so much that 'It is no longer needful to insist upon the necessity of aseptic and antiseptic procedures of strict cleanliness in air, person and environment'.[146] The improved prospects of surgical treatments and operations could have been due to many things: new surgical techniques, fewer last-ditch operations, more minor operations, better-run hospitals, cleaner and better fed patients, different patterns of injury and disease or changes in the virulence of pathogenic microorganisms. The great achievement of the Listerians was to claim and to be given almost exclusive credit for the improvement in hospital hygiene, the fall in surgical mortality, the increased scope of surgery and the relative rise of surgeons in the medical profession.

Opposition to antiseptic surgery was more difficult to maintain as the practice broadened and Listerians appropriated the term for all 'successful surgery'.[147] They even took on board the methods of their fiercest opponents; for example, Gamgee's 'dry dressings' (cotton wool lint) was presented

142 C. Keetley, *Index of Surgery*, London, Smith, Elder, 1881, 33.
143 J. E. Erichsen, *The Science and Art of Surgery*, Volume 1, ninth edition revised by Marcus Beck, Longmans Green, 1888, 3.
144 *BMJ* 1883, i: 855–60.   145 Clifford Allbutt, *BMJ*, 1882, ii: 621.
146 W. MacCormac, 'Old and New Surgery', *BMJ*, 1888, ii: 865.
147 Lawrence and Dixey, 'Practising on Principle', 206–7.

as fully antiseptic as it killed germs by drying, excluding air and drawing away pus. They sanctioned a wider range of antiseptic chemicals, allowed the spray to be optional and accepted the value of mixed practices.[148] Thomas Bryant of Guy's Hospital was one of many surgeons who argued that the diversity of precautions made the subject 'absolutely unintelligible', but such was the influence of the Listerians that he admitted making his point 'with some amount of trepidation'.[149] Other former critics of Listerism, such as Bantock, admitted that in the mid-1880s Listerian antiseptic surgery was the order of the day, though he took some satisfaction from the fact that strict adherence to the full rituals was declining, and that few surgeons were as scrupulous as Lister and his immediate circle.[150] Cheyne described the character of the new, more relaxed and inclusive Listerian practice in 1886. He wrote that there were in fact six forms of antiseptic wound management: first and foremost was Listerian 'asepsis', the gold standard of excluding microorganisms from the body. The five other methods – chemicals, drainage, irrigation, evaporation (as in the open treatment) and scabbing – were all said to be effective, but were endorsed with the qualification that they dealt largely with the consequences of established septic infections.[151] The distinction that he was trying to maintain was between *preventive* Listerian practice and the *curative* approach of other methods. However, the Cleanliness School reversed the point, saying that their practices were germ-free and preventive, whereas Listerism was first and foremost a method of wound treatment, killing septic bacteria in wounds.

Cheyne admitted that in many situations new Listerian prevention was impossible as surgeons had to deal with tissues that were already damaged and infected. It was with this type of injury that all surgeons now admitted the value of Listerism. The revised editions of Erichsen's and Holmes's textbooks, published in 1888, both described a six-stage process of wound treatment: (i) to arrest bleeding; (ii) to cleanse the wound; (iii) to close the wound; (iv) to establish drainage; (v) to ensure rest; and, finally, (vi) to prevent putrefaction by Listerian methods.[152] Erichsen's volume stressed that 'ferments' were one of several factors necessary to produce putrefaction, and that surgeons should try to manage other factors, such as dead matter, oxygen, water and temperature. Holmes's volume acknowledged the continuing dispute between the Cleanliness and Listerian groups, but recommended that surgeons judiciously combine both plans, as they were different means of achieving the same end. With operative surgery, all sides recognised the importance of scrupulous attention to the patient's skin, the surgeon's hands,

148 On the variety of techniques, see: J. Wood, "The Bradshawe Lecture on Antiseptics in Surgery', *BMJ*, 1885, ii: 1095–7, 1147–9.
149 *BMJ*, 1885, i: 351.   150 *BMJ*, 1887, i: 334.
51 Cheyne, 'Antiseptic Surgery', in Heath, *Dictionary*, 71.
52 See: T. Holmes, *A Treatise on Surgery: Its Principles and Practice*, revised by T. Pickering Pick, London: Smith Elder, 1888, 31, 309. Erichsen, *Science and Art*, 309.

instruments, sponges and ligatures, and dressings, but differences remained on when, where and how to use antiseptics, or soap and water, or the alternative of heat.

Through the 1880s, the influence of bacteriology in surgery began to be felt outside of debates over wound management and operative procedures. Manufacturers of surgical dressings were quick to see the marketing potential of antiseptic products. Bleached cotton wool as a surgical dressing had come into vogue because of its successful use in the Franco-Prussian War. In Britain it was promoted by Gamgee, who stressed its virtues in keeping wounds dry and rested, protected from disturbance.[153] However, manufacturers selling these products aimed to appeal to all groups. For example, they maintained that the properties of absorbency and purity, so attractive to the Cleanliness School, made cotton wool ideal for holding the wet antiseptics of Listerians. Surgical gauzes treated with antiseptics such as boracic acid, alembroth (double chloride of mercury and ammonia) and cyanide, as well as carbolic acid, began to be marketed. Local chemists and national companies offered a range of antiseptics, many of which were endorsed by famous surgeons. Such products were a primary conduit of disseminating bacterial knowledge to general practitioners, though the rising number of doctors with dual qualifications in surgery and medicine meant that many would have learned of antisepsis in their medical education. Such new products enabled general practitioners to use antisepsis in the minor operations they performed in their 'surgeries' or patient's homes and as wound dressings. Antiseptics continued to be used, as they had before Lister, as a treatment for burns, skin complaints and venereal diseases, especially gonorrhoea.[154] In the case of topical applications, new treatments were relatively easy to adopt and adapt into clinical practice. New rationales for older uses were clear in nonoperative procedures; for example, introducing antiseptics into the urethra for venereal diseases became an antigerm rather than antiinflammatory treatment. Beyond surgery, obstetricians were routinely using antiseptics to prevent and treat puerperal fever, including taking care to wash their hands and use clean instruments and towels.[155] There was also discussion about abandoning the term puerperal fever altogether and regarding the disease as a particular form of streptococcal infection.[156]

By the late 1880s, the details of antiseptic methods ceased to be a topic for discussion in the medical press or at medical meetings. Surgeons focused on new operations and procedures, happy to repeat the trope that Listerism

---

153 W. J. Bishop, *A History of Surgical Dressings*, Chesterfield, Robinson and Sons, 1959, 63–80. Gamgee was, of course, contrasting his emphasis on rest and dry dressings with the constant changing of wet dressings under Listerism.

154 J. Hutchison, 'Gonorrhoea', in Treves, *System of Surgery*.

155 I. S. L. Loudon, *Childbed Fever: A Documentary History*, London, Garland, 1995, xlix–liv.

156 Between 1850 and 1900, childbed or puerperal fever was desexed, changing from a disease specific to birthing women to another form of septic infection.

had made surgery safe and expanded its scope.[157] However, few of the new invasive and reconstructive treatments were pioneered by Lister's circle.[158] Lister's own practice was reparative rather than operative, and while he introduced many new techniques, he did not pioneer any major invasive procedure. Other surgeons did cut deeper into more parts of the body, more often, though the main areas of growth in surgical practice were in minor operations and procedures such as appendectomies. Among the increasingly routine procedures were the removal of tumours; repair of the stomach wall for hernias; removing diseased organs such as the gall bladder and spleen; fixing 'wandering' organs, notably the kidney; and generally adopting more radical measures for older operations, such as lithotomy.[159] Surgeons spoke of their progressive colonisation of the major body cavities, from abdomen to chest and then to the brain and spinal cord.[160] Bacterial aetiologies were also used to justify more radical excisions, for example, with tubercular joints and infected wounds.[161] The removal of tonsils, teeth and the appendix was understood to be either excising infected organs, or as a prophylactic, removing organs that were fertile soil for infection.

After Cheyne swapped his bench for the bedside and operating table, he became decidedly ambivalent about the tension between laboratory and clinic. In 1889, he spoke of there having been a reconciliation, between those who had overestimated the importance of the infecting organism and clinical observers who had stressed other factors. The antiseptic theory he now articulated made 'pyogenic organisms' the essential cause of sepsis, but he qualified this with the condition that the actual production of the disease 'much depends on other conditions', such as the species of organism, their number and concentration, their virulence, where they infect the body, general and local condition of the body, especially the presence of other disease, and 'local and seasonal conditions'.[162] This made pyogenic bacteria much less formidable enemies than Lister's original panspermic germs. Indeed, Cheyne concluded that it was 'comparatively easy' to keep germs out of operative wounds, and that in wound management surgeons now had the

57 The subject was mentioned for the first time in many years in a review of surgery for 1889 only to say that antiseptic surgery was 'universally recognised and practised', though the details varied. *BMJ*, 1889, ii: 1545.

58 One Listerian who was a major innovator in operative surgery was William McEwen in neurosurgery. See: A. K. Bowman, *The Life and Teaching of Sir William McEwen*, London, W. Hodge and Co., 1942.

59 A review of surgery in 1884 noted as the most striking changes: 'a more correct judgement of the claims of certain bold and heroic operations' and 'a still further extended application of operative surgery to regions and organs hitherto regarded as solely the province of the physician. *BMJ*, 1884, ii: 1294. Also see: F. A. Humphry, 'The Medical Aspect of Surgery', *BMJ*, 1886, ii: 307.

60 W. Stokes, 'The Altered Relations of Surgery to Medicine', *BMJ*, 1888, i: 1197–1202.

61 J. Burney Yeo, 'Clinical Lectures on the Treatment of Disease', *MTG*, 1884, ii: 772; A. E. J. Barker, 'Tubercular Joint-Disease and its Treatment by Operation', *BMJ*, 1888, i: 1202, 1259–65, 1322–5.

62 Cheyne, *Suppuration*, 66–85.

technologies to 'step in with vigorous action without any fear of doing harm'. However, he was also beginning to use military metaphors alongside those of seed and soil, though stressing defence over attack. Thus, he wrote of the need 'to prevent the enemy entering', 'to do battle with them outside the body' and not to 'trust to the efficacy of the tissues to repel their attacks'. This line of argument was undoubtedly influenced by the work of the Koch School that showed that the balance of forces between seed and soil could be very one-sided in favour of the seed, particularly with very virulent bacteria.

ASEPTIC SURGERY

During the 1890s three groups of surgeons laid claim to be the inventors and custodians of aseptic or germ-free surgery. First, and of longest standing, were the Listerians, who continued to say that Listerism had always aimed to create germless wounds. Second, the Cleanliness School were clear that their practice of absolute purity and had always denied germs opportunities to develop.[163] Third, there was a new group of no-germ surgeons whose practice had its origins in Germany. The essence of their approach was to make the whole surgical environment germ-free or aseptic. Included within this aim was the patient's skin; surgical instruments; ligatures; dressings; the surgeon's hands; and the tables, floors and walls of the operating room. Some supporters of the new asepsis were arguing that it was imperative to have a specially designed work space for operations, as well as special dress, for example, rubber gloves, boots and face masks. A key marker for this approach was that it used heat, either boiling, steam, or the dry heat of autoclaves, rather than chemical antiseptics. The new aseptic surgery stressed, as apparently had old-style Listerism, the battle against the seeds of septic infection. Its advocates took the injunction to treat surgical operation as a 'bacteriological experiment' literally, as they tested the sterility of everything from the patient's skin to the washings from the operating table with microscopy and cultures. The standard story has been that asepsis developed from Listerism; however, recently a number of historians have argued that the Cleanliness School was its true progenitor.[164] It was certainly the case that the new aseptic surgery was a departure from the eclectic Listerism of the late 1880s, and that Lister and many of his allies opposed the new aseptic surgery. However, I want to support the older idea of a continuity between Listerism and asepsis, though on wider grounds than previously.[165]

163 Bantock, *BMJ*, 1900, I: 806.
164 N. J. Fox, 'Scientific Theory Choice and Social Structure: The Case of Joseph Lister's Antisepsis, Humoral Theory and Asepsis', *History of Science*, 1988, 26: 368. Fox maintains that asepsis was not a development of Listerism, 'but an entirely novel process, based *on a completely different theory*'.
165 Pennington has also criticised the idea of a non-Listerian pedigree for asepsis. H. Pennington, 'Listerism, its Decline and Persistence: The Introduction of Aseptic Surgical Techniques in Three British Teaching Hospitals', *MH*, 39: 39–47.

The new aseptic surgery was pioneered in Germany and came mainly from two sources: the laboratory and the factory. Koch's school had little time for 'seed and soil' notions, and made germs powerful invading agents that had to be tracked down and combated at all costs.[166] Also, in large part due to Koch's own influential work on disinfection, German surgeons extolled the virtues of heat sterilisation over chemical antiseptics.[167] This commitment spawned a small manufacturing sector whose sterilising equipment was bought by a few British hospitals and public health authorities. Pennington has shown, in a comparison of three British hospitals, that asepsis was taken up unevenly and piecemeal, and that surgeons used chemicals and heat in many combinations.[168] Thus, even with the most fundamentalist heat sterilising, aseptic surgeons still used chemicals for cleaning their skin and that of their patients, and during actual operations. There were many enthusiasts for asepsis, and Listerians were forced to respond to the challenges they made against antiseptic surgery. The leading theorist of the new aseptic surgery in Britain was Charles Barrett Lockwood (see Figure 14). He had qualified MRCS in 1878, and had worked as a surgeon and demonstrator in anatomy before turning to bacteriology after working with Klein at St. Bartholomew's Hospital. Lockwood established a small bacteriological laboratory in the museum and, with Vincent Harris, taught the first course in practical bacteriology at the hospital in 1889.[169] This class was taken over by Kanthack in 1893 as, like Cheyne and Ogston before him, Lockwood pursued a clinical career, specialising in appendectomies and cancer. In 1891 he was made a surgeon at St Bartholomew's, replacing Lister's last great metropolitan opponent – William Savory.

Lockwood's initial studies of wounds were funded by a research grant from the BMA and focused on comparisons between the bacteriology of septic and nonseptic operative cases. He then moved on to explore the infective power of the skin, sponges and towels under different conditions.[170] His work was unusual for Britain, as surgeons were generally content to talk of ferments and germs instead of 'streps' and 'staphs', and were rather complacent about their practical and professional 'progress'. Lockwood argued that his studies showed that wounds healed faster and with fewer complications when they were completely free of septic microorganisms. He also confirmed the superiority of (dry) heat over (wet) chemicals for disinfection, and recommended the use of

66 J. A. Mendelsohn, *Cultures of Bacteriology: Foundation and Transformation of a Science in France and Germany, 1870–1914*, Unpublished PhD thesis, Princeton University, 1997, 255–63.
67 T. D. Brock, *Robert Koch*, Madison, WI, Science Tech, 1988, 105–13.
68 Pennington, 'Listerism', 39–43, 46–7.
69 E. C. O. Jewesbury, *The Life and Work of C. B. Lockwood, 1856–1914*, London, H. K. Lewis, 1936.
70 C. B. Lockwood, 'Preliminary Report on Aseptic and Septic Surgical Cases', *BMJ*, 1890, ii: 943–7; idem., 'Further Report on Aseptic and Septic Surgical Cases, with Special Reference to Infection from the Skin', *BMJ*, 1892, i: 1127–37; idem, 'Report on Aseptic and Septic Surgical Cases', with Special Reference to the Disinfection of the Skin, Sponges and Towels', *BMJ*, 1894, i: 175–83.

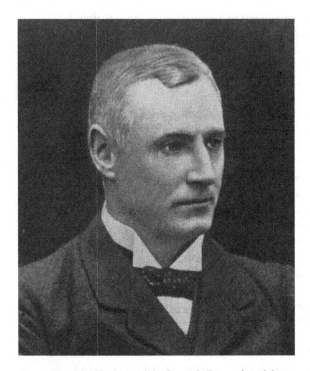

Figure 14. Charles Barrett Lockwood (Reproduced by courtesy of the Wellcome Institute Library, London)

bacteriological testing to monitor the efficacy of different methods. All of this
was said to require that surgeons adopt rigorous procedures for ensuring sterility, a point that Lockwood reinforced with the familiar suggestion that an
aseptic operation was 'a delicate bacteriological experiment'.[171] Surprisingly,
he argued that aseptic procedures made surgery 'more simple and rational'
rather than more complicated. However, most surgeons saw aseptic surgery as
complex, technically demanding and expensive. Lockwood's biographer recognised his modernist commitments, observing that 'his conception of the
coming doctor was one who would have his dwelling in a small apartment
adjoining a huge laboratory, and who would carry with him test tubes and antitoxins when he set out to visit his patients by aeroplane'.[172] In 1894, Cheyne,
after reasserting a Listerian pedigree for the new system, said that while 'theoretically perfectly correct', it was unnecessary. Cheyne was confident that the
range of antiseptic methods and what surgeons now knew about the receptiv-

171 C. B. Lockwood, 'A Brief Note on Aseptic Surgery; Advocating the More Frequent Use of
      Scientific Tests', *QMJ*, 1895–96, 4: 118.
172 Jewesbury, *Lockwood*, 77.

ity of the body had made surgery as safe as was practically possible. He pre-dicted that the new aseptic surgery would become a 'surgical curiosity' as it was irksome and gave no better results than the existing antiseptic methods.[173] The new asepsis was recognised as popular in Germany and the United States, but was said to be ill-suited to British voluntary hospitals because of its cost and the high turnover of staff made it difficult to ensure that assistants built up the necessary levels of expertise.

An important principle of aseptic surgery was that the 'resistance of the healthy living tissues to bacterial invasion cannot be relied upon'.[174] This view did not simply represent scepticism about immune responses as such; Lockwood also argued that the problem was that immunity was 'beyond the control of the surgeon, while asepsis is not'. Thus, asepsis gave surgeons the certainty and control that allowed them to accept full technical and moral responsibility for the patient and their treatment.[175] This made surgeons heroic both practically and morally, a position that befitted their professional self-image as the coming men of medicine. Given this ideology, it is paradoxical that Lister spent most of the 1890s involved in two main projects: spreading the word about the new ideas on chemical and cellular immunity, and extolling the value of simplified versions of his methods. At the International Medical Congress in 1890, Lister made his famous admission that he was ashamed' ever to have recommended the use of the spray. His confidence that surgeons could do without it came from his belief that most air-borne bacteria were attenuated and hence harmless, and from Metchnikoff's ideas on how phagocytes defend the body against the assaults of bacteria.[176] Lister's faith in the body's powers of resistance was evident at the end of the year, when he personally visited Berlin to learn of Koch's new Tuberculin remedy for tuberculosis, which was understood to act by boosting immunity.[177] The relative failure of Tuberculin did not dent Lister's faith in the powers of soil over seed, and by 1893 he was combining humoral and phagocytic notions to bolster his wonder at the 'power of nature's defences against the microbes'.[178] He also quoted the value of antitoxins and antisera, though he

73 W. W. Cheyne, *The Treatment of Wounds, Ulcers and Abscesses*, Edinburgh, Young J. Pentland, 1894, 57–60. For other critics of asepsis on practical grounds, see: *BMJ*, 1892, i: 327; W. W. Cheyne, 'Wounds and Contusions' in Treves, ed., *System*, 221.

74 Lockwood, *Aseptic Surgery*, Edinburgh, Young J. Pentland, 1896, 96.

75 S. White, 'Aseptic Surgery', *QMJ*, 1899–1900, 8: 14–25. White observes that teachers used to not recommend Listerism, but they insisted that failure to resort to these measures was tantamount to professional negligence.

76 J. Lister, 'An Address on the Present Position of Antiseptic Surgery', *BMJ*, 1890, ii: 377–9. Tait responded to Lister's remarks with a vitriolic attack in which he accused Lister of starting a 'school' and following every new theoretical speculation or laboratory finding in the field. He suggested that Koch's work had not as yet had the slightest practical importance and was dismissive of phagocytes. *BMJ*, 1890, ii: 728.

77 *Lancet*, 1980, ii: 1257–9.

78 *BMJ*, 1893, ii: 277.

ignored the specific examples that surgeons might have used, notably anti-streptococcal and antistaphylococcal sera.[179] The new knowledge of immunity was used to justify the simplification of antiseptic methods, especially the abandonment of the spray and return to favour of carbolic acid, albeit in weaker dilutions.[180] The contrasts that Lister drew between antiseptic and aseptic surgery were largely matters of detail: chemicals versus heat in sterilisation methods; antiseptics versus water and saline for irrigation and washing; simple versus elaborate techniques, though the sting was in the tail – a secure, proven practice versus an unproven method with lower margins of safety.

That antisepsis and asepsis were alternatives rather than opposites was confirmed in textbook advice on surgical techniques. Rose and Carless, in their influential *Manual of Surgery*, which went through an edition a year between 1898 and 1902, easily combined the two methods, though they recommended the latest versions of antisepsis rather than asepsis because it was more reliable and easier to practice.[181] In the management of injuries and infected wounds, they said that there was no choice – antiseptic methods had to be used as tissues were already likely to be infected. However, with operative wounds a number of approaches were possible from the broad spectrum of antiseptic methods. The choices made by surgeons had to depend on where in the body they were operating, the condition being treated, what procedure was being used, how long it would take and the staff and resources available. The authors described a seven-stage routine to establish 'the strictest antisepsis for the external parts, but asepsis for the interior of the wound'.[182] First, the surgeons had to wash and scrub their hands with soap and boiled water, followed by immersion in antiseptic lotion. Second, all instruments had to be sterilised in strong carbolic lotion, and, if time allowed, these were also boiled in the same solution. Next, sponges, dressings, ligatures and sutures were to be purified, with different substances used for each. Fourth, the site of the operation had to be made safe, with the skin of the patient treated in the same way as the surgeon's hands, and surrounded with antiseptically treated towels and macintoshes. After the operation the exposed tissues and wound had to be irrigated with antiseptics (or sterile saline) before closure, and then covered with an antiseptic dressing. They offered no alternative to the application of chemicals for germ-free surgeons' hands, ligatures and the patient's skin. The use of rubber or silk gloves was seen to offer little additional protection to the patient, but were thought to be beneficial in protecting surgeons from infection. The nonirritant advantages of heat-sterilised

179 L. Cobbett, 'Anti-streptococcal Sera', *Lancet*, 1898, i: 986–92.
180 J. Lister, 'An Address on the Antiseptic Management of Wounds', *BMJ*, 1893, i: 161–2, 277–8, 337–9; idem, 'The Essentials of Antiseptic Surgery', *BMJ*, 1893, ii: 1014. Idem., 'On the Simplification of the Antiseptic Treatment', *GMJ*, 1894, 41: 434–9.
181 W. Rose and A. Carless, *A Manual of Surgery*, London, Baillière, Tindall and Cox, 1898. The success of this volume was evident in the rapidity of new editions in 1899, 1900, 1901 and 1902.
182 Rose, *Manual*, 19.

swabs, towels and dry dressings (instead of sponges, macintoshes and wet dressings) were acknowledged, but Rose and Carless wondered if surgeons could be confident that sterilisation had been thorough and that there had been no subsequent contamination. The great advantage of chemicals was that they were long-lasting and that the experienced surgeon could rely on his sense of smell and feel the acid irritate his hands throughout the operation.

Between 1877 and 1900, Lister and his supporters changed the theory on which they justified their practice several times. The exciting agents of sepsis changed in form and function from 'germs' to 'bacteria' to micrococci, and then specific staphylococcal and streptococcal parasitic microorganisms. Their construction of how these agents acted changed many times, too. In the late 1870s and early 1880s, Listerians helped forge new understandings of septic infection; but after 1882 they were followers rather than leaders, selectively adopting and adapting ideas and practices from many specialisms and countries to legitimate their anticontamination methods. As the leading representatives of the modernising, scientific wing of surgery, Listerians were quite imperialist, maintaining their power by annexing alternative ideas and methods and exploiting them for their cause. In the mid-1870s, Listerians were still more concerned with showing that germs were real and with ensuring that they were killed than with understanding their nature. Their ideal was a germ-free microclimate around the wound or patient; hence I find no difficulty with the idea that aseptic surgery was a development of Listerism. Listerian antigerm practices were broadened in the 1880s, and incorporated many other methods that had been developed with quite different rationales and materials. However, the new aseptic surgery developed in the 1890s was a step too far for some Listerians, being rejected on practical grounds and for giving too much weight to germs and disease, and insufficient weight to the human body and health.

Exactly when Lister became interested in the germ theories of health is unclear, though the change of heart was quite marked. Until the mid-1870s Lister was widely understood to be a straightforward contaminationist; his panspermic germs were such powerful agents on dead or devitalised tissues that the entry of a single one could be fatal. Not only did they lose putative powers in the late 1870s and early 1880s, but human tissues gained powers. The first change was most evident when Listerians began to deploy and emphasise the distinction between putrefactive germs and infectious disease organisms, which previously had at best been implicit. The germlessness of living tissue and blood remained articles of faith. If the healthy body was otherwise, they had been wasting their time keeping germs out so assiduously. When forced to admit that septic microorganisms could survive in the body, Lister turned his attention to explaining how the body contained their

effects, hence his championing of Metchnikoff's ideas of scavenging leukocytes in the blood stream eating up septic micrococci and of chemical anti-
dotes to bacteria.

By 1900 the idea that antisepsis had revolutionised surgery was still being
promoted by Listerians, but contemporary assessments were usually more
modest. These placed antisepsis alongside a number of other factors that had
changed the practice of surgery, its position in medicine and its wider social
standing. Lister himself was the first to admit that his initial understanding
of septic infection had been crude, and that his practice had been refined
and improved with the advance of knowledge. What was accepted, by his
critics as well as his supporters, was that his ideas and methods had helped
to bring about a change in the culture of surgery.[183] First, Listerism had
shown and represented the need for 'greater care in all the details of hygiene'
and had persuaded all surgeons that sepsis could be avoided or combated.[184]
One surgeon wrote that Lister's practice carried the connotation of 'tran-
scendental cleanliness', a term that nicely captures the way that contemporaries thought the effects of Listerism had spilt over into improved ward
hygiene, better buildings with improved ventilation and even better nursing
care for patients.[185] Second, Listerians had widened the scope of the surgeon's
responsibilities. According to Sampson Gamgee in 1883, surgeons 'have ceased
to delegate the all important matter of dressing to comparatively unskilled
assistants, and have devoted themselves to it, with the painstaking care which
it deserves'.[186] This broader conception of the surgeon's role was congruent
with the earlier ideal of surgery becoming more medical in its work, style
and status. As early as 1876, Furneaux Jordan, Professor of Surgery at Queen's
College, Birmingham, observed that cellular pathology and the germ-theory
of disease had made surgeons 'subtle metaphysicians' while 'in practice they
aim to be superior dressers and ingenious mechanists'.[187] By 1900s surgeons
could claim to have their cake and eat it too, claiming to be both medical
sophisticates and heroic interventionists.[188] Third, antiseptic surgery, ever more
broadly defined, had demonstrated the importance of detail, precision, exactness and above all science in surgery.

183 An early statement of the Listerian history of surgery was John Chiene's article, 'Practice of
Surgery', *Encyclopaedia Britannica*, Vol. 22, London, 1887, 677–80; Cf. *BMJ*, 1888, ii: 295.
184 T. Holmes, 'Antiseptics', in Holmes, *System of Surgery*, 43; J. Wood, 'Bradshawe Lecture', 1097.
Stanley Boyd observed that 'every hospital shows the results of antiseptics, though Listerism may
not be practised'. S. Boyd, 'Hospitalism', in Heath, *Dictionary*, 740–1.
185 MacCormac, 'Old and New', 586
186 S. Gamgee, *On the Treatment of Wounds and Fractures*, London, Churchill, 1883, 298.
187 F. Jordan, 'On the Gradual Decrease in Operative Surgery', *BMR*, 1876, 5: 25.
188 Editorial, 'On the Relations of Modern Surgery to Medicine', *BMJ*, 1887, i: 118; *BMJ*, 1889, ii:
362.

6

From Heredity to Infection: Tuberculosis, Bacteriology and Medicine, 1870–1900

In the summer of 1882, W. M. Crowfoot, a provincial surgeon, remarked that the influence of germ-theory had been stronger in surgery and sanitary science than in medicine.[1] He speculated that this was largely because no one had come up with ways to kill or alter germs in the body without damaging healthy tissues. He might also have added that physicians tended to assume that most medical diseases had internal and often spontaneous origins, hence they only thought of external factors as predisposing rather than exciting causes. Crowfoot's comments were prompted by Robert Koch's claim in April 1882 to have identified the microorganism that was the essential cause of consumption. Some doctors at the time claimed, as have many historians since, that Koch's new aetiological construction of consumption was revolutionary.[2] Koch asserted that consumption was a contagious disease, with a specific, bacterial cause, rather than a constitutional condition, with hereditary origins. Of course, the new model for consumption exemplified the switch from physiological to ontological models of disease. Historians have mostly gone along with the assessment that there was a major discontinuity in 'theories' of consumption after 1882, but they have maintained that there were continuities of management and treatment practices; indeed, it is often stated that effective intervention was denied to doctors until the innovation of streptomycin and related drugs in the 1940s.

In this chapter I argue that these assessments of 'theories' and 'practices' need to be revised. First, I point to significant continuities in the medical understanding of consumption because of different responses across medicine, and because the dominant seed and soil metaphor allowed constitutional notions to be refashioned in terms of the vulnerability of the human 'soil' and then immunities. Second, I show that there were significant innovations in management and therapies, as doctors tried to attack the seeds of disease and, more importantly, to boost the condition of the

W. M. Crowfoot, 'The Germ-Theory of Disease', *BMJ*, 1882, ii: 554.

J. M. Grange and P. J. Bishop, 'Über Tuberculose: A Tribute to Robert Koch's Discovery of the Tubercle Bacillus', *Tubercle*, 1982, 63: 3–17. Cf. *BMJ*, 1882, i: 624.

human soil so that it could better resist the growth and effects of *Tubercle bacilli*.

I begin with a discussion of changes in the understanding and management of consumption from the 1860s to 1880, a period of considerable turbulence rather than one of enduring traditions as often assumed. I then explore the contrasting reception of Koch's work between clinicians, pathologists and public health doctors, particularly on how his findings were used to legitimate different approaches to the prevention and treatment of consumption. As germs arrived relatively late in medicine, and then only as well-defined bacteria rather than vague germs, an important part of this story is how physicians had to adapt to meanings and exemplars that had been negotiated in surgery and public health. I suggest that consumption was remodelled slowly in medicine and that attempts by MOsH to add it to their responsibilities were half-hearted and had not succeeded by 1900. However, I argue that Koch's practices were as important in medicine as his new theory. Rapid and radical changes resulted from the manner in which the germ practices that Koch developed were used as the basis for creating the discipline of bacteriology. By the mid-1880s, theorising about germs had been replaced by a research programme based on standard methods, an expanding group of practitioners, cognitive exemplars and the promise of clinical benefits. In this context, I test Clifford Allbutt's assertion in 1882 that 'Germ theory had become germ fact'.[3] In the final two parts of the chapter I discuss how the new practical, cognitive and ideological resources of bacteriology were adopted and adapted to produce new initiatives in the clinical management and above all the prevention of consumption. In this context, it should not be forgotten that the *Tubercle bacillus* appeared for the first time only a year after Pasteur's first public demonstrations of new preventive experiments with his new vaccines and the optimism that was built up around changing the human soil to make it immune to all contagious and infectious diseases.

CONSUMPTION AND TUBERCULOSIS, 1870–1882

Consumption was the largest single recorded cause of death in Britain in the nineteenth century and wrought an annual death toll of over 50,000 in England and Wales through the 1870s. A further 20,000 people died annually of nonrespiratory forms of tubercular diseases, such as scrofula, tabes mesenterica and tubercular joints.[4] As a chronic disease, where the patient declined towards death over an average of four to five years, from the

---

3 C. Allbutt, *BMJ*, 1882, i: 618; The Birmingham surgeon T. H. Bartleet similarly suggested that germ-theory had become 'Germ Law'. Cf. *BMR*, 1881, 10: 90.

4 The mortality rate in 1870 was 240 per 100,000 living. Put another way, there were 54,231 deaths from consumption out of a total of 515,229 deaths overall.

50,000 annual deaths we can estimate at least 200,000 active cases of the pulmonary form at any one time; thus, at least one in every hundred citizens, or one in every forty adults between the ages of twenty and sixty was a sufferer at any time. Given this level of incidence, which was highest in towns where doctors were also concentrated, there is little doubt that physicians, general practitioners and other healers saw and treated many consumptives. Most clinical experience of the disease was gained in the consulting room or the patient's home, not in hospitals or in the dissecting room. Consumptives were excluded from voluntary hospitals because they were incurable, while in Poor Law Infirmaries, which sufferers would only reach in the final stages of the illness, medical attention was perfunctory. A small number of voluntary chest hospitals, mostly in London, had been founded to offer care to this neglected group of patients, but the number of beds available was tiny. The leading metropolitan institution, the Brompton Hospital, became the focus for the development of clinical, if not pathological, knowledge and was home to a merging group of specialists in the disease.[5]

Consumption was the popular term for the disease, but doctors preferred the term 'phthisis', no doubt keen to confirm their learning and exclusivity. The terms of consumptive, scrofulous and tuberculous were alternative labels for sufferers and the presumed condition of their body that led to the disease; for example, they had a scrofulous diathesis or tuberculous constitution. Culturally, consumptives and their families carried the stigma of an inherited taint', with connotations of weakness and undesirable qualities.[6] Sometimes clinicians spoke of a person's diathesis or constitution as if tubercular disease was programmed into the system to emerge at a set time.[7] However, it was more common for doctors to regard a diathesis in terms of tendencies or proclivities that could remain latent, or would become manifest only in certain circumstances, for example, when tissues weakened and degenerated following other diseases, or with life-style and environmental changes. Indeed, a person's constitutional was not fixed, nor was it wholly hereditary. A weak (or strong) constitution could also be acquired through the influences of the environment, diet, behaviour and other illnesses. Epidemiological studies had shown consumption to be prevalent in certain occupations: publicans and those who worked inside or in dusty conditions had the highest incidence. In towns, male mortality was significantly higher than female, though in the countryside rates were equal; so was it a disease of the indoors? The incidence of the disease was highest amongst the poor, whose living conditions and life-style were thought to lower vitality and allow any diathesis to express

M. Davidson and F. G. Rouvray, *The Brompton Hospital: The Story of a Great Adventure*, London, Lloyd Luke, 1954.

K. Ott, *Fevered Lives: Tuberculosis in American Culture since 1870*, Cambridge, MA, Harvard University Press, 1996, 9–52.

F. B. Smith, *The Retreat of Tuberculosis*, London, Croom Helm, 1988, 25–55.

itself. Certainly, by the last quarter of the century the earlier romantic associations with genius and heightened sensibilities had been replaced by links with debility and degeneration.

The dominant medical account of consumption in the 1860s was based on Laennec's classic studies.[8] He had defined consumption as one of a number of tubercular afflictions that were recognisable postmortem by the presence of small swellings or nodules, in which grey-yellow masses were deposited (tubercles) and which over time became enclosed in hardened (caseous) deposits. His observation that tubercles had a common structure led him to regard all tubercular diseases as unitary, be they manifest as scrofula in the lymphatic system, tabes mesenterica in the abdomen, tubercular meningitis in the central nervous system, surgical tuberculosis in the joints, miliary tuberculosis in other organs or consumption in the lungs. The nodules were seemingly formed as existing tissues and organs were broken down and 'consumed', for example, producing cavities in the lungs or 'disorganised' joints. As new growths, tubercles were understood either to spread locally by infiltrating surrounding tissue, or to be disseminated to other sites in the body, in a way analogous to metastases in cancer. Laennec's view stood the first test of cellular pathology when Lebert found common 'corpuscles' in his microscopical studies of tubercular lesions in the 1840s.[9]

Laennec had matched the destruction of lung tissue to the characteristic clinical signs of the disease: a wracking cough (which removed debris from the lungs), general lethargy and wasting (due to poor respiration resulting from the reduced size of the lungs) and eventually haemoptysis (coughing blood) as blood vessels in the lung burst. He made these connections through his pioneering use of auscultation, that is, listening to the sounds of the body through a tube, and later bi-aural stethoscopes. From the rattles, wheezing and echoes heard, doctors learned how to create 'sound pictures' that were imaginatively correlated with anatomical changes that were checked against postmortem findings. However, older methods, such as percussion (tapping the chest), noting chest movements and above all observation of a person's demeanour continued to be valued. One reason for this was that the onset of consumption was insidious and had often reached an advanced stage before symptoms appeared. Early diagnosis required great acumen and the prognosis always demanded sensitive handling, as it usually meant a protracted illness and eventual death. These features and its prevalence in young adults made doctors, if not patients, alert to any tiredness, loss of appetite, loss of weight, indigestion, night sweats and 'diminished general health and deteriorated

8 R. Maulitz, *Morbid Appearances: The Anatomy of Pathology in the Early Nineteenth Century*, Cambridge, Cambridge University Press, 1987, 71–80, 94–100.
9 F. von Niemeyer, *Clinical Lectures on Pulmonary Consumption*, London, New Sydenham Society, 1870.

constitutional vigour'.[10] The combination of the old and the new methods was said by the mid-1860s to have allowed 'in the great majority of cases . . . an exactitude and certainty of which the modern cultivators of medicine may well be proud'.[11] The increased use and visibility of this auscultation was important culturally for medicine, as the lancet, an instrument of heroic intervention, gave way to the stethoscope, a device of diagnosis and prognosis, as the popular icon of medical practice.[12]

While Laennec's ideas were dominant, there remained an alternative, if minority, pathological model based on the ideas of his French contemporary, Broussais. This supposed that tubercles were neither unitary, specific nor primary. Rather, they were nonspecific and secondary, the possible result of any tissue becoming inflamed. In the 1860s, Virchow and other proponents of cellular pathology, using microscopes rather than the unaided eye and knife, offered support to Broussais. Virchow claimed to have distinguished true grey tubercular lesions from other processes producing caseous nodules, and argued that consumption and scrofula were quite different diseases. What became known as the 'German School' regarded tuberculosis as one possible result of inflammation, not a new growth of a specific nature. Further histological studies led to the increasingly fine differentiation of lesions and to calls for the term 'tubercle' to be dropped altogether. An immediate target was Lebert's corpuscles, which were said to have been imaginary, but the big prize was the unity of the disease – the defining feature of the so-called French School.

Uncertainties about the pathogenesis and status of tubercles were further compounded in the mid-1860s, when Villemin claimed that tuberculous lesions could be produced by the inoculation of tuberculous tissue into susceptible animals. The analogues that his vivisection suggested were the passage of glanders from animals to humans, and the transmission of syphilis from person to person. However, Villemin's laboratory procedure was said to produce only 'artificial tuberculosis', and it was difficult to see how tubercular matter might find its way from deep inside one body to the interior of another in ordinary conditions. Historians have been interested in Villemin's work because of its seeming anticipation of modern views; a recent assessment actually says that 'he got it right' and bemoans the fact that British doctors continued to dismiss his results for the next two decades'.[13] This reading of events is mistaken empirically and theoretically. Villemin's experiments were certainly not dismissed. They were repeated by Wilson Fox and Andrew Clark, and in state-funded research by John Burdon

0 J. Hughes Bennett, 'Phthisis pulmonalis', in J. Reynolds, *A System of Medicine*, Volume 3, London, Macmillan, 1871, 554–67.
1 Ibid., 555. Also see: *BMJ*, 1866, i: 12; *MTG*, 1865, ii: 689.
2 S. J. Reiser, *Medicine and the Reign of Technology*, Cambridge, Cambridge University Press, 1978, 30–44.
3 Smith, *Retreat*, 35.

Sanderson.[14] Their results were published and debated in Britain and elsewhere, but only, of course, in terms of prevailing pathological models, not,
unsurprisingly, in terms of yet to be invented bacterial pathologies.[15]

The idea that tubercular disease was 'infective', in the sense of the dissemination of tubercles *within* the body – self-poisoning as some put it – was
nothing new; after all, the disease was still classified with cancer. However,
'infective' in the sense of the external transmission or communication of
disease from person to person was quite another matter. In the late 1860s
and early 1870s, hardly anyone interpreted Villemin's work to suggest that
tubercular diseases were ordinarily contagious. If any implications for human
heath were drawn, it was by veterinarians and MOsH, who warned about
the dangers of ingesting meat and milk contaminated with tuberculous
matter. In Britain this whole paradigm was associated with William Budd,
not Villemin. In 1867, arguing in his familiar analogical style, Budd pointed
to similarities between consumption and a disease like typhoid fever, especially their specificity, their clinical manifestations, their casting off *materies
morbi*, their infectiousness and their pattern of incidence. He added to this
his own personal experiences of the disease spreading in families. Coming
from such a well-known figure, these claims provoked a reaction. John Simon
was quite receptive to the idea. In his commentary on Sanderson's inoculation experiments in the Medical Department's Annual Report for 1869, he
speculated that both tuberculosis and cancer might be zymotic diseases. This
led Lionel Beale to write to Sanderson that Simon must have been 'Some
wicked little microzyme . . . pirouetting in . . . the cortical portion of his
cerebral convolutions'.[16] Almost all of the comments by clinicians on Budd's
proposition were dismissive.[17] The attack was led by Richard Payne Cotton,
Physician at the Brompton Hospital, and Samuel Wilks (1824–1911), Senior
Physician at Guy's Hospital.[18] Cotton offered detailed evidence that only a
handful of Brompton staff had ever succumbed to consumption, and that
his own rude health was testimony to the noncontagiousness of the disease.
He reiterated that clinical experience had shown repeatedly that a particular
diathesis was the main aetiological factor. Cotton had his own pathological
analogue, namely, that tubercles were the product of consumption just as sugar

14 Dr. Wilson Fox also repeated Villemin's work independently; see: W. Fox, *On the Artificial Production of Tubercle in the Lower Animals*, London, Macmillan, 1868; J. B. Sanderson, 'Report on the
   Inoculability and Development of Tubercle', *Tenth Report of the Medical Officer of the Privy Council
   for 1867*, BPP, 1867–68, [4004], xxxvi, 413; idem, 'Further Report on the Inoculability and Development of Tubercle', *Eleventh Report of the Medical Officer of the Privy Council for 1868*, BPP,
   1868–69, [4127], xxxii, 91–125.
15 In 1873, the Pathological Society of London discussed the 'Pulmonary Phthisis' over three
   sessions, the sessions being led by Wilson Fox. 'Anatomical Relations of Pulmonary Phthisis to
   Tubercle of the Lung, *TPSL*, 1873: 24, 284–8. Beale and Bastian spoke, the former suggesting
   that Tubercles were bioplasm, Ibid., 315.
16 Beale to Sanderson, 16 November 1869, UCL, Sanderson Papers, 179/1 22–23.
17 *Lancet* 1867, ii: 451–2.   18 *Lancet*, 1867, ii: 550–1, 594–5.

was of diabetes. He argued that consumption was clinically quite unlike zymotic diseases, which were specific and ran a predictable course, while consumption was one of the most variable of all diseases, liable to wax and wane erratically. On top of this, epidemiological data showed that mortality for consumption was reasonably constant month to month, which suggested that whatever was producing the disease was not external.[19] Wilks noted that Budd was assuming that diseases were 'entities' and could 'attach themselves to healthy individuals from without', whereas received wisdom was moving towards the fact that 'they are manifestations of some prior constitutional peculiarity'.[20] The important point retrospectively was that the contagiousness of consumption had been debated and, at least in clinical medicine, dismissed.

The replication of Villemin's experiments in Britain produced significant new findings. Sanderson's results attracted the most attention. He was not content just to inoculate tubercular matter; he also tried pus and other substances, even leaving cotton setons in wounds as controls. He found that tubercles could sometimes form around the site of any inoculation or injury, which in his mind lent support to Virchow and the teaching of the German School. If tubercles were the result of inflammation in certain types of tissue, then it followed that tuberculosis was a nonspecific process. However, most clinicians stuck with Laennec's ideas, which they matched to their own clinical experience. Sanderson, who was an Assistant Physician at the Brompton, recognised the conflict but sided with the nonspecific, inflammatory viewpoint for clinical as well as pathological reasons.[21] He claimed that as long as consumption was seen to arise spontaneously rather than from injury, there would be a tendency merely to nurse patients. On the other hand, if physicians could rid themselves of the idea that tubercles had some 'specific malignity' and approach lesions as the 'unabsorbed residue of common inflammatory processes', then active treatment would be feasible.[22] Another advantage of the new model was that it removed one of the contradictions between Virchow's ideas and clinical experience, namely, how an affliction that presented clinically as a wasting disease could have its pathogenesis in the formation of new tissue.[23] Sanderson even suggested that tuberculosis was analogous to septic poisoning, as in both conditions adjoining tissues lost their vitality and decomposed.

During the 1870s, Thomas H. Green, another pathologist with a part-time appointment at the Brompton, became the leading British authority on the pathology of consumption. He was a graduate of University College

19 A. Hardy, *The Epidemic Streets: Infectious Disease and the Rise of Preventive Medicine, 1856–1900*, Oxford, Clarendon Press, 1993, 227.

20 Lancet, 1867, ii: 110, 134, 774. Also see: S. Wilks, 'Address in Medicine', *BMJ*, 1872, ii: 146–53.

21 *BMJ*, 1869, ii: 274.

22 Sanderson, 'On the Inoculability' 91–109.

23 Bennett, 'Pulmonary phthisis', 551–4.

Hospital, London, who had studied in Berlin and was Assistant Physician, Lecturer on Pathology and Superintendent of Post Mortem Examinations at Charing Cross Hospital, London. In 1871, Green published the first edition of what became one the most popular pathology textbooks of the late Victorian period. The changing accounts of tuberculosis in Green's writing and lectures reflect changes in thinking in Britain about tuberculosis and wider changes in pathology. In the first edition of his textbook, Green included tubercle under the section 'New Formations', though in a footnote he observed that it 'probably would have been more correct to have described tubercle amongst the *inflammatory* new formations'.[24] In the next edition, in 1873, tuberculosis was moved to the section on inflammation and its pathology now demanded two chapters rather than one. In published lectures in 1874, Green firmly sided with Virchow and Sanderson, even supporting the abandonment of the term 'tubercle' altogether.[25] As we might expect from an English pathologist at this time, Green concentrated on tissue changes and morbid histology, interpreting physiological actions by their anatomical results. His account of the pathogenesis of tubercular disease was congruent with the work being done by clinicians in differentiating the many different types of pulmonary consumption: acute, scrofulous, tuberculo-pneumonic, catarrhal, fibroid, heamorrhagic, laryngeal and chronic.[26] Some doctors spoke of this classification as typical of the 'British School', which was based on solid anatomical work and clinical experience, without the speculative excesses of the two Continental schools. Green's approach also revealed the concerns of a clinician, not least in how tubercular disease differed from other inflammations of the lung. By 1878, he was suggesting that different lung diseases resulted from the strength and duration of inflammation; for example, croupous pneumonia came from a brief but intense irritation that affected the blood and then the whole body. Consumption resulted from chronic inflammation that remained localised in the lungs. The key variable was the 'intensity' of the inflammation, which was determined by two factors: 'severity of injury, and susceptibility of tissue injured'.[27]

Green's views on the aetiology of consumption were expressed only briefly. Pathology had moved back from the results of disease to a concern with processes, but the final step back to a detailed consideration of causes had still to be made. Unsurprisingly, he favoured an inclusive, multifactorial account. The first component was an 'inherent weakness of the lungs . . . in

24 T. H. Green, *An Introduction to Pathology and Morbid Anatomy*, London, Henry Renshaw, 1871, 145.
25 'Anatomical Relations', *TPSL*, 1873, 24: 284–388.
26 W. Ewart, 'Pulmonary Cavities', *Lancet*, 1882, i: 515; S. Coupland, 'Tubercle', *BMJ*, 1882, i: 186–7; C. T. Williams, 'Phthisis', in R. Quain, ed., *Quain's Medical Dictionary*, London, Longmans Green, 1882, 1176–80.
27 T. H. Green, *The Pathology of Pulmonary Consumption: Three Lectures*, London, Henry Renshaw, 1878, 69. Unlike Burdon Sanderson, Green felt able to accommodate constitutional and diathetic ideas with inflammation.

most cases an inherited one'. This openness could be unique to the lungs,
or be part of 'a general weakness of the tissues', and might develop after
a respiratory or debilitating illness, for example, bronchitis, pneumonia or
pleurisy.[28] His second aetiological component was 'injuries', of which he listed
three kinds: (i) indirect injuries, like chills on the surface of the body; (ii)
direct injuries to the bronchi, like catarrh and pneumonic products spreading into the lungs; and (iii) infection by tuberculous matter from nodules that
had evolved *de novo* in other parts of the body, not from outside. The role
of one much cited factor in the disease – air – was explained in several ways.
Either rebreathed or devitiated air weakened the body by starving it of
oxygen, or its high carboniferous content irritated the alveoli and some
of this 'carbon' was possibly encrusted in tubercular deposits. Despite the
suggestions of Budd, Villemin and veterinarians, Green made no mention of
contagion.

This reshaping of consumption as an inflammatory affliction did not
produce a return to depletive, antiphlogistic treatments. Indeed, the very
opposite occurred. Given that the disease only became manifest in a weakened individual or devitalised tissues, treatments concentrated on strengthening and stimulating the patient with tonics. While some clinicians argued that
consumption was not a disease at all, but 'a mere mode of dying', and that
all medicine could do was 'prolong a life naturally drawing to its close', the
majority of doctors became more optimistic about arresting, if not curing,
the disease.[29] The bases for such hopes were many. First, it ought to be possible to remove irritants or counter their effects to reduce inflammation. Such
treatments would benefit from early diagnosis and steps to prevent irritation
from becoming chronic. Microscopy might be used to differentiate consumption from chronic pneumonia and pleurisy by looking in sputum for
fragments of the aureolar and elastic tissues derived from the disintegration
of the lungs'.[30] Second, regimens could be prescribed to revitalise the patient
by 'improving faulty nutrition' and, if an inherited phthisical constitution
could not be remade, then at least it might be compensated for.[31] The best
forms of restorative, antiinflammatory treatment were set out by John Hughes
Bennett: a good diet, cod-liver oil, exercise, a pure atmosphere and bathing,[32]
in other words, stimulant, phlogistic, or 'sthenic treatments, aided by climate
hygiene and medicine'.[33] For a short time cod-liver oil was somewhat of a

28 Green, *Pulmonary Consumption*, 77–9. Cf. A. B. Shepherd, *Goulstonian Lectures on the Natural History of Pulmonary Consumption*, London, Smith Elder, 1877; P. Gowan, *Consumption: Its Nature, Symptoms, Causes, Prevention, Curability and Treatment*, London, Churchill, 1878.
29 *BMJ*, 1867, ii: 137.
30 H. Williams, *Requiem for a Great Killer: the Story of Tuberculosis*, London, 1973. Williams entitled Chapter 7 'The Period of Physical Examination,' with the subtitle – 'Most of the Nineteenth Century'.
31 Hughes Bennett, 'Phthisis pulmonalis', 571.   32 Ibid., 571–9.
33 J. Henry Bennet, 'The treatment of pulmonary consumption', *BMJ*, 1867, ii: 137.

panacea, being described as 'an article of commerce on an enormous scale', and it was said by some physicians to have brought a therapeutic revolution.[34] Drugs were used largely to manage symptoms, especially the cough and expectoration. The variability of the disease, the patient's background, their temperament, their surroundings and their income meant that there was no formula; everything depended on the judgement of the doctor.[35]

A separate line of therapy was the use of specific antiinflammatory and antiseptic treatments. Principally these involved inhalations (with the vapours of carbolic acid, creosote, pine oil and hydrogen sulphide) and sending sufferers to mountainous climates.[36] At this time antiseptics were mainly used as deodorants because the breath of consumptives was offensive, though it was hoped that their acrid smell would stimulate expectoration, thereby removing irritants. However, some practitioners did see this approach as antiseptic in the Listerian sense, especially following Sanderson's speculations about parallels between tuberculosis and the septic poisoning of pyaemia. Their hope was that antiseptics would halt the absorption of poisons into the body and generally act as antiputrefactants.[37]

The role of climate in the development and management of consumption became a highly complex matter for physicians because success depended on matching the patient to a place and regimen. In the 1870s, the high Alps, sea voyages and distant deserts became more fashionable than the resorts of the Mediterranean. Pemble has suggested that cultural, moral and religious factors, as well as medical ones, produced this change.[38] However, there was no medical consensus on why cold temperatures, high altitude, dry air, or any climate for that matter, might help the consumptive. Physicians largely thought in terms of the sedative or tonic influence of the environment on the constitution. A patient with active disease might be recommended a long sojourn in a sedative, Mediterranean climate, both to lower the system and to avoid irritating chills. On the other hand, early or quiescent cases were recommended the bracing air of the Alps, either to stimulate the whole system or to elicit specific effects such as improved lung expansion and pulmonary circulation.[39] One practical reason for a move away from Mediterranean resorts was the hostility shown to consumptives by local people and medical practitioners, as in southern Europe there was a strong belief that

34 E. A. Parkes, 'Address in Medicine', *BMJ*, 1873, ii: 143.
35 *BMJ*, 1866, ii: 12–13.
36 *BMJ*, 1876: 273. Yeo also mentioned the use of hypophosphites and local rest. The latter required the use of strapping and other mechanical restraints to reduce respiratory movements, which it was said would in turn reduce the pulmonary circulation and hence the absorption of inflammatory products. *Lancet*, 1880, ii: 871.
37 Williams, 'Phthisis', 1181.
38 J. Pemble, *The Mediterranean Passion: Victorians, and Edwardians in the South*, Oxford, Clarendon Press, 1987.
39 Reduced air pressure at high altitudes would also lead to an expansion of the lungs and ozone might act as an antiseptic.

consumption was contagious. British and other northern European doctors routinely dismissed such ideas as ignorant and typical of the backward medical professions of southern Europe. Writing in Quain's *Dictionary of Medicine* in 1882, C. T. Williams, Senior Physician at the Brompton, summed up prebacillus therapeutics as a three-pronged strategy: (1) medicinal – to improve nutrition, reduce inflammation and relieve symptoms; (2) dietetic and hygienic – to build up the patient; and (3) climatic – to help breathing and stimulate the system.[40] None of these offered a 'cure' as such; rather, they aimed to arrest the disease by aiding the patient's ability to counter a disease whose hereditary character was 'too well known to be required to be more than stated'.[41]

TUBERCULOSIS AND THE BACILLARY THEORY

While clinicians played down the significance of the experiments of Villemin and others, MOsH worried about the possible dangers to humans of eating milk or meat from tuberculous animals.[42] Within public health medicine there was growing awareness of the decline in mortality from tubercular disease, which had fallen from 259 to 188 deaths per 100,000 population over the period 1865 to 1880, a drop of twenty-seven percent that was similar to the fall in zymotic diseases. Leading MOsH attributed the decline to 'inclusive' sanitary improvements, especially improved ventilation and hygiene, removing predisposing causes, but they were beginning to advocate 'exclusive' measures that targeted milk and meat supplies.[43] The Public Health Act, 1875, contained clauses that enabled MOsH to seize unsound meat as a public nuisance and control dairies. For example, in April 1877, the MOH for Rotherham seized a carcass because it contained tubercles, which he said were 'the active agent which produces disease in humans'.[44] Many veterinarians also believed that tuberculosis was contagious, the most notable being George Fleming, who was disappointed when the new Contagious Diseases (Animals) Act, 1878 (CD(A)A), did not schedule tuberculosis for stamping out.[45] Initiatives by MOsH and veterinarians drew strength from continuing European experimental work on the inoculation of tuberculous matter and, in the late 1870s, from reports that the 'virus' of tuberculosis had been isolated. In

40 Williams, 'Phthisis', 1181–3.   41 *BMJ*, 1880, i: 704.   42 *BMJ*, 1880, i: 707, 1602; ii: 388, 472–3.

43 A. Ransome, *Consumption: Its Causes and Its Prevention*, Manchester and Salford Sanitary Association, 1882.

44 *VJ*, 1877, 5: 67. The case was lost on 'insufficient evidence', largely because medical opinion was divided. Two MOsH from rural authorities spoke for the defence, while the prosecution relied on experts from the nearby towns of Rotherham and Sheffield.

45 G. Fleming, 'The Transmissibility of Tuberculosis', *BFM-CR*, 1874, 54: 461–86; T. Walley, 'Tubercle', *VJ*, 1878, 6: 184; G. Fleming, *VJ*, 1880, 9: 74–95, 303. Nonetheless, new Dairy, Cowshed and Milkshop Orders gave MOHs powers to control milk supplies. See the discussion between Prof. Axe and J. Greaves, *VJ*, 1878, 6: 282; 1878, 7: 52.

Germany, Klebs and Cohnheim reported finding possible causative microorganisms in tubercular lesions from experiments said to be more exacting than those of Villemin, as they inoculated minute amounts of material to reduce the possibility of contamination by septic or other infective matter.[46] They used microscopy to identify the 'virus', which Klebs found to be a micrococcus and Cohnheim named *Monas tuberculosum*.[47] This work was controversial in Germany as it reinstated the unity of tuberculosis and went against the teachings of Virchow and Niemeyer. Yet the results were widely publicised and discussed, being typical of the speculative germ 'discoveries' of the period.[48] Klebs and Cohnheim promoted the radical implications of their views, arguing that tuberculosis would be defined differently, as a preventable contagious disease, and that control could be based on laboratory methods, with diagnoses made from material taken from patients.[49] Klein recognised the challenge to existing views of such work when he observed in 1881 that new views reduced the constitution merely to the 'delicacy and vulnerability of the tissues. . . . a secondary or accidental condition'.[50]

The last extended discussion of tuberculosis in Britain before Koch's now famous lecture in March 1882 was in Glasgow in February and March 1881.[51] This heated debate revealed divisions amongst pathologists, and between clinicians and pathologists.[52] The leading Scottish pathologists, Joseph Coats and David Hamilton, while no experimentalists, had sided with the German School that the disease was 'always the result of irritation'.[53] Coats, following Cohnheim, argued that the specific irritant was a 'self-propagating virus . . . introduced from without or formed within the body'. However, he qualified this by saying that 'all persons and all tissues are not equally susceptible to the virus, just as all people are not equally susceptible to the viri of typhus or any infectious disease'.[54] His final thoughts at the end of a protracted debate were 'that pathology undoubtedly points to a virus as the cause of consumption, and clinical facts point to the state of the system as at the bottom of it'.[55] Hamilton, who followed Niemeyer's teaching, maintained that

46 *BMJ*, 1880, i: 704. Cf. H. Cullimore, *Consumption as a Contagious Disease*, (a translation of Professor Cohnheim's pamphlet, 'Die Tuberklose vom Standpunkte der Infections-Lehre'), London, Baillière, Tindall and Cox, 1880. For the clinical case for contagion, see: *Lancet*, 1881, ii: 825–6.
47 On other organisms described at this time, see: R. Saundby, 'Recent Researches on Tubercle and their Bearings on the Treatment of Consumption', *Practitioner*, 1882, 29: 178–83.
48 *MTG*, 1880, ii: 38–9, and *Lancet*, 1880, ii: 860–1.
49 *MTG*, 1880, ii: 38–9. On opposition to 'the renewed, – daily renewed and totally unproven views' about consumption and infection, see: *Lancet*, 1881, ii: 1108.
50 E. Klein, 'Aetiology of Miliary Tuberculosis', *Practitioner*, 1881, 27: 83.
51 J. Coats, *Discussion on the Pathology of Phthisis Pulmonalis*, Glasgow, A. MacDougall, 1881.
52 A typical view from a clinician was that tuberculosis was a physiological state rather than an entity: '[Tubercle is] not an accidental product evolved in the individual, but an expression of a subtle organic dyscrasia operating in the individual. It is not so much a factor in the downfall of the physiological status of the individual, as it is proof of a previously operating decay in the organism.' A Turnbull Smith, *GMJ*, 1881, 15: 110.
53 *BMJ*, 1880, ii: 388.   54 *GMJ*, 1881, 15, 269.   55 *BMJ*, 1881, i: 818.

the irritant was nonspecific, and that the capacity for tubercle formation was inherent in certain types of cell. As well as the continuing divisions in pathology, the discussions also showed clinicians under pressure from pathologists to abandon the idea of a purely diathetic origin and accept some version of the irritation–inflammation model, not least for the therapeutic possibilities that it opened up.[56]

Koch's now famous paper, 'On the Aetiology of Tubercular Disease', was read to the Physiological Society in Berlin on 24 March 1882 and published on 10 April. First notices appeared in Britain on 22 April in an editorial in the *Lancet* and, in a now typical flourish, in a report in the *Times* by John Tyndall, supported by a 'Leading Article'.[57] Tyndall emphasised two points – Koch's claim that tubercular diseases were communicable, and how the results were a triumph for experimental medicine. As was noted in Chapter 5, the timing of Koch's announcement was opportune, coinciding with the inauguration of the Association for the Advancement of Medicine by Research (AAMR) and the reflections on the state of British science prompted by the death of Darwin. Koch's findings gave Tyndall powerful ammunition to attack antivivisectionists and those medical practitioners who were resistant to laboratory medicine. He observed that Koch's methods, especially the inoculation of animals, had been difficult to use in Britain since 1875, though before then Sanderson, Fox and others had been at the forefront of research using inoculation methods. Tyndall also demoaned the absence of a British equivalent of the state-funded research institute in which Koch now worked, or of university science departments more generally.[58]

Medical reactions to Koch's claims were mixed. At one extreme, it was said that his claims were 'revolutionary' and that there was no precedent for 'so sudden and complete casting aside of tradition'.[59] Against this, many pathologists maintained that the 'virus' had been expected and that it could be easily adapted to prevailing doctrines.[60] In Britain, the *Tubercle bacillus* suffered from Tyndall's endorsement and because it promised to reopen pathological issues that had only recently been settled.[61] The main objections to Koch's ideas, according to Julius Dreschfeld, the German-born and -trained Professor of Pathology at Owen's College, Manchester, were: '1. The fact that tubercle is

6 One clinician argued that it was time to fight back and 'override the pure pathologist'. *GMJ*, 1881, 15: 280.
7 *Times*, 22 April 1882, 5; *Lancet*, 1882, i: 655–6; *MTG*, 1882, i: 411–2; *BMJ*, 1882, i: 624–5.
8 *MTG*, 1884, i: 533. In a chauvinistic move, in the summer of 1882 the *Practitioner* reprinted Sanderson's 1872 paper on the inoculation of tubercular matter and implied that it was a precursor of Koch's bacterial model. *Practitioner*, 1882, 29: 186–70, 266–78, 352–60, 401–25.
9 *BMJ*, 1882, ii: 624.
10 B. G. Rosenkrantz, 'Koch's Bacillus: Was There a Technological Fix?', in E. Ullman-Margalit, ed., *The Prism of Science*, Dordrecht, Reidel, 1986, 147–60.
1 *BMJ*, 1882, i: 186. Robert Saundby referred to the history of tubercle as 'a history of controversy'. R. Saundby, 'Recent Research', 180.

hereditary; 2. That phthisis is not easily communicable from man to man; 3. That inoculation experiments on animals do not allow conclusions to be drawn as to their causal agency in man.'[62] It is worth noting that the existence of the bacillus itself seems not to have been an issue; the important question was whether it was a cause, concomitant or consequence of the disease. The bacillus was soon around for all to see.[63] Cheyne, Klein, E. M. Nelson, G. A. Heron, Heneage Gibbes and Alexander Ogston, amongst others, showed *Tubercle bacilli* to audiences at metropolitan and provincial medical meetings during 1882[64] (see Figures 15 and 16). In his Croonian Lectures on Consumption in March 1883, the physician James Pollock took his audience through a separate lecture on 'the whole theory of the induction of diseases from germs introduced from without' before discussing the *Tubercle bacillus* and consumption in detail.[65] Whatever its status with medical understandings of consumption, the *Tubercle bacillus* was being used as a vehicle for the wider promotion of bacterial theories of disease.

Most physicians seem to have accepted the 'reality' of Koch's *bacillus* but debated its meaning, trying to synthesise its properties with existing ideas on pathogenesis and their clinical experience. The commonest way of harmonising the *bacillus* with 'the fact of heredity' was to suppose that 'physico-chemical changes must precede botanical aggression'.[66] In other words, for consumption to develop degenerative changes arising from a tubercular constitution, poor general health, or the predisposing effects of another chest disease had to have made the lungs 'open' to infection.[67] T. H. Green expressed the accommodation as follows: 'two conditions . . . are necessary in order to produce the disease: the presence of the *Tubercle bacillus*, and some abnormal state of the pulmonary tissue'.[68] Seed and soil notions were adapted to the inflammation model, with the *bacillus* acting as a specific or general irritant. Brompton physicians, like C. T. Williams, were comfortable with this account, though Williams widened the range of predisposing factors:

If we are to accept the bacillary theory at all, we must suppose that the various and well known predisposing causes of phthisis, such as dampness of soil, bad ventilation, bad confinements, and other debilitating conditions, must act by preparing a fit soil for the bacil-

---

62 J. Dreschfeld, 'Micro-organisms in Their Relation to Disease', *BMJ*, 1883, ii: 1055–8.

63 'Bacilli in Tuberculosis', *Lancet*, 1882, i: 797. Koch's assistant, Goltdammer, came across to help Watson Cheyne, who himself made a visit to Koch's laboratories to learn bacteriological techniques and to confirm that the bacillus was the causal agent. W. W. Cheyne, 'Report to the AAMR on the Relation of Micro-Organisms to Tuberculosis,' *Practitioner*, 1883, 30: 240–320. But compare: H. Gibbes, 'Bacteria and Micrococci: Bacilli in Tuberculosis, *PMSL*, 1881–3, 6: 314–20, and J. L. Stevens, 'The Tubercle Bacillus and its Relations to Phthisis Pulmonalis', *GMJ*, 1883, 19: 348–54.

64 *Lancet*, 1882, ii: 1094; *BMJ*, 1882, ii: 735.

65 J. E. Pollock, 'Croonian Lectures: Modern Theories and Treatment of Phthisis', *MTG*, 1883, i: 261–2, 320–2, 378–80, 431–3, 577–9, 605–7.

66 *BMJ*, 1885, i: 897.   67 *BMJ*, 1885, i: 889.

68 T. H. Green, 'A Lecture on the Tubercle-Bacillus and Phthisis', *BMJ*, 1883, i: 194.

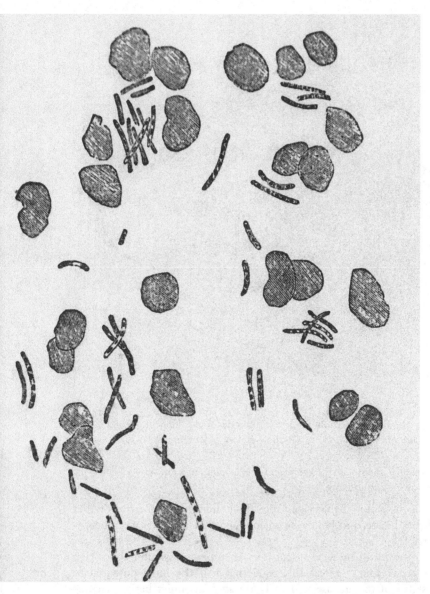

Figure 15. Human tuberculous sputum, stained after the Ehrlich–Weigert Method (×700) (From E. Klein, *Micro-Organisms and Disease*, London, Macmillan, 1884, 36)

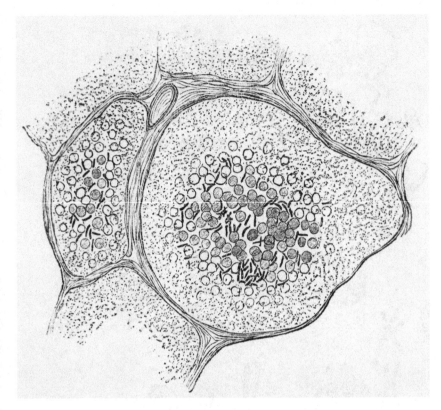

Figure 16. From a section through a tubercle of the lung of a child (×350)
(E. Klein, *Micro-Organisms and Disease*, London, Macmillan, 1884, 39)

lus either by bringing about some low inflammatory condition . . . or by weakening the resisting powers of the constitution.[69]

However, Williams believed that *bacilli* spread secondary inflammations rather than caused the disease, and hence he maintained that nonbacillary tuberculosis was possible.

The major novelty in medical discussions on tuberculosis after the spring of 1882 was contagion.[70] It was this issue that had the most potential to change the status of the disease and to bring about conflict between clinicians and laboratory scientists.[71] Also, if the disease was contagious, then it

69 *Lancet*, 1883, ii: 176; G. A. Heron, 'Some of the More Recent Facts and Observations Concerning the Bacillus of Tubercle', *BMJ*, 1883, i: 805–7.

70 For opposing views, see: R. Shingleton Smith, 'The Proofs of the Existence of Phthisical Contagion, *BM-CJ*, 1883, 1: 1–41; E. Markham Skerritt, 'Clinical Evidence Against The Contagiousness of Phthisis', Ibid., 48–70.

71 J. Burney Yeo, *The Contagiousness of Pulmonary Consumption and its Antiseptic Treatment*, London, Churchill, 1882; C. T. Williams, 'The Contagion of Phthisis', *BMJ*, 1882, ii: 618–21; W. Pirrie, 'Infectiveness of Tubercle', *Lancet*, 1882, ii: 171.

was perhaps no longer a medical problem, but instead one for sanitary authorities and MOsH. For some people even talk of contagion was dangerous, as they brooded on the social consequences of 'phthisiso-phobia' and worried that consumptives would be treated like lepers.[72] What was medicine coming to, they asked, if 'science should thus come to override sympathy'? The diagnosis of consumption already signalled a termi-nal illness and brought the stigma of an inherited taint, so there had to be very good reasons for adding the possibility of sufferers being socially ostracised.

In January 1883, opinion on the contagiousness of consumption was explored in two surveys. These were made under the auspices of a new move-ment that sought to distill clinical opinion in 'collective investigations'. In part this movement was an attempt to bolster the authority of clinicians, against the laboratory and experimental investigators, by systematising clinical experience.[73] The first survey, taken amongst members of the Cambridge Medical Society, revealed that thirty-four out of thirty-eight doctors had never seen any instances of communicability. A larger national survey was also organised by the National Collective Investigations Committee, with the support of the BMA. This committee already had a poll underway on whether diphtheria was 'catching', so the contagiousness of phthisis was an obvious follow-up.[74] In January 1883, the *BMJ* published a form that practitioners were asked to fill in and return, giving their answer to the question: 'Have you observed any case or cases in which Pulmonary Phthisis appeared to be communicated from one person to another?'.[75] By the end of the year, 1,078 replies had been received, of which sixty-two percent said 'no' and twenty-four percent 'yes', leaving fourteen percent unde-cided or equivocal.[76] The 'don't knows' are the most interesting as they show typically complex, clinical views about germs and contagion. To begin with, contagion was given a broad meaning. It was used for direct person-to-person transmission; indirect transmission by the inhalation of contaminated dust or the ingestion of contaminated food; and transmission from husband to wife by sexual intercourse was also talked about, sometimes as a form of hereditary transmission'. Echoes of Beale and Dobell were evident in other suggestions that *bacilli* were ubiquitous in the body and that latent germs developed tubercular characteristics when an inherited or acquired susceptibility became manifest.[77] There remained a minority who contended

Lancet, 1883, ii: 991; 1884, i: 482; *BMJ*, 1885, i: 213.

W. Gull, 'An Address on the Collective Investigation of Disease', *BMJ*, 1884, ii: 305–8; T. J. Maclagan, 'On Methods of Therapeutic Research', *BMJ*, 1884, ii: 260–1.

The Cambridge Medical Society organised its own poll in January 1883. *BMJ*, 1883, i: 77.

BMJ, 1883, i: 20.

BMJ, 1883, ii: 983. These results were comparable to the smaller Cambridge survey in January, which showed that fifty-six percent of medical men had never encountered any hint of conta-gion. *BMJ*, 1883, i: 77.

BMJ, 1882, ii: 621.

that tubercle lesions, and hence *bacilli*, could arise spontaneously and that such 'germs' only became infective within the body, being unable to survive outside.[78] The aetiology of the disease was elaborated as a very variable thing, and there was little or no sense that one had to accept the *bacillus* as the necessary or single causal. This meant that doctors could accept the *Tubercle bacillus* as just another factor in the pathogenesis of this most variable and capricious of medical afflictions.[79]

Amongst pathologists, many of whom were developing bacteriological interests and skills, the *Tubercle bacillus* was very readily accepted.[80] Given Koch's past successes with anthrax and septic micrococci, it was entirely plausible that he had isolated the 'virus' that had eluded Klebs and Cohnheim.[81] Green immediately accepted that Koch's *bacillus* was the 'injurious influence' that either caused the inflammation that led to tubercle formation or produced tubercular lesions directly.[82] Joseph Coats, in his *Manual of Pathology*, published in 1883, incorporated 'the recent discoveries of Koch, already confirmed by several others' as proven.[83] One reviewer attacked Coats for his rapid acceptance and was confident that the *bacillus* would not be 'the whole story'.[84] In a rejoinder, Coats said that he had drafted the section on tuberculosis in February 1881, over a year before Koch's work appeared, and yet 'Koch's facts could thus be inserted without dislocating anything'.[85] However, not all pathologists took the *bacillus* in their stride. Some were suspicious because the tubercular pathology had a history of being swayed by 'every wind of doctrine' and where no idea lasted more than four or five years.[86] Why should 'bacterial pathology' be any different?[87] David Hamilton complained about the 'exaggerated and illogical conclusions now so freely drawn from Koch's important discovery'.[88]

The *Tubercle bacillus* was announced immediately after the publication of Pasteur's studies on the attenuation of germs and his first trials with protective vaccines.[89] Three main points were taken from this work in Britain: first, that it made vaccination against smallpox as a 'modern' germ practice; second, that it held out hopes for 'vaccines' against all zymotic diseases; and, third, that notions of the fixity of bacteria and the specificity of associated diseases needed to be

78 Green, 'A Lecture', 194.   79 *BMJ*, 1885, i: 129.
80 Worth noting are the remarks of William Ewart a fortnight before Koch's lecture in Berlin, in which he said that he still trusted to the naked eye and the coarser anatomy it revealed. *Lancet*, 1882, i: 383.
81 Green, 'A Lecture', 195.
82 T. H. Green, 'Lectures on Phthisis', *Lancet*, 1882, i: 813.
83 J. Coats, *A Manual of Pathology*, London, Longmans Green, 1883, 164.
84 *BMJ*, 1883, ii: 878–9.   85 Ibid., 997.   86 S. Coupland, 'On Tubercle', *BMJ*, 1882, i: 186–7.
87 David Hamilton remained loyal to the ideas of Virchow and Niemeyer that tubercles formed only when certain types of cells were altered. D. J. Hamilton, *On the Pathology of Bronchitis, Catarrhal Pneumonia, Tubercle and Allied Lesions of the Human Lung*, London, Macmillan, 1883.
88 Quoted in the *Practitioner*, 1883, 30: 203.
89 G. L. Geison, *The Private Science of Louis Pasteur*, Princeton, NJ, Princeton University Press, 1995, 145–76.

ooked at again.[90] The first point was included in the *Times* editorial that accompanied Tyndall's letter in April 1882. Although the differences between Pasteur and Koch were emerging, the editorial writer, no doubt briefed by Tyndall, put the work of the two together to create a unified and optimistic picture of bacteriological and medical advances to come:

t is characteristic of many of the disease-producing bacilli, and probably all of them, that they can be so altered by cultivation as to produce a mild disease instead of a severe one, and that the designed communication of the former will afford protection against the latter. PASTEUR has lately shown how completely this may be accomplished in the case of the bacillus which causes splenic fever in cattle; and vaccination itself is now regarded merely as inoculation with the smallpox bacillus, after it has been modified in its character by being cultivated in the bodies of the bovine race. The experiments of Dr KOCH .. seem as yet to have been carried no further than to the repeated cultivation of the tubercle bacillus in it original virulence; but they will speedily be followed, as a matter of course, by attempts at cultivation in diminished intensity . . . At this point, therefore, we come into manifest contact with the high probability that the thousands of human lives which are now sacrificed every year to the disease produced by bacilli may at no distant period be protected against these formidable enemies.

t is interesting and significant how germ theories and germ practices were quickly portrayed as offering so much.

BACTERIOLOGY AND LABORATORY MEDICINE

The *Tubercle bacillus* arrived at a time when the identification of possible causative agents of contagious, infectious and other diseases was becoming routine. However, many of these turned out to be 'bogey-germs' that were set up, only to be knocked down again and forgotten'.[91] In 1883 Dreschfeld was able to list ten diseases 'in which it is fully established that the microorganism is the causal agent', two diseases where it was 'less fully proved' and another twenty-two where microorganisms had been found but where there was little evidence of a firm causal link with disease.[92] This was the maximal claim; sceptics accepted that only two diseases were 'fully proven to be caused by a bacterian parasite' — anthrax and fowl cholera.[93] On his return from his AAMR-funded tour in the spring of 1883, Cheyne tried to add a third certainty when he confirmed that the *Tubercle bacillus* was 'definitely . . . the cause of acute tuberculosis'.[94] The laboratory evidence on its own was impressive, especially coming from an authoritative investigator, but doctors were perhaps more impressed by the congruence between the reported properties

T. D. Brock, *Robert Koch: A Life in Medicine and Bacteriology*, Madison, WI, SciTech, 1988, 117–39. *BMJ*, 1883: ii: 829.   92 Ibid., 1055.   93 *MTG*, 1883, ii: 515.

Practitioner, 30, 1883: 301, 315–9. Also see: *BMJ*, 1883, i: 527. In the spring of 1883, the journals reported what they termed the 'German tubercle-bacillus wars', where the Austrian Spina directly challenged Koch's ideas and technique.

of the *bacillus* and their clinical experience of the disease syndrome. The disease developed slowly – the *bacilli* divided slowly; the disease produced cavities in the lungs and caused a severe cough – the *bacilli* digested tissue and produced debris in the lungs; sufferers were lethargic and lost weight – the *bacilli* used up nutrients and oxygen, compromising respiration and vitality; the bacilli had a tough waxy coat and were hard to destroy – the disease was largely incurable and chronic. A significant change from the 1870s was that discussions of germ theories of disease were now concentrating on the 'theories of disease' element, and not on whether germs were 'theoretical' or 'real' – 'ancestral' or *de novo*. Attempts were made to agree on a general theory, for example, that bacterial germ-diseases were 'caused by the presence in the system of minute germs or spores, which form no natural part of the body, but which, by their growth and multiplication in the body, give rise to the phenomena of disease'.[95] Putrefactive germs, *contagium viva* and fungoid body's were all lumped together as 'bacteria', alien invaders that damaged the body's structure or function. Why the word 'bacteria' dominated is unclear. It may have been due to the adoption of the term in Germany, or perhaps because since its first use in the 1840s it had been applied mainly to microorganisms with putrefactive and morbidific properties. Bacteria were still seen as parasites, and discussions of parasitic diseases included bacteria amongst the smaller parasites.[96]

Many of the new bacterial aetiologies, unlike germ claims in the 1870s, were for diseases of major medical and political significance.[97] Consumption was the single largest cause of death in industrialised countries, while other candidates for bacterial aetiologies were serious local, national and imperial problems, such as typhoid fever, smallpox, cholera and malaria. Medical authorities anticipated that further important diseases would be shown to be 'bacterial', and would become open to new methods of prevention, control and treatment. For example, in 1883, the Grocer's Company tried to stimulate the search for the germ of smallpox by offering a 'Discovery Prize' of £1,000 for the first person to devise 'the method by which the vaccine contagion may be cultivated apart from the animal body'.[98] While the establishment of aetiologies was important, the methods by which disease-agents were fashioned and displayed were of greater immediate significance. Koch's techniques in microscopy, solid culture methods for growing bacteria on agar plates and inoculation procedures offered new opportunities for medical research and possible new approaches for diagnosis, prognosis and guiding treatment. One doctor in 1883 suggested that the microscope could spot

95 Crowfoot, 'The Germ-Theory', 551.
96 Accounts of parasites were added to the 1896 edition of Crookshank's textbook. E. M. Crookshank, *A Textbook of Bacteriology: Including Etiology and Prevention of Infective Diseases and a Short Account of Yeasts, Moulds, Haematozoa and Psorosperms*, London, H. K. Lewis, 1896.
97 W. D. Foster, *A Short History of Clinical Pathology*, Edinburgh, E. & S. Livingstone, 1961, 62–63.
98 *SR*, 1883, 4: 592.

ulmonary tuberculosis five weeks before the 'skilled ear', while others suggested that bacterial diagnosis based on microscopy, culturing or inoculations
nto vulnerable animal species would offer greater certainty in medical
work.[99] Monitoring the numbers of *bacilli* in sputum, and any variation in
heir activity and virulence over time, promised to be a pointer to the
rogress of the disease and hence the prospects of the patient. However, there
vere potential problems. For example, what to make of patients with clini-
ally indicated tuberculosis who did not have *bacilli* in their sputum, and
vhat of healthy people whose sputum contained *bacilli*? Which were the
most reliable, clinical or laboratory methods? In the 1880s the answer to this
question was relatively easy – clinicians decided. This was because for the
most part laboratory work was being performed on a do-it-yourself basis by
clinicians themselves. The conflict between bedside and bench that has
ecently so interested historians was a later phenomenon, which obviously
equired the institutionalisation of bacteriologists and laboratories as distinct
ultures, apart from clinical medicine.[100] Before the 1890s most bacteriolog-
cal work was performed in the corners of domestic rooms, doctors' surg-
ries or in 'microscope rooms' in hospitals. Indeed, there was as yet no vision
f clinical or service laboratories staffed by full-time bacteriologists; rather,
he expectation was that the microscope and culture plate would be used by
loctors as often as the stethoscope and thermometer.[101]

Before the introduction of Koch's ideas and methods, the science and tech-
ology of germs had been uncertain, in large part due to the lack of standard procedures.[102] Koch's methods set new standards in both senses of the
vord – better quality and more consistency. The success of these methods
nd their adaptability came from the fact that they were refined with a *bacil-
us* that was difficult both to grow in culture and to stain for microscopy. It
vas slow to propagate, fastidious about its culture medium and had a waxy
oat that dyes did not easily penetrate. However, the powerful images that
vere seen down microscopes and on culture plates, plus their wide dissem-
nation, meant that there was tremendous interest in emulating Koch's
vork.[103] Initially, there appeared to be few technical barriers to the spread of
he new germ technologies: microscopy was familiar and culture plates and
otato slices seemed simple enough. Doctors now realised that they were used
o handling germs as vaccine lymph, though in Britain animal inoculations

99 *MP*, 1883, ii: 160.
00 There is now an extensive literature on the conflict between bedside and bench. The seminal
article is: R. Maulitz, '"Physician versus Bacteriologist": The Ideology of Science in Clinical
Medicine', in M. J. Vogel and C. E. Rosenberg, eds., *The Therapeutic Revolution: Essays in the Social
History of American Medicine*, Philadelphia, University of Pennsylvania Press, 1979, 99–108.
01 *Practitioner*, 1886, 36: 120.
02 P. Gossel, 'A Need for Standard Methods: The Case of American Bacteriology', in A. E. Clarke
and J. H. Fujimura, eds., *The Right Tools for the Job: At Work in Twentieth Century Life Sciences*,
Princeton, NJ, Princeton University Press, 1992, 287–309.
03 E. M. Crookshank, *Photomicrography of Bacteria*, London, H. K. Lewis, 1887.

were not an easy option. As soon as Koch's work was published, attempts were made to speed up and simplify his methods for clinical use.[104] Advice on bacterial microscopy and culturing was rapidly added to medical and pathology textbooks. The new 1882 edition of Bristowe's *Theory and Practice of Medicine* contained an appendix on bacterial techniques. The following year, Heneage Gibbes brought out a second edition of his *Practical Histology and Pathology*, which contained advice on: 'How to choose a microscope, how to seal a preparation jar, how to find Tubercle-bacilli in the breath of patients and a multitude of like points'.[105] It is often overlooked that Klein's influential *Micro-organisms and Disease* was first published in the spring and summer of 1884 in the *Practitioner*, a journal aimed at the general practitioner.[106] Klein began with an account of microscopy and culture techniques, arguing that it was crucial that methods were well understood so that the uneven quality of the work in the burgeoning field could be assessed by all. He gave details on the best types of microscopes, the preparation of specimens, the best dyes and fixing agents and recipes for different culture media.[107] It was not uncommon for authors to recommend particular makes of instruments and to name suppliers. The first volume from Lister's department, by Edgar Crookshank in 1886, was significantly titled a *Manual of Bacteriology*, and again began with technique.[108] The interest in techniques was evident in the new bacteriological section of the sixth edition of Green's pathology textbook in 1884, which closed with an account of 'Methods for Demonstrating Micro-organisms'.[109] Woodhead and Hare's *Pathological Mycology*, published in 1885, was subtitled 'Methods' and for many years was regarded as giving the clearest exposition of bacterial technique.[110] Cheyne published his practically oriented *Public Health Laboratory Work* in 1884, two years before his collection of seminal studies in *Recent Essays on Bacteria in Relation to Disease*.[111]

The anticipated adoption of bacteriological methods into general and hospital practice did not happen. Once the novelty of seeing the microbial world first-hand had gone, the practical value of the new bacteriological skills to ordinary practitioners seemed meagre, especially when compared to the time,

104 Foster, *Clinical Pathology*, 60, and *BMJ*, 1882, ii: 142.
105 H. Gibbes, *Practical Histology and Pathology*, London, H. K. Lewis, 1883.
106 E. Klein, 'Micro-Organisms and Disease', *Practitioner*, 1884, 32: 170–86, 241–64, 321–52, 401–26; 1884, 33: 21–40, 81–112, 161–80, 241–57. E. Klein, *Micro-Organisms and Disease*, London, Macmillan, 1884.
107 *Nature*, 1884, 31: 49–50.
108 E. M. Crookshank, *Manual of Bacteriology*, London, H. K. Lewis, 1886. Also see: idem., 'Microbes and Disease', *BMJ*, 1886, ii: 407.
109 Green, *Pathology*, sixth edition, 1884, 474–538. The previous edition in 1881 had no such chapter.
110 G. S. Woodhead and A. W. Hare, *Pathological Mycology: An Enquiry into the Aetiology of Infective Diseases*, Edinburgh, Young J. Pentland, 1885.
111 W. W. Cheyne, *Recent Essays by Various Authors on Bacteria in Relation to Disease*, London, New Sydenham Society, 1886.

effort and money they had to put in.[112] It proved hard to learn technical procedures from manuals, however well written, and courses were slow to start up. The first formal course was started at King's College in 1886, typically as an extramural programme aimed at qualified doctors as much as students. The first bacteriology courses were predominantly practical and technical, leaving it to the practitioners to incorporate what they learned into their work and established ideas about disease. The extent to which ordinary doctors used the new bacteriological techniques is difficult to gauge, but observations were soon made that dependable results required regular practice, and that this was hard to develop as the number of diseases where methods were useful clinically, say in diagnosis, was small. Doctors found that the microscopic examination of fresh specimens for diagnostic purposes was unreliable, and that accuracy required either staining with dyes and fixatives, or culturing, with its requirements for sterilisation, special culture media and incubators. Given doctors' confidence in their existing methods of diagnosis, bacteriological methods were largely used to confirm clinical judgements or used in doubtful cases. All of this meant that there was not the volume of work for expertise to be developed and maintained.

This lack of demand was also a factor in hospitals. Before 1890 the only institutions with fully experimental laboratories for bacteriological work were at King's College Hospital, St Thomas's Hospital, the Royal College of Physicians, Edinburgh, and the Brown Institution, London.[113] These facilities had mostly been established for research or teaching. It was not until the mid-1890s that the demand for clinical diagnostic pathology was sufficient for dedicated agencies to be started. The most important in Britain was the Clinical Research Association (CRA), set up as a private venture in 1894 by a group of doctors at Guy's Hospital to offer diagnostic laboratory services to hospitals, local authorities and individual practitioners.[114] The CRA charged a subscription fee and then payment for service, collecting and reporting on most specimens by the post. In the first year, 2,000 doctors joined the association, suggesting a significant demand for laboratory services; but on average each sent in only three specimens for testing.

The plans to develop clinical pathology in part derived from a reorientation in the work and interest of pathologists from the dead to the living. As was clear with the changing pathological understanding of tuberculosis, pathologists had long been exploring the pathogenesis and disease processes.[115] Pathologists were the medical specialists best placed by expertise and opportunity to pursue bacteriological work, because of their skills in

---

112 *Lancet*, 1886, ii: 215–6.   113 Based on the issue of vivisection licences.
114 *Guy's Hospital Gazette*, 1893, 7: 127; 1894, 8: 311; 1896, 10: 243. *The Clinical Research Association Limited*, London, Ash and Co, 1901.
115 S. Jacyna, 'From Laboratory to Clinic: The Impact of Pathology on Surgical Diagnosis in the Glasgow Western Infirmary, 1875–1920', *BHM*, 1988, 62: 384–406.

microscopy, the handling of morbid specimens and prior studies of inflammation. Many pathologists had used their extended repertoire and the demands for teaching to convert their hospital and university appointments from part-time to full-time, and there was optimism in the late 1880s that pathology was at a new dawn as the 'science of disease'.[116] The novel features of the subject meant that there was no clear line between research and routine investigations, so there were many opportunities for doctors to make a name in the new science. While pathologists took to bacteriological work because of its technical demands, they did little to simplify or demystify the subject; indeed, the reverse was true. By the end of the 1880s the days of the dabbler in bacteriology were numbered, as the expense and technical demands of maintaining equipment, reagents and, for serious work, licensed animals. It was not only protobacteriologist surgeons, such as Cheyne and Ogston, who pursued other careers; for example, C. A. Ballance and Victor Horsley became distinguished neurologists. The first generation of full-time bacteriologists who found posts after 1890, like Klein and Greenfield earlier, began their careers as pathologists: Frederick Andrewes, David Bruce, George Dean, A. A. Kanthack, Sidney Martin, Robert Muir, C. S. Roy, Armand Ruffer and Almroth Wright. The title of the first British journal specifically devoted to bacteriology, *Journal of Pathology and Bacteriology*, founded by German Sims Woodhead in 1892, implied that the subject was subsidiary to, or a branch of, pathology.

Pathologists carried over into bacterial work their interest in disease processes, which in the case of bacterial diseases were represented as deviations from normal function caused by an external agent. Direct analogies continued to be drawn between the actions of bacteria and those of parasitic fungi and worms on the one hand, and chemical poisons, such as snake venom, on the other.[117] Also, there continued to be debates over making infectious diseases entities, but as we have seen the external agent was never the whole story, and in most cases the body's variable physiological reaction to germs continued to define the disease syndrome. For example, the action of the *Tubercle bacillus* was thought to be similar to micrococci, that is, they produced chemical toxins (ptomaines) that caused the softening and disintegration of nearby tissue and the subsequent systemic effects. There were also physical and biological effects, for example, *bacilli* blocked and altered the microcirculation, thereby devitalising tissues, and competed for nutrients and oxygen.[118] While doctors could accept that the *Tubercle bacillus* might initiate disease, the disease syndrome was largely determined by the body's response.

116 W. Aitken, 'On the Progress of Scientific Pathology', *BMJ*, 1888, ii: 348–59; W. H. Dickinson, 'On the Uses of Prospects of Pathology', *BMJ*, 1891, ii: 247–50. W. D. Foster, *The History of Pathology as Profession*, London, Royal College of Pathologists, 1978.
117 *BMJ*, 1882, ii: 554; *MTG*, 1883, ii: 515–7.   118 *BMJ*, 1883, ii: 1059.

THE *TUBERCLE BACILLI* AND CLINICAL MEDICINE

Contemporary press comments on the impact of Koch's claims about consumption on clinical medicine suggested that it was modest. An editorial in the *Medical Times and Gazette*, after a meeting of the Royal Medical and Chirurgical Society in London in 1884, observed that '[The] discovery and even the full acceptance of the aetiological doctrine associated with Koch's tubercle bacillus leaves the subject of tubercular phthisis as regards its diagnosis, prognosis and treatment, exactly where it was before'.[119] This view has been echoed recently in historical discussions where it has been suggested that the 'therapeutic consequences of germ theory were very limited'.[120] Much here depends on the meaning of therapeutic consequences. Certainly the 1880s and 1890s did not see effective cures judged by the modern standards set by antibiotics; however, after 1882 there were major changes in general strategies for managing the disease, as well as specific innovations.[121]

The greatest influence of bacterial pathology was the way in which it was used to persuade doctors and the public that tuberculosis was curable, or at least could be 'arrested'.[122] If the disease was 'caught', rather than inherited or arose spontaneously, then in the first instance there were greater possibilities of prevention. As well as preventing the 'seed' reaching the body, physicians suggested trying to limit its effect on the body by hardening the lungs.[123] There was already evidence from postmortems that in many people tubercular infection was 'contained' in caseous lesions.[124] If this was the case, then the normal pattern was for most people to overcome infection. This phenomenon was explained in many ways. Some bacteriologists supposed that the virulence of the *bacilli* was reduced in the body, or that in such cases relatively few organisms had reached vulnerable tissues. The most common view, however, was that the body actively 'resisted' infection, which meshed with clinical experience of the susceptibility of different people to the disease. Openness to infection was not fixed and the age-specific incidence of the disease was well-known, as were differences between the sexes, between

119 *MTG*, 1885, i: 153.

120 *MTG*, 1885, i: 94; ii: 326; *Lancet*, 1885, ii: 1040; J. H. Warner, *The Therapeutic Perspective: Medical Practice, Knowledge and Identity in America, 1820–1885*, Princeton, NJ, Princeton University Press, 1986, 258–83.

121 S. West, 'The Bacilli of Tubercle Found in the Contents of Cavaties and not in Lung Tissue', *TPSL*, 1883, 34: 16–28; *BMJ*, 1883, i: 195, 254. W. F. Bynum, *Science and the Practice of Medicine*, Cambridge, Cambridge University Press, 1994, 226.

122 *MTG*, 1885, i: 384–5; S. Jaccoud, *The Curability and Treatment of Pulmonary Phthisis*, London, Kegan Paul, Trench, 1885; C. J. B. Williams and C. T. Williams, *Pulmonary Consumption: Its Etiology and Treatment, with An Analysis of 1,000 Cases to Exemplify its Duration and Modes of Arrest*, London, Longmans Green, 1887.

123 *MTG*, 1885, i: 95.

124 *BMJ*, 1885, i: 1885; J. Kingston Fowler, *The Localisation of Phthisis, in relation to Diagnosis and Prognosis*, London, Churchill, 1888.

occupations and between races; moreover, other diseases seemed to predispose to consumption.[125] Clinically, all of this was used to suggest that, if the effects of other diseases could be minimised and the lungs and other tissues strengthened, then it might be possible, not only to reduce the openness in the uninfected, but in those people already infected, to tip the balance in favour of the soil countering the growth of the seed. Another idea was that people with high metabolic rates did not suffer from consumption, because they used up all available nutrients and literally starved the *Tubercle bacilli* to death, hence the advice to move to mountain climates where respiration rates rose. At the other extreme, it was suggested that the body's ability to localise infection depended on directing physiological energy; hence the basis of rest therapy, as in surgery, was to allow the sufferers to concentrate their vitality on countering the *bacilli*.

Some clinicians did try direct attacks on the *bacilli*, applying antiseptics directly to lesions in the lungs by inhalation, irrigation or injection.[126] Despite studies that showed that less than one percent of the creosote and other vapours inhaled from antiseptic masks reached lesions in the lungs, inhalation therapy had a considerable vogue.[127] New antiseptic rationales were invented for hygienic and climatic treatments in terms of the properties of alpine air, sunlight or low temperatures. The physician's task was to help 'by placing persons under circumstances in which they are less liable to become infected, and when infected, more able to limit the progress, and to effect a more or less perfect and more or less permanent cure'.[128] Exercise was recommended to promote deeper breathing and pulmonary circulation, which would stimulate overall vitality and perhaps prevent the *bacilli* from lodging in the apices of lungs. Climate was talked about less in terms of the overall environment and more about the specific properties of the air. In these terms, high altitudes had several advantages: low temperatures that would kill *bacilli* in the air; low atmospheric pressure that would deepen breathing; low levels of aerial pollution; low levels of soil moisture and dry air; and strong sunlight to kill germs.[129] Weber initially termed this 'the hardening open-air treatment', his belief being that sun and wind would toughen the lining of the lungs just as they did the skin.[130]

125 There was an explanation for the localisation of tubercles in the upper part of the lung; this was the part that moved least in ordinary breathing, where vitality was lowest and where bacilli would most easily lodge.

126 *BMJ*, 1885, i: 1038.

127 *MTG*, 1885, i: 153; *BMJ*, 1885, i: 518. A. Hill Hassall, *The Inhalation Treatment of Diseases of the Organs of Respiration, including Consumption*, London, Longmans Green, 1885.

128 H. Weber, 'The Hygienic and Climatic Treatment of Chronic Pulmonary Phthisis', *BMJ*, 1885, i: 517–8.

129 Ibid., 690.

130 *BMJ*, 1885, ii: 657; and *Lancet*, 1888, i: 1037. Walther's regimen stressed large intakes of food and discipline, respectively, aimed at improving the body's ability to resist the bacillus and hygienic life-styles. These institutions can appear to present a form of nature therapy, living lives of

Despite Tyndall's hopes in 1882 that a tuberculosis vaccine would be produced, the prospects for this in the 1880s were not good. To begin with, tuberculosis was not a disease where one infection conferred immunity to further attacks; if anything, sufferers became more vulnerable over time. Hence, neither of the earlier models of immunity – those of exhaustion or antidote – had much to offer, which revived earlier ideas that tuberculosis was similar to septic diseases. As noted above, the large numbers of spontaneous cures were explained by suggestions that sufferers had not received the critical number of bacteria necessary to establish infection, or that their tissues had a vital resistance or immunity that was either inherited or acquired.[131] Laboratory research had shown that different animals had different susceptibilities to the *Tubercle bacillus*, a situation that was apparently paralleled in human racial groups, families and individuals. Many clinicians were happy to leave it at the level of notions of 'vital resistance', but pathologists and bacteriologists wanted to know the mechanism, not least so that they could use it to produce artificial immunity or an effective biological antidote. One of the new explanations of immunity in the mid-1880s, Metchnikoff's phagocytic theory, where white blood cells sought out and ingested invading microorganisms, was used in new explanations. Physicians now pictured *Tubercle bacilli* in a Darwinian struggle for existence against the cells of the body, or had a militaristic vision of invading germs and bodily defences. However, other doctors continued with more ecological ideas, especially in the plans for bacteriotherapy, where the aim was to find bacteria that were directly antagonistic to the *Tubercle bacilli* and inject them into patients.[132]

The success of Pasteur with his rabies vaccine in 1886 raised hopes again that other protective vaccines would be produced. The Pasteurian programme was based on the attenuation of bacteria by two methods, either weakening their virulence by passage through other animal bodies (e.g. the smallpox and anthrax model), or by killing bacteria in controlled ways so that whatever factor (probably chemical) that the human immune response reacted to remained potent enough to stimulate an immune response (e.g. the sheep pox). The former method produced 'live' vaccines while the latter 'killed' vaccines. However, the rabies vaccine also seemed to be able to cure the disease, as the modified 'virus' seemingly led the body to develop powers to counter

regulated rest and exercise outdoors in rural locations and also included hydropathy and other treatment systems.

131 T. Harris, 'The Curability of Phthisis', *BMJ*, 1889, ii: 1385–8; J. Swanson, *Consumption: A Curable Disease*, Glasgow, W. & R. Holmes, 1890.

132 This approach was also based on the clinical observation that people with tuberculosis did not suffer from certain other diseases, and that certain diseases, for example, septic infections, seemed to 'protect' against tuberculosis. *BMJ*, 1885, ii: 403. Also see: L. G. Stevenson, 'Antibacterial and Antibiotic Concepts in Early Bacteriological Studies and in Ehrlich'C Chemotherapy', in J. Pascandola, ed., *A History of Antibiotics*, Madison, WI, University of Wisconsin Press, 1980, 43–50.

the effects of the true 'virus' already in the system. The assumption was that this must be due to some chemical process whereby the products of the modified 'virus' either neutralised the toxins of the true 'virus' or inhibited the ability of the true 'virus' to produce toxins. This model of poison and antidote was being explored in laboratories around Europe, and in the late 1890s there were many reports of the isolation of toxins, most of which were albuminoses or proteids (what are now called proteins).[133] The next step was to determine if there were specific substances that the human body produced to counter toxins, and to see how specific these were. Researchers and clinicians realised that if these substances could be isolated and then produced in reasonable quantities, either synthetically or harvested from immune people or animals, then medicine would have antibacterial therapies, or rather antibacterial toxin therapies.[134] In 1889, Behring and Kitasato announced the isolation of diphtheria toxins, and in 1891 they reported the existence of specific antitoxins in the blood of infected sufferers. In Britain, Sidney Martin, Leonard Wooldridge and Ernest Hankin tried to isolate the active chemical component in various Pasteurian vaccines. What appeared to be a promising research programme and possible research school produced very little, because of the loss of key researchers.

Wooldridge died in 1889 and Hankin took up a post in India in 1894.[135] Martin's time was taken over by the Royal Commission on Tuberculosis, which took evidence and made investigations between 1890 and 1893, reporting in 1895, and then his move to a hospital post in 1896, as Professor of Pathology at University College Medical School.[136]

The other line of enquiry with therapeutic promise, which Lister had mentioned in 1884, was whether there was some physiological property of blood, lymph or other tissue that inhibited the growth of microorganisms or directly killed them. The optimism around the preventive, protective and curative products in the later 1880s was not just born of the presumed power of laboratory science; it was also grounded in bacterial theories of health. As Sheridan Delépine explained in 1891, doctors had learned from the many instances where 'causes do not always bring about . . . results', which pointed to the

133 S. Martin, 'The Chemical Products of the Growth of Bacillus Anthracis and their Physiological Action', *PRSL*, 1890, 48: 78–80; E. H. Hankin, 'A Bacteria-Killing Globulin', Ibid., 93–107; *BMJ*, 1890, ii: 65, 1494.
134 One approach developed in France was to inject goat's or dog's blood or serum into patients. Both animals had relative immunity to the disease, and hence the hope that whatever property of their blood that gave this refractoriness would also work in humans. *Therapeutic Gazette*, 16 March 1891; *Lancet*, 1891, i: 559–61; *BMJ*, 1891, ii: Suppl., 61.
135 Leonard Wooldridge (1857–1889). For his work see: L. C. Wooldridge, *On the Chemistry of the Blood and Other Scientific Papers* (arranged by Victor Horsley and Ernest Starling), London, Kegan, Paul, Trench, Truebner, 1893.
136 S. Martin (1860–1924). His last major work on the topic was: S. Martin, 'Croonian Lectures on the Chemical Products of Pathogenic Bacteria', *BMJ*, 1898, i: 1569–72, 1644–6; ii: 11–15, 73–6.

healing powers of nature.[137] Nikolai Gamaleia, working through the Pasteur Institute in Paris, had found the supposed pneumococcus germ in the mouths of the healthy and the sick. Thinking along familiar Pasteurian lines, he suggested that the germ was benign in the mouth but became pathogenic if and when it found its way to the distinctive physiological conditions of the lung.

HUMAN AND BOVINE TUBERCULOSIS

The campaign by MOsH and other public health officials against meat and milk contaminated with tubercular matter, which began in the late 1870s, was given new impetus by the identification of the *Tubercle bacillus* in 1882, although as important were the International Medical Congresses in 1881 and 1884, and the International Veterinary Congress in 1883, at which British medical and veterinary practitioners learned of the ambitious continental plans to control and eradicate bovine tuberculosis. The common response of veterinarians during the 1880s in any discussion of bovine tuberculosis and its threat to humans was to suggest that the disease should be added to the provisions of the next CD(A)A, with a view to stamping it out. The threat of contaminated meat and milk posed slightly different problems. MOsH had responsibility for abattoirs and meat markets, being able to condemn grossly contaminated meat, though with milk their powers were more limited. Fears about the milk supply as a conduit of contagion were long-standing, with childhood infections such as scarlet fever and diphtheria, and with adult diseases such as typhoid fever.[138] Until the late 1880s, MOsH tried to secure a pure' supply of milk by 'inclusive' measures, such as cleaning up dairies and milk distribution, rather than the 'exclusive' methods that targeted infected animals or their produce.[139] However, child health was a growing issue in medicine, in large part due to the persistence of high infant mortality rates, and in the 1890s the vulnerability of children to infected milk became a major issue.[140] On the question of milk safety, public health officials were caught between the chemically oriented public analysts, who were concerned with added substances and dilution, and the Veterinary Department, who did not regard bovine tuberculosis as a problem at all. However, legislation was framed as early as 1882 to move responsibility for the control of dairies from the Veterinary Department to the Medical Department of the Local Government Board, and this became effective in 1886. Locally, the legislation was little used, as urban MOsH could only police town dairies and had no control over the supplies coming from surrounding rural areas. There were

37 S. Delépine, 'On the Development of Modern Ideas on Preventive, Protective and Curative Treatment of Bacterial Diseases, and on the Immunity or Refractoriness to Disease', *Lancet*, 1891, i: 241–4.
38 H. E. Armstrong, 'Infectious Diseases and the Milk Supply', *BMJ*, 1883, ii: 570.
39 A Wynter Blyth and A Spence, *TSMOH*, 1885–86, 73–91.
40 G. S. Woodhead and J. M'Fadyean, 'Tubercle in the Dairy', *BMJ*, 1887, ii: 673.

three solutions to this problem canvassed amongst MOsH: either extend the powers of MOsH to cover all suppliers to their district; or to halt the contamination at the source by stamping out the disease in the national herd; or make the final product safe by boiling milk, or even adding antiseptics, at the distribution centre or in the home.

The powers of MOsH with meat were clearer, and this is where their efforts were concentrated in the 1880s. A small group of MOsH mounted a campaign for tighter controls in the medical, veterinary and public health press and, perhaps more effectively, in local magistrate courts. Many of the prosecutions brought against abattoirs were vigorously contested as meat traders and butchers stood to lose condemned carcasses without any compensation. Usually they tried to evade prosecution on legal technicalities; if that failed, they claimed that they bought meat in good faith from farmers and had no way of knowing whether a beast was tuberculous or not. In rare cases medical evidence was challenged, with the meat trade arguing that they were the real experts on the soundness of meat and could judge its safety by its look and smell. They also maintained that diseased carcasses could be made safe by excising affected parts, assuming that tuberculosis was a localised disease. Against this, MOsH relied increasingly on microscopy to identify contaminated tissues, assuming that tuberculosis was an infective and systemic disease, where minute tubercles could spread anywhere in the body. They recommended that the whole carcass be condemned if any tubercles were found. In court, both sides drew on professional experts, with no simple division of veterinarians siding with butchers and medical men with sanitary authorities. The outcome of cases was unpredictable and unsatisfactory to all sides, especially as it seemed that the real culprits – stock breeders and farmers – were escaping altogether. In fact, the butchers' organisation campaigned for the inclusion of tuberculosis in the CD(A)A, hoping either that the problem and economic losses would be passed back to farmers, or that compensation would be paid as with other scheduled diseases. Medical practitioners were less interested in stamping out and argued that the best practical measure would be to close private slaughter houses and replace them with public abattoirs, inspected by MOsH. These claims had symbolic as well as practical import.[141] Private slaughter houses represented the antithesis of everything that MOsH stood for: they were smelly, unsanitary, unregulated and profit-driven, providing the means for spreading all manner of disease. In their place municipal abattoirs would be clean, efficient, scientifically regulated, service-oriented – working models of preventive medicine.

The pressure from MOsH for action on tubercular meat mounted and led in 1888 to the Departmental Committee then investigating bovine pleurop-

---

141 Part-time MOsH often lost business in private practice from bringing such prosecutions. *BMJ*, 1882, ii: 542.

neumonia to be asked also to look into tuberculosis. The Committee's Report concluded that the solution to bovine tuberculosis lay both in stamping out the disease by adding it to the CD(A)A and in better hygiene on farms, principally improving the ventilation of cow sheds.[142] It was a popular belief in farming that bovine tuberculosis had flourished recently due to the increasing practice of keeping stock indoors, which in the view of the committee devitiated the air, lowering the vitality of the livestock, rather than aiding the dissemination of *Tubercle bacilli*.[143] Before the government had time to respond, a succession of 'Dead Meat Dramas' in the courts came to a head in a test case brought by J. B. Russell, MOH for Glasgow, in April 1889.[144] Glasgow was an obvious site for a show trial; it had an active MOH, a reputation as the centre of the trade in unsound meat and the place where relations between the medical and veterinary professions were closest.[145] The Glasgow case hinged again on whether a carcass was safe after the excision of affected parts, or whether the whole carcass should be condemned. Pathologically, the question was whether tuberculosis was a local or general disease. For the prosecution, Russell called, amongst others, Professor Tom M'Call (Principal of the Glasgow Veterinary College), Professor John M'Fadyean (New Veterinary College, Edinburgh), Dr. Joseph Coats (Pathologist, Western Infirmary, Glasgow) and Dr. Maylard (Surgeon, Sick Children's Hospital, Glasgow). They argued that tuberculosis was a systemic bacterial disease and that if any traces were found the whole beast should be condemned. The defence relied mainly on English MOsH – Goldie (Leeds), Gibbon (Holborn), Arthur Hill (Birmingham) and Mason (Hull) – who argued, also relying on bacterial ideas, that tuberculosis was localised.[146] Russell won the case, which seemed to set a precedent and strengthened demands for effective national action, though an editorial in the *BMJ* was unhappy that pathological questions should be decided in courts of law.[147]

Following the Departmental Committee's Report, the Glasgow case and other lobbying, the Board of Agriculture asked its leading veterinary advisor, G. T. Brown, to draw up Draft Orders for the inclusion of tuberculosis in the CD(A)A. This Brown did, but with his draft to his superiors he added a paper saying that any legislation on this matter was unworkable. He set out four problems: first, that the disease was difficult to diagnose in cattle; second, that

42 *Report of the Departmental Committee appointed to inquire into Pleuropneumonia and Tuberculosis in the United Kingdom*, BPP 1888, [C. 5461], xxxii, 267.
43 This view echoed medical ideas that pulmonary tuberculosis was a disease of the 'indoors', precipitated by breathing rebreathed air, with low oxygen levels and high carbon levels. Of course, such ideas were useful to those supporting the open-air treatment.
44 The phrase 'Dead Meat Drama' was used in a headline in the veterinary press. *VR*, 1, 1888–89, 307.
45 T. Walley, 'Animal Tuberculosis in Relation to Man', *EMJ*, 1887–88, 33: 984–997, 1078–89.
46 *PH*, 1889–90, 2: 75.
47 *BMJ*, 1889, ii: 990; 1890, i: 728. Only Thomas Hime, MOH for Bradford and a Pettenkofer supporter, argued publicly that the Glasgow verdict had been wrong.

the levels of compensation would be difficult to assess as they could be made either on the value of the sick beast or its assumed value if healthy; third, that the cost in compensation was likely to be prohibitive, and, fourth, that there was no support for the scheme from farmers. Cattle were not dropping dead in large numbers on farms; they may not have been putting on as much weight as they should, nor might they be producing as much milk, but these were accepted losses that were already factored into the economics of farming. As the disease was not scheduled in the CD(A)A, the Agricultural Department did not recognise that it was within its remit. Thus, the department was only too happy to hand the problem over to the Medical Department, on the tacit understanding that rather than be tackled at the source in the national herd, it would be tackled at the end of the food chain by inspection, hygiene and public education.

Rather than give the problem to one department, the government thought about creating an interdepartmental committee to deal with the problem, before finally settling in 1890 on a Royal Commission – by then a recognised way to delay action on a problem.[148] The Commission was given a narrow remit that concerned only the safety of food, not the position of the disease in livestock or issues around processing and handling. Work began in the usual fashion, with interviews of representative and expert witnesses, though the Commission also supported experimental investigations. These were conducted by German Sims Woodhead, John M'Fadyean and Sidney Martin. The work was completed fairly quickly, although the results were not officially published until 1895. However, important findings were released. In the Glasgow case and after, leading veterinary and medical opinion had favoured the condemnation of whole carcasses rather than excision. In their investigations Woodhead and M'Fadyean changed their minds, maintaining that the dangers of tuberculous meat were less than previously supposed.[149] Martin suggested that the main threat from meat actually came from the contamination of sound flesh by the knife used to remove tubercular organs or tissues. Woodhead reported later that normal cooking temperatures readily destroyed *Tubercle bacilli*.[150] Butchers were pleased and argued that the work of the Royal Commission vindicated past practices, while veterinarians smugly reflected that the medical profession had once again got it wrong with an animal disease.[151] Coincident with the experimental work of the Royal Commission came Koch's announcement of the Tuberculin remedy for tubercular disease, the value of which for cattle was investigated by M'Fadyean. As will be shown in the next section, the therapeutic value of

148 *Royal Commission Appointed to Enquire into the Effects of Food from Tuberculous Animals on Human Health*, BPP, 1895, [C.7992], xlvi, 11.
149 J. M'Fadyean and G. S. Woodhead, 'On the Communicability of Tuberculosis from Animals to Man', *BMJ*, 1891, ii: 412–3, 635–6. Sanderson gave the opening address at the section on Tuberculosis, see: *BMJ*, 1891, ii: 403–6.
150 *JCPT*, 1896, 9: 77.   151 *VR*, 1895–96, 8: 577.

Tuberculin for human disease was soon dismissed, though doctors found that it had some value in diagnosis, as when injected under the skin people with tubercular disease or arrested cases developed a rash. The same test was adopted for animals.

By the mid-1890s, M'Fadyean, by then Principal of the RVC in London, had changed his whole approach to the problem.[152] He now stressed bovine tuberculosis as an agricultural problem and suggested that future historians would be puzzled at how the problem in livestock had been ignored while so much fuss had been created about the small, though not insignificant risk that the bovine disease posed for humans. M'Fadyean went along with the views that reported as little as one percent of total human tuberculosis deaths were due to bovine sources, though the figure for childhood infection was higher.[153] However, he thought that it was impossible 'for any sane person' to advocate the inclusion of tuberculosis in the Diseases Animals Act, which replaced the CD(A)A, because of the cost and logistics of replacing over half the national herd.[154] Instead he advocated a voluntarist solution, where diseased livestock would be identified by Tuberculin tests, after which it would be left to the self-interest of cattle breeders and owners to achieve the progressive elimination of diseased stock.

The narrow terms of reference given to the Royal Commission in 1890 meant that after it finally reported in 1895, a second Commission had to be appointed to make policy recommendations on the findings. This Second Commission reported in 1898, supporting a voluntarist approach. However, before any measures were implemented, new uncertainties were added when, in 1901, Robert Koch told the British Congress on Tuberculosis that human and bovine tuberculosis were distinct diseases and, hence, that the disease in bovines carried no threat to humans. Although his views were immediately challenged by British veterinarians and doctors, his authority was such that the government appointed another Royal Commission, which this time took ten years to report and delayed future effective action on the problem until well into the twentieth century.

'BACTERIOLOGY ON TRIAL': TUBERCULIN AND AFTER

The willingness of British doctors and veterinarians to challenge the views of Koch's in 1901 was unsurprising, as his authority had been damaged in 1890 by the failure of his much-hyped Tuberculin cure. Tuberculin was a biological product made from extracts of culture plates on which the *Tubercle bacillus* had been grown. Koch's remedy was trailed in August 1891 at the International Medical Congress in Berlin and used by

---

52 See the editorials in M'Fadyean's *Journal of Comparative Pathology and Therapeutics*. *JCPT*, 1893, 6: 353; 1895, 8: 141.
53 *JCPT*, 1897, 10: 63.   154 *JCPT*, 1899, 12: 57.

the German government to enhance the standing of the country and its advanced medical science. The supposed basis of the treatment, though Koch admitted that he did not fully understand the mechanism, was that Tuberculin killed (necrotised) infected tissues and denied the *bacilli* the substrate it needed to grow. The simplest version of its action given by Koch was that it 'starved out' the *bacilli*. Koch's announcement of a cure for such a major disease caused a sensation. Leading medical men and patients flocked in the hundreds to Berlin. At the time, as one of the world's most successful medical scientists, it was entirely believable that Koch had made such a breakthrough. Rabies had recently been conquered by Pasteur, and other antibacterial remedies were being promoted. None other than Joseph Lister took his niece to Berlin to be treated, and on his return he reported that the effects of Tuberculin were 'simply astounding' and that 'the world would be startled by the magnificence of these researches'.[155] However, other doctors were more sceptical, and when the initial euphoria turned to doubt they argued that, along with Koch's remedy, 'bacteriology itself was on trial'.[156]

The rapid rise and demise of Koch's Tuberculin treatment has been discussed many times, and there is no need to tell the story again here.[157] Instead, I will focus on what the episode tells us about the position of bacteriology in British medicine in the early 1890s, nearly ten years from the coming of the *Tubercle bacillus* and the emergence of bacteriology. The reports from visits to Berlin of Lister and Conan Doyle have been widely cited; however, the number of British visitors was very large indeed. Individuals and representatives of provincial medical societies from across the country visited Berlin, and by the end of the year the remedy had been discussed at meetings in Birmingham, Bristol, Newcastle, Edinburgh, Glasgow, Manchester and Sheffield, as well as in London.[158] The management committee of the new Conjoint Laboratories of the Royal Colleges in London arranged to send their new director, German Sims Woodhead, on a fact-finding mission to Berlin, assuming that if the treatment lived up to expectation, their new laboratories would be the best placed to produce Tuberculin for the British market.[159] The various medical meetings focused on clinical assessments, the most common verdict being that the remedy had been 'tried and found wanting'. There were some reports of successes, but these diminished over time. Indeed, the number of reports where Tuberculin worsened the condition of the patient grew.[160] At the end of 1891, Tuberculin was said to be

155 *Lancet*, 1890, ii: 1184, 1244, 1257.   156 *Lancet*, 1890, ii: 933.
157 The best recent discussion is in G. Feldberg, *Disease and Social Class: Tuberculosis and the Shaping of North American Society*, New Brunswick, NJ, Rutgers University Press, 1996, 55–80.
158 *Lancet*, 1890, ii: 1248, 1282, 1294, 1303, 1357.
159 Royal College of Physicians, Minutes of Laboratory Committee, 19 November 1891. Days later the plan was abandoned when unfavourable reports of the treatment began to filter through to London.
160 BM-CR, 1891, 9: 185, 297.

'much abused but little used'. However, some doctors hoped that it might prove useful in lupus (tuberculosis of the skin) and in surgical tuberculosis (infected bones and joints).[161] In these conditions the disease was localised and it seemed possible that necrotised tissue could 'fall away' or be cut out. One worry with the treatment of pulmonary disease was that necrotised tissue 'falling away' into the lung might actually spread the infection within the respiratory system and then via the blood stream to the whole body.[162]

Despite the 'shattered hopes and expectations', Koch and bacteriology more generally, emerged relatively unscathed from the episode. Many tuberculosis specialists continued to use the remedy and report successes in selected cases. A succession of 'new' Tuberculins was marketed throughout the 1890s, each supposedly more efficacious or purer than the original. The product was used more and more in diagnosis, though there was debate about whether the skin reaction was merely an allergic reaction showing that the *bacillus* had been present in the body, or whether it indicated immunity. Publicly, medical practitioners found three scapegoats for the episode: the media, the public and the German government. The press was said to have misrepresented Koch's cautious claims and created huge public expectation. The public had then demanded treatment before adequate testing and the refinement of dosage had been established. Finally, the German government was blamed for forcing the premature release of the substance, and then for insisting that its composition remain a state secret, denying other researchers the opportunity to develop and test the treatment. Within medicine, bacteriologists and supporters of laboratory medicine maintained that clinicians had been too hasty and had not used the remedy in controlled and responsible ways. On the other side, the bacteriosceptic wing of the profession were content that, after all the fuss, the laboratory had produced no advance on the ordinary methods they had built up over many years from clinical experience. In fact, physicians began to claim that they were increasingly able to cure or arrest disease.

'CURABLE AND PREVENTABLE'

What were the 'ordinary methods' for managing and treating pulmonary tuberculosis in the early 1890s? There were many approaches, and the essence of successful treatment was to match a selection of these to individual patients and their illness. If the disease was in its earliest stages, then radical or 'offensive' treatments could be tried, though with patients in an advanced condi-

61 W. W. Cheyne, 'The Value of Tuberculin in the Treatment of Surgical Tuberculosis', *BMJ*, 1891, i: 951, 1043, 1070, 1097–1101.
62 Lister was not worried by this, arguing that dead tissue would be absorbed in similar fashion to the way catgut ligatures were absorbed.

tion more moderate, 'defensive' measures were recommended. The range of antibacterial treatments was enormous, with substance such as creosote, iodoform and guaiacol introduced into the body orally, by inhalation, by injection, by irrigation and even 'per rectum'.[163] The treatment of choice was 'rest and a change of air', though this was now always combined with symptomatics and some antiseptics. The earlier the disease was caught the more rest, or more radical change of circumstances, was recommended, though economics and family circumstances often circumscribed a patient's options. The most common pattern of treatment was a combination of 'hygienic' measures, which followed the accumulated experience that consumptives did best with a 'change of air', rest, good diet and clean living. In a sense, this regimen tried to give individuals the conditions that doctors thought were responsible for the long-term mortality decline in the population as a whole. In terms of bacillary theory, the intention was to achieve a 'strengthening of the resisting powers of the tissues' and to reduce further infection with *bacilli*. Clinicians' optimism had been boosted by further evidence that the disease was curable. To spontaneous cures and those following treatment were added reports from pathologists that less than half of the people infected with the *Tubercle bacillus* developed full-blown consumption. Reviews of postmortem findings showed that the bodies of over a quarter of people dying from nontubercular diseases showed signs of healed or dormant tubercular lesions.[164] Once alerted to this finding, pathologists found that yet more dormant lesions and Tuberculin skin tests of the general population revealed infection rates to be as high as ninety percent amongst adults in some cities. Whether the majority of these were instances of spontaneous cures or merely latent, arrested disease was much debated. Doctors asked if there were people whose body had adapted to the infection and who carried the disease, spreading it to others while they tolerated the disease.[165] The general point taken from such concerns was that, with most people, most of the time, the balance force was with the power of the human soil to resist the growth of the seeds of tubercular disease.[166]

For the wealthy, the preferred treatment was to enjoy a change of air in alpine resorts. However, in Germany in the 1880s a number of doctors brought the treatment down from the mountains and downmarket, offering the regimen in more accessible and cheaper places, and on a different basis. They downplayed the value of air as such, and instead promoted the virtues

163 R. Shingleton Smith, 'Phthisis', *Medical Annual*, 1892, 366–84. J. E. Squire, 'The Influence of Bacillary Theory of Tuberculosis on the Treatment of Phthisis', *BMJ*, 1896, i: 208; idem. *The Hygienic Prevention of Consumption*, London, C. Griffin, 1893.
164 Harris, 'Curability of Phthisis', 1385–6; J. F. Coats, 'The Spontaneous Healing of Tuberculosis', *BMJ*, 1891, ii: 933–8; J. K. Fowler, *Arrested Pulmonary Tuberculosis*, London, Churchill, 1892.
165 *BMJ*, 1895, ii: 1358; Lancet, 1895, i: 119.
166 *PRM-CS*, 3 (N.S.), 1896: 27 *et seq*.

of life in forests in the open air and of the systematic application of hygienic rules. They also began to claim that this treatment was truly curative, especially with early cases. In the mid-1890s, instead of making the pilgrimage to Berlin for Tuberculin, many British doctors, especially those suffering from tuberculosis themselves, went to the forest areas of Germany to try the 'open-air' or sanatorium treatment. Many doctors were 'cured' and were so impressed with the therapy that on their return to Britain they established private sanatoria on the same principles.[167] The main model for British doctors was Dr. Otto Walther's sanatorium at Nordrach in the Black Forest. His regime had four main elements: living day and night in the open air, 'overfeeding', rest with some controlled exercise, and strict discipline. Walther did not allow drugs, but monitored a patient's temperature and sputum bacteriologically. It might be thought that the sanatorium treatment represented a return to nature and holistic therapies, and reaction against bacteriology and laboratory medicine. This may have been part of its attraction, but overall its legitimation and meanings were mixed.[168] In 1898, William Calwell characterised it intriguingly as 'the open-air life of the savage, combined with the hygienic comforts of our own age, and systematised with military precision'.[169] Another view was that in sanatoria 'a fierce battle is waged between science and the *Tubercle bacillus*', though it seems that the key to a victory lay not in laboratory science, but in scientific methods of management, as the patient was required to have 'the constant personal supervision of the physician [with] firm enforcement'.[170] The supporters of sanatoria were keen to stress that their institutions were not isolation hospitals; they were curative institutions that worked by strengthening and hardening the patient 'to resist the invasion of the *Tubercle bacillus*'. They also placed the patient in a germ-free environment, but that was for the patient's benefit, not that of the society.[171]

After 1896, those promoting the development of sanatorium treatment in Britain were absorbed into a wider movement to control the disease, in what was the first large-scale campaign to mobilise medical, voluntary and state agencies against a single disease in Britain. National associations against consumption had been founded in continental Europe during the 1890s, with those in Austria and Germany established largely to extend the sanatorium treatment to the working class. The British campaign started after discussion at the Annual Meeting of the BMA in the summer of

67 M. Worboys, 'The Sanatorium Treatment for Consumption in Britain, 1890–1914', in J. V. Pickstone, ed., *Medical Innovation in Historical Perspective*, London, Macmillan, 1992, 47–71.

68 C. Allbutt, *BMJ*, 1898, ii: 1149–50.

69 W. Calwell, 'The Hygienic Treatment of Consumption independently of Sanatoria', *BMJ*, 1898, ii: 947.

70 *BMJ*, 1897, i: 1164.

71 R. Thorne Thorne, *The Administrative Control of Tuberculosis*, London, Baillière, Tindall and Cox, 1899.

1896. A loose federation of interested parties came together, which, as well as clinicians, included veterinarians, MOsH and lay people. The National Association for the Prevention of Consumption was established in November 1898 with the combined ideals that consumption was both 'curable and preventable'. The elite metropolitan physicians who led the association were able to ensure royal patronage for the Association and a high public profile.[172]

The Association planned to work in three specific areas: to educate the public on prevention; to remove the threat to humans from bovine tuberculosis; and to promote the establishment of sanatoria, especially for the working class. It was significant that the NAPC's proposals did not suggest that consumption join the roster of contagious and infectious diseases to be combated by notification, isolation and disinfection. This reflected continuing uncertainties amongst public health doctors about whether consumption was ordinarily contagious-infectious and whether notification was workable. These issues had been debated and tried in northwest England as a result of the efforts of a group of MOHs including James Niven, Arthur Ransome and John Robertson. In Manchester, Arthur Ransome had championed the idea that consumption was not communicated person-to-person directly by breath, but rather by dried sputum in dust.[173] Following the ideas of Cornet, he supposed that the *bacillus* could lay dormant in the environment and might even have to undergo some Pettenkofer-type developmental changes that depended on specific environmental conditions. However, he took hope from evidence that the *bacillus* was vulnerable to sunlight and ordinary sanitary measures. In the early 1890s, Ransome and other MOsH argued that the disease had still to be fought by 'inclusive' measures, backed up by more 'exclusive' measures, such as notification. However, local authorities were reluctant to make tuberculosis notifiable, and general practitioners worried about losing patients to MOsH and about the consequences of the state endorsing the idea that consumption was contagious. Ransome in particular sought to counter what he regarded as the 'scare' stories that the disease was highly contagious. He worried that if such views were broadcast, the problem would be more difficult to manage, as sufferers would be neglected by their families and forced onto the streets or into Poor Law hospitals.[174] However, by the end of the 1890s there was a vocal minority, notably James Niven in Manchester and Arthur Newsholme in Brighton, who were forcefully putting the case for notification and other 'exclusive' measures, and who were critical of the priorities of the clinicians

172 L. Bryder, *Below the Magic Mountain: A Social History of Tuberculosis in Twentieth Century Britain*, Oxford, Oxford University Press, 1988, 16–22.
173 A. Ransome, *The Causes and Prevention of Consumption*, London, Smith, Elder, 1890; idem., *A Campaign Against Phthisis*, Manchester, John Heywood, 1892.
174 A. Ransome, 'The Consumption Scare', *Medical Chronicle*, 1895, 2: 241–9.

heading the NAPC, whose policies were dominated by the promotion of the sanatorium treatment.[175]

An argument can be made that consumption was the medical condition most altered by the adoption of germ aetiologies and pathologies, changing in a short period from an inherited constitutional affliction to a specific, contagious disease. Indeed, this was a switch that was an exemplar of ontological conceptions of disease displacing physiological conceptions. The argument in this chapter has been that changes were more complex, showing as many continuities as changes. Medical understanding and management of the disease was in flux before the arrival of the *Tubercle bacillus*, and this state of affairs continued in its wake. There was no closure of medical opinion before 1900 that consumption was a specific, contagious disease. That said, the role of the *Tubercle bacillus* in the disease was accepted quite rapidly, in large part because by 1882 the important questions were no longer about the very existence of disease-germs, but rather about the role of different 'bacteria' in different diseases and pathological processes. Thus, what continued to be at issue were theories of disease and health, and in the case of tuberculosis, why most infected people remained healthy. These issues remained the subject of complex negotiations and debates that arguably became less rather than more settled over time. Despite aetiological and pathological uncertainties, I have shown that the clinical management of the disease was reshaped after 1882, with new therapeutic regimes aimed either at limiting the effects of the tubercular seed or at strengthening the human soil. The disease was also claimed to be preventable by public health doctors and clinicians, though they had quite distinct visions of how this might be achieved.

The *Tubercle bacillus* was the germ around which bacteriology was established, largely by pathologists. The cluster of technical innovations in microscopy and culturing developed by Koch to study this uncooperative germ were refined and used to study other diseases as pathologists, often restyled as bacteriologists, brought other important medical conditions into the canon of bacterial afflictions. Early bacterial methods seemed robust and simple, and enthusiasts thought that they could be readily learned and transferred within the medical profession, allowing pathogenic bacteria to be observed and manipulated by anyone with the time, resources and expertise. However, the expected widespread adoption of bacteriological practices into everyday clinical work did not materialise, in part because the techniques were not robust and simple, in part because bacteria were complex organisms, in part because high technical standards were created, and in part because few practitioners, apart from researchers, needed to undertake the

75 'The Prevention of Tuberculosis', *BMJ*, 1898, ii: 1891–2, 1899–1903. J. Niven, 'Tuberculosis', *Practitioner*, 1889, 43: 223–40. Idem., 'On the Notification of Tuberculosis', *Medical Chronicle*, 1897, 7: 1–15; S. Delépine, 'The Prevention of Tuberculosis', *PH*, 1898–99, 11: 469–78.

number of tests necessary to establish appropriate levels of expertise. Bacteriology classes were started in a small number of centres in the mid- to late 1880s, run mainly by surgeons or pathologists. These classes stressed the technical character of the bacteriology, as they offered training in the skills that were so difficult to communicate through text. However, initially they taught what were research methods, as clinical pathology had yet to be invented and routine laboratory tests had still to be developed. Nonetheless, and as in surgery, the growth of bacterial pathologies in medicine led to greater interest in the investigation of antibacterial therapies despite the failure of Tuberculin. Clinicians had few successes administering antiseptics into the body, though they tried, especially with the lungs and digestive system. This left them with the alternative approach of countering bacteria indirectly by mobilising the healing powers of nature in science-based treatments like Tuberculin, antisera and sanatoria.

The arrival of germ theories of tubercular disease in the late 1870s and early 1880s was inseparable for the creation of germ theories of health. The seed and soil metaphor was central to the reconstruction of tubercular aetiologies and pathologies, not least because it enabled clinicians to square the circle of contradictory views of young and old, pathologists and clinicians and MOsH. If consumption was contagious, it was very, very contingently so. Moreover, the high prevalence of the disease meant that many of those contingencies were within the body rather than environmental. Indeed, tuberculosis provides perhaps the best example of the change in the presumed nature of 'germs' from *c.* 1870 to *c.* 1900, analogous to that in surgery. In 1870, disease-germs were seen as protean panspermic microorganisms that arose and spread in the environment and could overpower the body. By 1900, *Tubercle bacilli*, now well-defined organisms, were a danger from intimate contact with other people and from within the body, where they might live for years, even a lifetime. Interestingly, the theories of immunity that developed after 1890 were not widely applied to tuberculosis. Its pathology was not easy to accommodate with metaphors of attack and defence, at least not the rapid pace of modern warfare, though notions of seiges and 'hundred year wars' would have been more appropriate. Theories of health had to explain the clinical experience of cures, plus the findings of postmortems and Tuberculin skin tests, that infection amongst European adults was almost universal. Yet, the disease only killed one in seven adults, so how did the great majority of adults survive infection? The best answer was because of some hereditary predisposition, or through strength acquired by hygienic living.

Indeed, the intensive and systematic application of the conditions that produced the natural arrest of the disease was the essential characteristic of the sanatorium treatment, which was said by some physicians to be the specific remedy for consumption. It is intriguing that the disease which is often said to have been most changed by reductionist, laboratory-based, medical science in the 1880s should at the turn of the century be fought by a holistic therapy based on methods that anticipate scientific management rather than modern scientific medicine. Laboratories, X-rays and other symbols of scientific medicine were often part of the sanatorium package, but its core was the enhancement of the healing powers of nature.[176]

176 Worboys, 'Sanatorium Treatment', 59–66.

7

Preventive Medicine and the 'Bacteriological Era'

Historians of public health have often referred to the period 1880–1900 as the 'bacteriological era'.[1] Their claim is that in the last two decades of the nineteenth century the science and technology of germs was used to transform the aims and methods of public health work from an 'inclusive' concern with the environment to an 'exclusive' focus on disease agents, people and their interactions. I have already argued that this transformation began earlier than 1880, and in this chapter I will suggest that while germs and bacteria were used by various groups to promote 'exclusive' approaches during the 1880s and early 1890s, it was only after 1895 that bacteriologists played a major part in public health. The broad shift in public health from inclusive to exclusive measures was accompanied by other changes, the most important of which was that MOsH took more specific approaches, using a different mix of measures for each disease. Thus, MOsH saw themselves as practising 'preventive medicine', not sanitary science. The main policies developed in the 1880s were a triumvirate of notification, isolation and disinfection, which were supplemented in the 1890s by laboratory diagnosis, preventive vaccines and curative products. Bacterial accounts of epidemics and zymotic diseases were principally interpreted to support the contention that every infection had its origins in a prior human case, though many MOsH tenaciously held on to the possibility of de novo origins in the environment, for example, with Pettenkofer-type germs developing pathogenicity outside of the body. The shift from environment to people as the main sources of infection meant that it became imperative for public health agencies to know who was infected with preventable diseases and where they were, so that cycles of transmission could be halted. Public health authorities, as they now significantly styled themselves, rather than sanitary authorities, also targeted particular channels of transmission and the points of passage between bodies where bacteria were vulnerable to natural and artificial disinfectants. This is

1 G. Rosen, *A History of Public Health*, Baltimore, MD, Johns Hopkins University Press, 1993 edition, 270–471.

not to say that sanitary practices ceased or were downgraded; indeed, attempts to solve problems such as water purity, sewage treatment and food safety gained new impetus from bacteriology.[2]

Accounts of changes in public health after 1880 that accord a pivotal place to bacteriology have been largely developed for the United States.[3] There has been some reluctance to apply the term to Britain, as public health professionals and agencies have been seen as less interested in new disease theories and slow to adopt laboratory methods. This situation has been explained in various ways, most notably by the continuing power of the 'Sanitarian Syndrome' and the relative backwardness of British bacteriology and science more generally.[4] Many MOsH and local authorities also maintained that they needed good reasons to change from the measures that had given the country one of the lowest mortality rates in the industrialised world despite high levels of urbanisation. Many doctors argued that other countries needed new scientific methods, backed up by strong state powers, because their sanitary conditions were so poor, whereas Britain would continue to be best served by common sense and experience, enabling legislation, and persuasion. As I have shown in Chapter 4, the 'British way' in public health medicine was already a mix of inclusive and exclusive measures, though after 1880 the balance undoubtedly shifted towards exclusivity and person-centred approaches. It is important to remember that this shift occurred largely in public health medicine; inclusive measures continued to be pursued by sanitary engineers, civil engineers and nuisance inspectors. At one level the change was a political one – sanitary work became more technical, routine and remote from public affairs – whereas the new preventive medicine continued to deal with local crises, and, because MOsH focused more on people and their behaviour, their work increasingly impinged on social policy and politics. The MOsH were also well-organised, with a vocal leadership that found itself speaking for the whole institution of public health. However, they still had to fight the idea that hygiene and sanitary reform were seen as mostly about 'structural works', such as water supplies and drainage.[5] The MOsH used the improving ideologies of modern science and technology to enhance their authority and link their aims with wider welfare priorities. Porter has argued that the MOsH leading this enterprise, notably Arthur Newsholme, George Newman and Sheridan Delépine, used the ideological resources of bacterial germ theories to carve out a new and distinctive professional identity for public health doctors.[6] However, Porter plays down the

C. Hamlin, *A Science of Impurity: Water Analysis in Nineteenth Century England*, Bristol, Adam Hilger, 1990.
D. Porter, *The History of Public Health and the Modern State*, Amsterdam, Rodopi, 1994, 236–9.
L. G. Stevenson, 'Science Down the Drain: On the Hostility of Certain Sanitarians to Animal Experimentation, Bacteriology and Immunology', *BHM*, 1955, 29: 1–26. R. MacLeod, 'The Frustrations of State Medicine, 1880–1899', *MH*, 1967, 11: 15–40.
E. Seaton, 'A Report on the Present State of Knowledge Respecting the Etiology and Prevention of Diphtheria', *BMJ*, 1894, ii: 573–77, 577.

Table 4. *Comparison of Death Rates from Major
Infectious Diseases, 1881–90 and 1891–1900 (Death Rates
per 100,000)*

Disease	1881–90	1891–1900
Tuberculosis	180	140
Scarlet Fever	167	84
Diphtheria	69.0	13.6
Measles	39.2	39.9
Typhoid fever	20	17
Smallpox	4.6	1.3
Cholera	0	0

Figures from A. Hardy, *The Epidemic Streets: The Rise of
Preventive Medicine in London, 1850–1910*, Oxford, Oxford
University Press, 1993.

influence of bacteriology on public health practice. I broadly concur with the arguments recently made by Simon Szreter and Anne Hardy that bacterial theories and practices were used to redirect and improve the efficacy of public health medicine after 1880, with the qualification that the bacteriological laboratory only played a significant role after 1895.[7]

This chapter considers in turn the major public health diseases of the period, as defined by legislation: smallpox, cholera, diphtheria, typhoid fever and scarlet fever. I use each to highlight at least one changing feature of public health policy and practice. Still referred to at times as zymotic diseases, these ailments had the highest profile in public health, though they were not necessarily those with the highest mortality and morbidity (see Table 4).

In the 1880s, the desire to control smallpox was the major impetus for the construction of isolation hospitals, which became the physical embodiment of the contagious powers of bacteria and of personal infection. As smallpox declined, MOsH gradually extended the range of diseases admitted, so that by 1900 isolation hospitals were effectively children's infectious disease institutions. MOsH also tried to make their hospitals germ-free environments and centres for clinical care and research. With smallpox, as well as with a number of other infections, MOsH and bacteriologists had to live with the fact that,

6 D. Watkins, *The English Revolution in Social Medicine, 1889–1911*, Unpublished PhD Thesis, University of London, 1984. J. M. Eyler, *Sir Arthur Newsholme and State Medicine, 1885–1935*, Cambridge, Cambridge University Press, 1997; D. Porter, *Health, Civilisation and the State: A History of Public Health from Ancient to Modern Times*, London, Routledge, 1999, 139–46.
7 S. Szreter, 'The Importance of Social Intervention in Britain's Mortality Decline', *SHM*, 1988, 1: 1–37; A. Hardy, *The Epidemic Streets: The Rise of Preventive Medicine in London, 1850–1910*, Oxford, Oxford University Press, 1993, 289–94.

as late as 1900, there was no agreement on the nature of its specific germ. That this was not more troublesome is interesting, as smallpox was associated with the exemplary germ practice of vaccination. The cholera threat in 1883–85 was seen as the first test of the new bacteriology in Britain and its empire. However, the purported 'discovery' of the germ of cholera by Koch in 1883–84 was double-edged for British public health. It promised to allow more accurate epidemiological mappings of epidemics and better diagnosis of individual cases, but it was also used internationally to advance the case for quarantines. However, the status of Koch's cholera vibrio was contested in Britain and its empire between 1883 and 1895, with British doctors adopting a complex Pettenkofer-type aetiology, which I explain by reference to the peculiarities of British bacteriology and the influence of colonial, especially Anglo-Indian, doctors. Paradoxically, despite the sceptical attitude towards any specific bacterial cause of cholera, the epidemic threat in 1893–94 saw the first systematic use of laboratory diagnoses in British public health. The opening at the same time of the grandly titled, but modestly funded, British Institute of Preventive Medicine (BIPM) will be used to explore the state of bacteriological research in Britain in the early 1890s. If any event can be said to have ushered in the 'bacteriological era' in British public health, it was the adoption of the diphtheria antitoxin from 1894. The incidence of diphtheria had risen in the early 1890s and became a priority for MOsH, especially in London, where mortality rates were high. Antitoxins were an entirely new weapon in public health medicine, a specific remedy that had the potential to make isolation hospitals curative institutions. Antitoxins, as well as new vaccines, required laboratory personnel and facilities for development, production and testing, so the second half of the 1890s saw a rush to found laboratories, which came from diverse initiatives. Within two years such laboratories were also being used to monitor typhoid fever outbreaks with the Widal Reaction, a diagnostic test based on determining whether a person's blood serum showed an immune response to an extract of the causative *bacillus*. Typhoid fever had continued to be important within public health because of the persistence of serious local epidemics and the opportunities that these gave for new forms of interventions, including an anti-typhoid vaccine after 1896. The largest single problem at the end of the century, defined by notifications and hospital admissions, was scarlet fever. Yet, this was another of the great zymotic diseases where the role of a specific bacterium remained uncertain. Various candidates had been nominated, but no consensus had emerged. Indeed, with this disease, the enthusiasts of the new preventive medicine were being challenged over the value of one of their prized practices, with claims that isolation was unnecessary and even dangerous.[8]

I make no judgements on the impact of germ theories or practices on mortality or morbidity rates, though I do suggest that they suggested and legitimated different approaches.

PUBLIC HEALTH 1880–1900

When elite doctors reflected on medical progress at Queen Victoria's Diamond Jubilee in 1897, they highlighted the decline of mortality in the second half of the century.[9] They claimed that it was largely due to sanitary reform, which they portrayed as a movement led by the medical profession. In particular they noted the decline in national epidemics, notably of smallpox and cholera, and suggested that the fall in mortality from consumption was also due to improved hygienic conditions. Even clinicians admitted that prevention rather than cure was the great achievement of the Victorian era.

Patterns of mortality and morbidity changed between 1860 and 1880, and changed again by 1900; however, real epidemiological trends were less important than the shifting perceptions and priorities within public health. In 1860, the aim of public health departments still reflected the origins of the enterprise as a response of the crisis of urbanism and the need to control epidemics, fevers and zymotic diseases. By 1900, the targets were specific diseases, and in an unforeseen and still little acknowledged change, medical work focused on childhood infections. In the 1860s, the government had sought to resist cholera, in the main, by reducing the 'receptivity' of the country; by 1900 more attention was being paid to reducing the receptivity or vulnerability of individuals to infections, with general strengthening measures being supplemented by the promise of vaccines. Public health was repoliticised, away from the mainly liberal agenda of rights, responsibilities and the 'Condition of England', to the politics of expertise and the duties of the state to maintain the health of the nation or British race.[10] As mentioned above, the term 'preventive medicine' has been said to best capture this shift, though the label 'state medicine' continued to be used and older terms, such as hygiene, were recast in a modern scientific guise. While epidemic crises and medical breakthroughs were often a catalyst to specific changes, public health doctors increasingly saw themselves as playing a longer game of preventing disease by reforming individual behaviour, treating diseases and improving national efficiency.

Despite past successes and such future ambitions, the standing of public health doctors remained a matter of concern to the leaders of the medical profession as well as MOsH. The number of full- and part-time appointments had risen, but pay was still poor and tenure uncertain. MOsH were the poor relations of the profession in every sense, though there were many who were well-qualified, highly motivated and highly effective medically and politically. A marked change after 1880 was that the pursuit of legislation ceased to be a major aim. This is not to underestimate the influence of the implementa-

9 A Jubilee Edition was published on 24 June 1897. *BMJ*, 1989, i: 1521–672.
10 D. Porter, ' "Enemies of the Race": Biologism, Environmentalism and Public health in Edwardian Britain', *Victorian Studies*, 1991, 34: 160–78.

ion of the consolidating Public Health Act, 1875, but to note that only two
major new acts were passed between 1880, and 1900 – the Notification of
Diseases Act, 1889, and the Isolation Hospitals Act, 1893. Besides encoding
the new approach to disease control, these acts increased the opportunities
for conflict with general practitioners over the control of patients and con-
fidentiality, and with the public over the removal of children and the seizing
of household goods for sterilisation. Both acts were permissive, so the use of
notification and the diseases to which they applied varied between local
authorities. The main strategy for improving the professional and social position of MOsH was to back up the authority they enjoyed from being agents
of the state with that of specialist expertise.[11] This enterprise took MOsH on
to new ground, with advice extending to personal and social behaviour in
what would later be termed the medicalisation of everyday life.

The number of institutions offering Diplomas of Public Health increased
in the 1880s, and there was a campaign to improve the standard of teaching
of public health in medical schools, with bacteriological laboratory work a
particular feature. Special qualifications for appointments did not become
mandatory until 1892, but before then a new identity had been forged in
large part by the handing over of routine environmental and sanitary work
to engineers and administrators. This left MOsH with the medical, person-
centred and diseased-centred work. The break from the broad sanitary agenda
was evident in the founding of two journals largely aimed at MOsH: *Public
Health* in 1889 and the *Journal of State Medicine* in 1892. In 1887, the College
of State Medicine (CSM) opened in London to provide advanced teaching
for the Diploma of Public Health. It was a small enterprise with a part-time
staff of two, though it broke new ground by employing none other than
Edward Klein to teach bacteriology. Also in the late 1890s and early 1900s,
a new generation of public health textbooks was published, almost all of
which had long sections on bacteriology. The number of titles and reprint-
ings showed the increased demand from students taking the new postgraduate courses and the enlarged hygiene syllabuses in first degrees. Amongst
the most successful new titles were those by Louis Parkes, A. Winter Blyth,
B. Arthur Whitelegge, Thomas Stevenson and Shirley F. Murphy, and J. Lane
Notter and R. H. Firth.[12] The second volume of Stevenson and Murphy
opened with over 200 pages on bacteriology by Klein, essentially an abridged
version of his textbook. Also significant were the titles of some volumes,

1 D. Porter, 'Stratification and its Discontents: Professionalisation and Conflict in the British Public Health Service', 1848–1914', in E. Fee and R. M. Acheson, eds., *A History of Education in Public Health*, Oxford, Oxford Medical Publications 1991, 83–113.
2 Louis Parkes, *Hygiene and Public Health*, London, H. K. Lewis, 1889; A Winter Blyth, *A Manual of Public Health*, London, Macmillan, 1890; B. Arthur Whitelegge, *Hygiene and Public Health*, London, Cassell, 1890; T. Stevenson and S. F. Murphy, *A Treatise on Hygiene and Public Health*, Vols. 1 and 2, London, Churchill, 1892–94; J. Lane Notter and R. H. Firth, *The Theory and Practice of Hygiene*, London, Churchill, 1896.

especially the linking of the private and the public in Arthur Newsholme's *Hygiene: A Manual of Personal and Public Health* in 1892, and from the mid-1880s a number of public health bacteriology manuals appeared.[13] The older books based on sanitary science ceased to be revised. The last edition of Parkes's *Manual*, much revised but with its original structure in tact, was published in 1891; Wilson's *Handbook of Hygiene* last appeared in 1898.[14]

SMALLPOX, 1880–1900

Despite its declining incidence, smallpox remained the most political of public health diseases. Epidemics were major national and local crises that were blamed either on the failures of state medicine, or the public for neglecting vaccination, or the dangerous propaganda of the antivaccinationists. The latter group maintained pressure throughout the final quarter of the nineteenth century against compulsory vaccination and for the adoption of other means of control, principally isolation and sanitary improvements. However, the potent contagionism popularly associated with smallpox meant that isolation brought its own problems over the siting of hospitals. There were major smallpox epidemics in 1881–82 and 1884–85, along with localised and often severe outbreaks in other years. However, by the 1890s the long-term hope that the disease might be stamped out seemed possible as both overall mortality and the scale of individual outbreaks had diminished markedly. The medical profession tried to claim all of the credit for the achievement through its practices of vaccination and isolation, aided by general sanitary progress.[15] The combined effects of the decline in incidence, the introduction of notification, changes in admission criteria to hospitals and the building of isolation hospitals ensured that by the 1890s almost all smallpox cases were medically managed in isolation hospitals. The decline in the disease paradoxically strengthened the hand of antivaccinationists, who argued that vaccination was no longer necessary and that the disease was being successfully controlled by other methods.[16] Also, the developing knowledge of the 'bacteriology' of the disease brought more questions than answers.

Throughout the 1870s anxieties grew about the dangers that isolation hospitals posed to the public in surrounding areas. In the 1870s the panspermic

---

13 A. Newsholme, *Hygiene: A Manual of Personal and Public Health*, London, George Gill, 1892; H. R. Kenwood, *Public Health Laboratory Work*, London, H. K. Lewis, 1893; G. Newman, *Bacteria in Relation to the Economy of Nature, Industrial Processes and the Public Health*, London, John Murray, 1899.

14 J. Lane Notter, ed., *Parkes Manual of Practical Hygiene*, 8th edition, London, Churchill, 1891; G. Wilson, *A Handbook of Hygiene and Sanitary Science*, London, Churchill, 1898.

15 *SR*, 1881, 2: 346.

16 Political changes also aided the antivaccinationists. See: R. MacLeod, 'Law, Medicine and Public Opinion: The Resistance to Compulsory Health Legislation, 1870–1907: Part II', *Public Opinion*, 1967, 189–207.

visions of Tyndall and others had fed these fears; indeed, as Benjamin Ward Richardson continued to argue, a living virus was more potent than a mere chemical entity. In 1876, petitioning and legal challenges by local residents had led to the closure of the smallpox hospital in Hampstead, and in the early 1880s the Metropolitan Asylums Board (MAB) was under pressure to close its fever hospitals at Fulham, Deptford and Homerton. In other parts of the country, the not-in-my-backyard attitude was also in evidence; for example, in Berkshire in 1890 local residents allegedly took direct action and dumped a tented isolation hospital into the Thames.[17] Amongst MOsH, their own personal immunity to infection, despite constant exposure to the disease, was the best demonstration of the effectiveness of vaccination; hence, their response to criticisms over hospital locations was that any one who was vaccinated had nothing to worry about anyway. The loss of support for panspermism by 1880 meant that doctors became more concerned about transmission by contact, especially in filthy, ill-ventilated conditions, and between weakened bodies. However, epidemiological evidence, most notably over the Sheffield epidemic in 1881–82, swung back to support fears that smallpox hospitals were foci of infection.[18] The role of smallpox hospitals, as defined by the Public Health Act, 1875, was only to provide isolation for those people who could not be effectively isolated at home, that is, the poor, living in overcrowded conditions. It was up to local authorities how many beds to provide, whether to rely on temporary rather than permanent provision, and whether people should be compulsorily removed. Thus, the type of isolation and the extent of its use varied from place to place.[19] In towns such as Leicester, where antivaccination feeling was strong, isolation policies were highly developed.[20] Indeed, many of those who opposed vaccination on the grounds of freedom of the individual were prepared to accept the compulsory removal of the sick to hospital.[21] Elsewhere, especially in London, where the disease was more prevalent and the MAB a proactive agency, the siting of hospitals was often more controversial than vaccination.

Matters came to a head in London in the epidemic in 1881–82. To avoid local protests, the MAB took powers to establish a temporary tented hospital out of London, on the banks of the Thames at Long Reach near Dartford. During the epidemic ships were taken to Long Reach to house serious cases and staff – the images of hulks on a remote stretch of the

7 *PH*, 1890–91, 3: 8.
8 F. W. Barry, *Smallpox in Sheffield, 1881–82*, Sheffield, 1883; W. H. Power, 'Report on Later Observations (1881–84) of the Influence of Fulham Smallpox Hospital on the Neighbourhood Surrounding It', *Supplement to the Fourteenth Annual Report of the LGB, continuing the Report of the Medical Officer for 1884*, BPP, 1884–85, [C.4516], xxxiii, 55–90.
9 J. V. Pickstone, *Medicine in an Industrial Society*, Manchester, Manchester University Press, 1985, 156–73.
0 S. M. F. Fraser, 'Leicester and Smallpox: The Leicester Method', *MH*, 1980, 24: 315–32.
1 *Hansard*, 1889, 334, 1817–25, Halley Stewart (MP Spalding).

Thames, miles from habitations, told of a highly contagious disease that was ideally kept at a great distance.[22] Such was the crisis, that in December 1881 the question of the future of London fever hospitals was put to a Royal Commission.[23] Voluminous oral and written evidence was taken, but no new experimental studies were made.[24] The Final Report, issued at the end of 1882, accepted that smallpox hospitals might pose a danger from contagion to local communities and recommended a single, large smallpox hospital be built in a remote location for all London cases, which was established at Long Reach. The Commission also called for separate institutions for fever cases, the compulsory notification of all infectious diseases, and that isolation hospitals be taken out of the Poor Law system and made available to all citizens for public protection.[25] Although it was some time before the recommendations were acted upon, the Report gave the green light for the establishment of similar institutions across the country, such that between 1861 and 1911 the number of isolation beds in England and Wales rose from under 500 to over 30,000. The Commission was undecided on whether the slight risk of infection faced by those living adjacent to hospitals was caused by 'poison' radiating in the air, or it being carried into the community by hospital workers, or it coming from patients on their way to hospital. Fears with the latter led to the creation of an elaborate ambulance system in London, involving boats and covered narrow gauge railways at Long Reach. An intriguing feature of the Report, especially given that its members were mostly known germ sympathisers, not to mention the timing of its deliberations just after the International Medical Congress in London and the announcement of the *Tubercle bacillus*, was its lack of interest in the nature of the smallpox germ. Indeed, in 1882 Koch wrote that he had possibly observed the 'vaccine micrococci' in preparations of lymph. One of the few times questions about the intimate pathology of variola and vaccinia were raised by the Commission was in the evidence of Sir William Gull (1815–90). He was asked what determined the severity of the disease in individuals; his answer was that the virulence of the poison never altered, but that variations were due 'mostly to the constitution of the patient', that is, to the soil and not the seed.[26] On the nature of the poison, Gull deferred to Sanderson's ideas from the early 1870s, of

22 J. Burne, *Dartford's Capital River: Paddle Steamers, Personalities and Smallpox Boats*, Buckingham, Barracuda Books, 1989.
23 *Report of the Royal Commission on Smallpox and Fever Hospitals*, BPP, 1882, [C. 3314], xxxix, 1 The members included: Sir James Paget, John Burdon Sanderson, Alfred Carpenter, William Broadbent and Jonathan Hutchison.
24 Surprisingly, the Medical Department did not commission any scientific investigations of smallpox. However, Sanderson, who was a member of the commission, undertook new studies of disinfection at this time which had an indirect bearing on isolation.
25 G. M. Ayers, *England's First State Hospitals and the Metropolitan Asylums Board, 1867–1930*, London, WIHM, 1971, 69–94.
26 *Royal Commission on Smallpox*, Appendix, Par. 4352–4.

minute particles carrying the poison and perhaps being themselves the agent
of the disease.[27]

While Koch's larger research programme fed anticipation of the 'discovery', as seen in the Grocer's Company 'Discovery Prize, Pasteur was constructing smallpox as a germ disease in different terms, through his
appropriation of the term vaccination for all forms of protective inoculations
with altered germs.[28] The development of Pasteur's vaccine research programme has been discussed extensively by historians, but the consequences
of his work for Jennerian vaccination have been overlooked.[29] It is well
known that he appropriated the term vaccine by drawing a direct analogy
between the protection that a mild infection of cowpox gave against smallpox and how the inoculation of attenuated fowl cholera germs protected
against subsequent exposure to the disease. Pasteur qualified his analogy,
noting that the relationship between cowpox and smallpox was still disputed,
but then in a circular argument he used the mutable properties of fowl
cholera germs to suggest that cowpox was attenuated smallpox.[30]

In 1881, Charles Cameron, a leading Dublin sanitary reformer, MP and
supporter of germ theories of disease, observed that 'one protective virus had
been elaborated in the laboratory of nature' and the other by 'art'.[31] While
Pasteur was trying to naturalise his artificial attenuation methods, at the same
time he was associating an empirically derived, 'natural' phenomenon with
his own germ theories and laboratory science. It is interesting in this context
that the word 'inoculation' was subsequently used by bacteriologists for both
the seeding of culture plates and test tubes, and the insertion of morbid products and bacteria into animals in experimental studies. Pasteur's 'vaccination'
procedures suggested possible new experiments with smallpox, for example,
trying to 'culture' vaccinia and variola in different 'media', not just in tubes
and on plates, but in other animals such as horses and monkeys, and to
explore the relations between all pox diseases. The passage of different disease
poisons through different species in the hope of altering virulence or producing immunity was not a new practice; it had been tried with many veterinary diseases, for example, with whole animal studies of pleuropneumonia.
What was new, however, was the idea of doing this in a highly controlled
manner with laboratory products to give predictable results. By the 1890s,
it was commonplace to explain the mechanism of smallpox vaccination by
reference to Pasteurian and neo-Pasteurian ideas on attenuation and altered

7 Gull observed: '[T]hey call them bacteria. They are very minute, but Dr Sanderson will tell us
best; they are very minute, that I cannot conceive of their minuteness; they speak of them in
the fraction of one thousandth of an inch, so that they could easily float in the air.' Ibid., Par. 4363.
8 *SR*, 1883, 4: 592.
9 B. Latour, *The Pasteurization of France*, Cambridge, MA, Harvard University Press, 1988, 79–93.
0 L. Pasteur, 'The Attenuation of the Causal Agent of Fowl Cholera (1880)', in D. J. Bibel, ed.,
Milestones in Immunology: A Historical Exploration, Madison, WI, Science Tech, 1988, 21–2.
1 C. Cameron, 'Micro-organisms and Disease', *BMJ*, 1881, ii: 583–7, 585.

virulence. In his evidence to the Royal Commission on Vaccination in 1896, Woodhead explained how true cowpox vaccination worked by referring to Haffkine's new anticholera vaccine that he had recently produced by attenuating cholera vibrios. Politically, the association of vaccination with readily variable virulence was useful ammunition to the pro-vaccinationists in showing that cowpox and smallpox were likely to be closely related. One argument that had long been used against vaccination was that cowpox and smallpox were distinct diseases and offered no cross-protection. This was linked with the idea that Jenner and subsequent vaccinators had been inoculating with variola all along, or else they did not know at all what they were inoculating! However, antivaccinationists also worried, very publicly of course, that variable virulence might allow vaccinia to convert spontaneously to variola, with dire consequences for the vaccinated.

Given its medical and political importance, it is surprising that there were so few bacteriological studies of smallpox published in the wake of the new bacteriological techniques introduced after 1881. In the 1870s the large number of failed 'discoveries' had not caused problems for germ theorists; germs were still 'theoretical', the limits of microscopy uncertain and the use of liquid cultures made it hard to distinguish different types of germs. However, from 1882, the absence of the smallpox or cowpox germ might have been a problem. That it was not reveals much about the status and uses of bacteriological knowledge. Smallpox was a disease that was easily diagnosed, undeniably contagious and had a proven preventive technology; hence there was little to be gained practically from finding the virus. On the other hand, the clinical presentation of the syndrome was congruent with fermentative, zymotic pathologies, and the seeming minuteness of the smallpox germ and difficulty in observing it helped excuse the large number of other, yet undiscovered germs. That said, many 'discoveries' of the smallpox germ were claimed in the 1870s and 1880s, but all failed to achieve lasting or widespread acceptance. It is interesting to note the grounds on which 'discoveries' failed. The authority of the claimant was important; the findings of figures such as Sanderson, Cohn and Weigert were cited for many years even though they were not replicated by others.[32] On the other hand, Klein's work with sheeppox, published at the same time as his controversial typhoid work, attracted very little attention. A feature of all germ claims in the 1870s was their tentativeness over observational evidence and the experimenter's own difficulties in replicating findings. With pox diseases, experimenters usually reported single findings, or made assertions, like those in Sanderson's early work, which simply said that the contagion was particulate. Striking visual evidence was important when available, as with the two most widely accepted diseasegerms of the 1870s – the distinctive spirilla of relapsing fever and the parasite-like forms of the anthrax bacillus. Otherwise, analogical reasoning

---

32 See list in G. S. Woodhead and A. W. Hare, *Pathological Mycology: An Enquiry into the Etiology of Infective Diseases: Section 1 Methods*, Edinburgh, Young J. Pentland, 1885, 166.

continued to be used, especially with reference to fungal spores, plant seeds and the life cycles of parasites.[33] The improvements in microscopy during the 1870s and early 1880s showed that whatever 'particles' produced smallpox were extremely small or had some covert existence. The culturing of germs, especially the continuing use of liquid media for 'difficult' organisms, complicated matters by revealing a rich fauna in cowpox lymph and smallpox pustules. This raised new questions: was the 'vaccine virus' a single organism, or the product of combinations of germs? What other organisms were in vaccine lymph, and what were their effects?

In Britain, answers to some of these questions were provided in 1886 when John Buist (1846–1915), a physician at the Western Dispensary, Edinburgh, and a teacher of vaccination for the Local Government Board, published the results of his laboratory studies on the life history of vaccinia and variola.[34] By using Koch's plate culture methods he found three types of micrococci in vaccine lymph, and he singled out one as 'the bacteric form of the true contagium'. However, he stopped short of making it the specific organism of the disease – he had only found its 'bacteric form'; it might be pathogenic in some other state. Also, he was unable to produce the disease by inoculation of culture plate material in either animals or humans. Buist's claims to be the discoverer of the smallpox germ have impressed historians more than his contemporaries, who regarded his work as technically flawed.[35] The leading British vaccine researchers of the 1890s, Klein and Sydney Monckton Copeman, disregarded Buist's findings, believing that his cultures had been contaminated. Klein found minute bacilli in lymph when he returned to pox work in the 1890s.[36] He now argued that the reason no organism had been isolated from vaccine lymph was because it was only ever present there in its latent spore form. Klein developed elaborate methods for staining these spores' but could find no reliable method of cultivation. Copeman, who worked with Klein, tried culturing lymph in eggs and other living media, and while unable to isolate any organism did manage to maintain the vaccinating power of lymph in egg cultures.[37]

The culturing of vaccine lymph provided fertile research possibilities in two other directions. First, the failure to find tiny bacteria led researchers to look for other types of microorganisms and even for larger forms such as moulds (Blastomycetes), sporozoa and protozoa. In the early 1890s, there was short-

3 G. Harley, 'Some New Facts Conected (sic) with the Action of Germs in the Production of Human Diseases', *MTG*, 1881, ii: 570–3, 596–8, 651–3, 705–7, 732–4.
4 J. B. Buist, *Vaccinia and Variola: A Study of Their Life History*, London, Churchill, 1887.
5 S. M. Copeman, 'Bacteriology of Vaccine Lymph', *TESL*, 1891–92, 11: 70–80.
6 E. Klein, ' On the Etiology of Vaccinia and Variola', *Supplement to the Twenty-Second Annual Report of the LGB, containing the Report of the Medical Officer for 1892–93*, BPP 1894, [C.7412], xxxix, 693–7; idem, 'Further Observations on the Microbes of Vaccinia and Variola', *Supplement to the Twenty-Fourth Annual Report of the LGB, containing the Report of the Medical Officer for 1892–93*, 1895, BPP, [C.7906], li, 267–86.
7 S. M. Copeman, 'The Milroy Lectures on the Natural History of Vaccinia', *BMJ*, 1898, i: 1185–9, 1245–50, 1312–8.

lived excitement about the work of Ruffer and Plimmer, who not only supposed that smallpox was a protozoan disease, but also that cancer was the result
of protozoan infection.[38] The second area of work involved attempts to disinfect vaccine lymph of unwanted organisms. This effort was in part prompted by
the influence of antivaccinationist groups. While still campaigning mainly on
the principle of the freedom of the individual, they continued to exploit divisions within medicine, especially the value of isolation and the impact of
general sanitary improvements.[39] Another issue that they had long exploited
was public fears that inoculation might carry or induce other diseases, especially
syphilis, erysipelas, tuberculosis, glanders and whooping cough. By monitoring
medical journals, antivaccinationists mobilised bacteriological findings to their
cause, using the most obscure reports to muddy the waters and create uncertainties. For example, in 1892 there were suggestions in the medical press that
smallpox was a fungoid skin disease, which antivaccinationists used to question
the value of administering vaccinia to the blood.[40]

The medical profession had long advocated the use of lymph direct from
the calf as the safest procedure, but questions about tubercular infection by this
route grew in the 1890s along with the wider antituberculosis campaign. These
fears were stirred at the International Congress on Hygiene and Demography
in London in 1891 when Edgar Crookshank reported finding large numbers
of different bacteria in vaccine lymph. He was convinced that these were all
nonpathogenic, but the antivaccinationists spread alarm about the findings.[41]
Already in 1890, the *Vaccination Inquirer* had carried an article entitled ' "Vaccination" by a "Bacillus" '. The 'Bacillus' thanked the 'Modern Medicine Man'
for all of 'the varieties of inoculation' they now used, 'as it immensely
increases our facilities for bringing up our large families'.[42] One answer to
the problem of lymph contamination was to improve its disinfection. The
best methods to achieve this were discussed in another paper at the 1891
Congress by Copeman, who was by this time head of the National Vaccine
Establishment (NVE) in London. He advocated the use of glycerinated calf
lymph, which met all of the possible objections of the antivaccinationists over
deterioration and contamination with septic, tubercular and syphilitic germs.[43]

38 E. Klein, 'Report on Psorosperms in their Relation to the Etiology of Cancer', *Supplement to the
Twenty-Third Annual Report of the LGB, Containing the Report of the Medical Officer for 1893–94*, BPP,
1894, [c. 7538], xl, 479–93.

39 D. Porter and R. Porter, 'The Politics of Prevention: Antivaccinationism and Public Health in
Nineteenth-Century England,', *MH*, 1988, 32: 231–52.

40 *Vaccination Inquirer*, 1892, 14: 137. This news item was based on an article in the *Guy's Hospital
Reports*.

41 On W. J. Collins's questioning of Crookshank, see: *Fourth Report of the Royal Commission on Vaccination*, BPP, 1893, [C.6527], Par. 11.058–70. By this time Crookshank was questioning the value
of vaccination, largely on the grounds that cowpox and smallpox were distinct diseases, and that
vaccinia did not protect against variola infections.

42 *Vaccination Inquirer*, 1890, 12: 51–2.

43 S. M. Copeman and F. R. Blaxall, *Report on the Influence of Glycerine in Inhibiting Growth of Micro-
organisms in Vaccine Lymph*, London, Eyre and Spottiswoode, 1898.

Glycerine was an alcohol 'derived from animal and plant oils' that had been used as a mild antiseptic for many years. However, Copeman was using a much purer form of the compound and now presented glycerinisation as a bacteriologically based method. The antivaccinationists played Copeman's innovation in two ways. On the one hand, they accepted that glycerine had 'healing in its wings', but then asked what damage had been previously wrought by lymph that doctors had assured the public was safe. They gloated that medical progress had shown how little doctors had known previously, so what might future progress reveal about the current levels of ignorance and risk? Antivaccinationists also sought to erode the credibility of medical scientists by questioning whether an organic acid really had selective germicidal powers, and might it not diminish the power of the vaccinia organism.[44] The main response to these attacks, by Copeman and the Local Government Board, was to try to reduce their reliance on antiseptics, converting the National Vaccine Establishment into an aseptic environment, to establish a state-of-the-art laboratory to monitor the purity of lymph and to continue research to reveal finally the intimate nature of the contagion of smallpox.

CHOLERA, 1880–1900

A new pandemic of cholera developed in the early 1880s and reached the Mediterranean coast of Egypt in 1883, only months after the country had come under British rule. Governments in southern Europe saw the disease as a major threat and once again called for quarantines. British sanitary experts on the spot, as well as those in London and India, continued to resist these pleas, saying that quarantines were futile and even counterproductive.[45] Foreign Office staff saw their responsibilities in Egypt as saving lives and protecting trade; hence they sent twelve medical officers to establish hospitals, institute port inspections and improve sanitation. They also called on Surgeon-General William Guyer Hunter, from the Indian Medical Service, to report on the origins and spread of the epidemic. A different response came from Germany and France. Government commissions were dispatched to investigate the aetiology of the disease, in what was seen as an opportunity to show the power of the germ scientists and perhaps to gain a foothold in a strategically important area. None other than Robert Koch led the German group, while Isidore Strauss (1845–96) and Emile Roux (1853–1933) headed the team from Paris.[46] The Foreign Office report came out first and

---

44 *Vaccination Inquirer*, 1898, 19: 161–71.
45 There was speculation that securing the Suez Canal reduced the threat to Europe; the logic of this was that communication with India need no longer involve any reprovisioning at ports, and that without the ability to renew itself in the soil, the cholera-poison would not survive the direct journey to Europe.
46 W. Coleman, 'Koch's Comma Bacillus: The First Year', *BHM*, 1987, 61: 315–42.

was a classic statement of the Anglo-Indian medical view of cholera as a disease of 'locality'. Having collected epidemiological evidence and listened to local doctors, Guyer Hunter concluded that cholera was endemic in Egypt and that the latest outbreak came from the reactivation of poisons that had been in the soil since 1865. It was not a recent importation and hence would not have been prevented by quarantines.[47]

Needless to say the German and French reports addressed different audiences in quite different terms. Their work was concentrated in laboratories and was concerned with the identity of specific causative bacteria. Koch, fresh from his success with the *Tubercle bacillus*, reported in September 1883 that a small rod-shaped bacillus was the essential cause of cholera. The French researchers were unconvinced, especially as neither group managed to reproduce the disease by the inoculation of germs into animals. Research was soon halted by the decline of the epidemic, though undeterred, and with Indian government permission, Koch went on to Calcutta to continue his work. It is worth noting that, before leaving Egypt, Koch also collected epidemiological evidence on the question of importation versus local development, so that he could advise the German government on quarantines. The French Commission returned home having completed exhaustive laboratory investigations but without the prized 'cholera germ'. Koch found his *bacilli* again in India, only these were now described as comma-shaped. He was still unable to meet the requirements of his own third postulate of producing the disease experimentally by inoculation, so he had to maintain his aetiological claim on the basis of his first two postulates – constant association and isolation on culture plates.

Guyer Hunter's report did not completely ignore germ science and laboratory work, though rather than follow recent German and French findings, he trusted the authority of India's leading medical scientists, Timothy R. Lewis and D. D. Cunningham. They remained convinced that a specific cholera contagion had 'no existence' and continued to articulate their version of Pettenkofer's theory.[48] Sir Joseph Fayrer, formerly of the IMS and by this time a metropolitan authority on disease in India, said that '[H]e yielded to no one in his admiration of microscopic research, but he thought that research of other kinds, and over a wider field, was necessary before it could be proved that the all important element in the causation of cholera was a bacillus'.[49] The aetiology of cholera had crucial political implications for the British and Indian governments, as the impending meeting of the International Sanitary Commission was expected to take the 'discovery' of a specific germ as confirmation of the contagiousness of the disease and to call for quarantines.[50] British public health

47 *TESL*, 1883–84, 3: 43–64.
48 J. D. Isaacs, 'D. D. Cunningham and the Aetiology of Cholera in British India, 1869–1897', *MH*, 1998, 42: 279–305.
49 *BMJ*, 1884, i: 459.
50 N. Howard-Jones, *The Scientific Background to the International Sanitary Conferences, 1851–1938*, Geneva, WHO, 1975.

officials were now firmly committed to water-borne transmission, which they interpreted as requiring inclusive and person-centred exclusive measures, not quarantines. Thus, MOsH focused on two measures to keep the disease at bay: (i) inspection to keep cholera-carrying individuals and objects out of the country, and (ii) cleansing to ensure that sanitary conditions were maintained so that any cholera germs that did arrive would not find the environment or people receptive to their development.[51] They argued that if there was no 'explosive material' (insanitary conditions), then the 'match' (the imported germ) could not 'ignite' (to produce an epidemic).[52] To switch to the other favoured metaphor – seed and soil – MOsH argued that the only measures they could take before the 'seed' arrived was still to diminish the receptivity of the local 'soil'. In public health circles, there was great interest in the mixed reception that Koch received on his return to Germany.[53] He was lauded by the state and Berlin medical establishment, but amongst public health doctors his ideas were greeted with some scepticism, not least because of his unwillingness to compromise with Pettenkofer's ideas that the soil, literally, played some role in the establishment of epidemics. That said, all welcomed the fact that Koch himself did not support quarantines, though his reasons were that he favoured direct measures against the comma bacillus.

While British medical scientists were slow off the mark to exploit the laboratory research opportunities in Egypt and India, their opinions on the disease were valued. Both French and German commissions shared their findings with British medical scientists and sought their endorsement. Following his return to Europe, Koch sent some of his specimens to the Royal Medical and Chirurgical Society in London for examination and what he hoped would be confirmation of his aetiological claims. However, the experts consulted – Klein, Heneage Gibbes and Victor Horsley – were unconvinced.[54] Echoing criticisms made in Germany, they noted that many similar organisms were present in the gut and that Koch's aetiology rested only on constant association.[55] In addition, it was noted that neither Koch nor the French expedition had found the organism in the bloodstream of sufferers, so they had not accounted for the pathology and systemic effects of the disease. What should be done in the face of these uncertainties? Speaking at the BMA in Belfast in the summer of 1884, Charles Cameron argued that it was too early to act on Koch's work, especially as its accep-

1 T. Hime, 'Cholera', *SRec*, 1883, 4: 131. The anticholera measures recommended at a meeting of the Yorkshire Association of MOsH in September 1883 was typical: 'ventilation, cleanliness, thorough sanitary arrangements, a pure water supply, and efficient disinfection'. *TSMOH*, 1883, 131.
2 *BMJ*, 1884, i: 287. Of course, until infected people arrived ('the match') all that the MOHs could do was to remove the deadly conditions ('a powder magazine') and then prevent the match from sparking.
3 *MTG*, 1884, ii: 691. 54 *Lancet*, 1884, i: 625–6.
5 Klein was about to set out Koch's postulates in his series on 'micro-organisms and disease' in the *Practitioner*, a journal edited by his St. Bartholomew's colleague, T. Lauder Brunton. E. Klein, 'Micro-organisms and Disease', *Practitioner*, 1884, 32: 170–86, 241–64, 321–52, 401–26; 1884, 33: 21–40, 81–112, 161–80, 241–57.

tance might narrow sanitary intervention merely to prevent the ingestion of germ-bearing water.[56]

From the British perspective, the German and French commissions had brought heat rather than light to the subject of cholera; so in July 1884 the British government decided to send its own researchers to India, choosing Edward Klein, Heneage Gibbes and Alfred Lingard.[57] In the meantime, Lewis, now Professor of Pathology at the Army Medical School, Netley, used the summer vacation to travel to Marseilles, where cholera was still present, to test Koch's claims for himself. Using microscopy only, he found no evidence that the comma bacillus was present in all cases of cholera.[58] The earliest reports of the British Cholera Commission arrived in October 1884.[59] They stated that Klein had become so confident of the error of Koch's findings that he had drunk a solution containing the comma bacillus with no ill effects.[60] This previously unrecognised event may at last have given Klein a place in the germ Hall of Fame, with priority over Pettenkofer for this famous autoexperiment.[61]

An outline of Klein's report reached Britain in January 1885 and was unequivocal: 'The statement of Koch that "comma bacilli" are present only in the intestines of persons suffering from or dead of cholera is not in accordance with the facts'.[62] Klein was back in Britain in February and gave a full report of his work to the Royal Society.[63] He not only criticised Koch, he aligned himself with Pettenkofer-type aetiologies, concluding that 'the infective agent of cholera was extraneous to the body, that it had its breeding ground in a suitable soil, and that it produced a chemical virus which was the real cause of cholera'.[64]

The British medical elite took some pleasure from the fact that home-grown investigators were mixing it with Koch, though Klein's track record on germ pathologies did not inspire confidence. There was much comment that Koch had been too hasty; perhaps he too had succumbed to 'bacteriofröhe'. Nonetheless, his British followers felt that 'the eminent Teuton', having lost this battle, would still win the war.[65] Koch's work was vigorously

56 *BMJ*, 1884, ii: 237.
57 The investigation was also prompted by the pressure put on British delegates for the imposition of quarantines in imperial possessions at the International Medical Congress in Amsterdam.
58 *Lancet*, 1884, ii: 513.
59 *Lancet*, 1884, ii: 928, 1061. The 'honour of British science' was said to be at stake in these investigations and there were worries about Klein carrying the flag.
60 *BMJ*, 1884, ii: 675.
61 In fact, Pettenkofer first challenged Koch with this 'experiment' at the Berlin Cholera Conference in 1885. On the later episode see: R. Evans, *Death in Hamburg: Society and Politics in the Cholera years, 1830–1910*, Oxford, Oxford University Press, 1987, 497–8.
62 *BMJ*, 1885, i: 35–6. J. M. Cuningham, a well-known opponent of germ ideas and quarantines, said that their conclusions were 'altogether subversive of the statements advanced by Professor Koch'.
63 E. Klein, 'The Relation of Bacteria to Asiatic Cholera', *PRSL*, 1885: 154–7.
64 *Lancet*, 1885, i: 564.
65 A leader in the *BMJ* felt that it was too soon to say that the English Commission had dealt a coup de grâce. *BMJ*, 1885, i: 301, 674.

defended by Cheyne, in what was a battle with Klein for the leadership of nascent British bacteriology. The sides were quite revealing, Cheyne was quite isolated, with only Crookshank, his colleague at King's College, and Lister supporting his position. Klein, on the other hand, enjoyed the support of many MOsH, a government department and Sanderson, who referred to Koch's work on cholera as an 'unfortunate fiasco'.[66] Those interested in bacteriological questions worried about the damage caused by such public disputes. Even so, everyone was surprised when an ad hoc suggestion by Thomas Hime, the MOH for Bradford and a Pettenkofer follower, that the differences be referred to a Commission of Inquiry was actually taken up by the Royal Society.[67] In 1885, C. S. Roy, Charles Sherrington and Thomas Brown visited Spain, where cholera was still present, to look for the comma bacillus. They were unable to find it, but returned home suggesting that another agent, a fungus, was the cause. The importance of their work was not their specific findings, which few doctors or scientists took seriously, but that once again Koch's work was challenged by British experts.[68] However, an editorial in the *Lancet* questioned the satisfaction being drawn from all of these negative conclusions and worried about the absence of any plans to continue the research to find the true cholera-germ. This brought out once again the complaints about the neglect of laboratory research in Britain, due to the lack of state funds and the law that 'rendered perfectly legal the killing of rats and other vermin with the wanton intention of merely getting rid of them, while] rendered it a penal crime to inoculate a rat or a mouse with the object of saving human life'.[69]

The implications of the debate and the adoption of the Klein–Pettenkofer view for MOsH was clear. The uncertainty over the *bacillus* and its implications for the contagionist-localist debate meant that preventive measures should continue to be inclusive and exclusive. In fact, the LGB recommended what seemed a particularly well-judged compromise. On the one hand, authorities were asked first to concentrate on sanitary improvements to render the environment unsuitable for the disease-germ and to ensure that water supplies were uncontaminated. While on the other hand, MOsH were asked to use their inspection powers to monitor possible sources, especially shipping and people arriving at ports, as well as local diarrhoea outbreaks. However, the comma bacillus continued to be discussed, not as the cause of the disease but as a diagnostic indicator, and even Klein accepted that its presence (as a result) was evidence of the disease. This point had been urged as early as 1885 by George Heron and Thomas Hime, both of whom were

66 *Lancet*, 1885, i: 564–5; *BMJ*, 1885, i: 1076–7.   67 *BMJ*, 1885, i: 1270.
68 C. S. Roy, ' Preliminary Report on the Pathology of Asiatic Cholera (as Observed in Spain in 1885)', *PRSL*, 1887, 41: 173–81. The report was read in 1885 but not published until 1887. While welcoming the commission's anti-Koch position, Klein was sceptical of the commission's bacteriological skills and questioned their results.
69 *TSMOH*, 1885–86, 31. For earlier complaints, see: *BMJ*, 1885, i: 141.

sceptical of the causative standing of the comma bacillus. They argued that its potential as a diagnostic indicator made all-embracing quarantines totally unnecessary, as port and other inspections now could be pursued with the 'exactness of a scientific experiment'.[70]

With the support of Anglo-Indian doctors, Klein continued to lead British medical opinion against accepting a direct causative relationship between Koch's comma bacillus and Asiatic cholera.[71] Nonetheless, when the disease threatened again in 1892–93, he made many hundreds of diagnostic examinations of tissue and faeces for the LGB. There was some unease amongst Koch's supporters about a nonbeliever performing the tests, but his results were used to allay public fears and to save money on unnecessary precautions. A similar service provided by Delépine in Manchester was the beginning of permanent public health laboratory services in the northwest of England. Despite the proximity of east coast ports to Hamburg and other infected cities, Britain suffered only isolated cases and a local epidemic centred on Grimsby and Cleethorps. This wholly favourable outcome was portrayed by MOsH, chauvinistically, as another triumph for practically oriented British preventive medicine, in contrast to Germany, where no amount of advanced laboratory science had prevented the Hamburg catastrophe.

Medical and government interests in cholera in the 1880s and 1890s were as much imperial as British. The international pressures for quarantines and the problems that the disease caused the Raj ensured that the disease was the focus of continuing debate and research. As Harrison and others have shown, Anglo-Indian medical opinion remained decidedly localist and against contagion; however, this did not mean that it was opposed to bacterial germ theories or laboratory medicine.[72] Indeed, one consequence of the work of Klein's English Cholera Commission was the establishment of a laboratory in Calcutta for D. D. Cunningham to continue experimental work. Like Klein, he continued to argue that there were several *bacilli* associated with cholera and that their variable virulence depended on where they developed in the environment. It is not without irony, therefore, that it was Cunningham who provided Waldemar Haffkine, working from the Pasteur Institute in Paris, with the specimens from which he made his first anticholera vaccine in 1893. Moreover, the effectiveness of the vaccine, made from the comma bacillus, quickly came to be cited as the best evidence for specific causation. Haffkine demonstrated his methods in England in 1893 and was given the

---

70 *BMJ*, 1885, i: 706. G. A. Heron, 'The Cholera Bacillus of Koch', *TSMOH*, 1885–86, 17–32. It was argued that 'The establishment of a causal connection . . . is of far less practical importance than [Koch's] other achievement . . . a means of diagnosing Asiatic cholera'.

71 E. Klein, *The Bacteria in Asiatic Cholera*, London, Macmillan, 1889. As with his earlier volume, the text was first serialised in the *Practitioner* from October 1886 to June 1887. *Practitioner*, 1886, 37: 241–58, 334–50, 414–425; 1887, 38: 4–19, 104–25, 182–201, 267–80, 321–6.

72 M. Harrison, *Public Health in British India: Anglo-Indian Preventive Medicine, 1859–1914*, Cambridge, Cambridge University Press, 1994.

opportunity to undertake trials of his vaccine in India in 1894.[73] The results of the first use of the vaccine were mixed. They were treated sceptically by the leaders of the Indian Medical Service, though Haffkine enjoyed the support of Ernest Hankin, the former rising star of chemical pathology and the newly appointed Indian government bacteriologist, and William Simpson, the chief medical officer in Calcutta.

Haffkine had returned to India for further trials in 1896 when the plague arrived. Using now established Pasteurian techniques, he quickly produced an antiplague vaccine, though this was based on 'killed' organisms rather than 'live' attenuated ones, as with his cholera vaccine.[74] The epidemic, and especially Haffkine's vaccine, caused such shock waves that the Indian government established a Plague Commission to investigate the disease in India and report on the best means to control it. One member of the commission was Almroth Wright, who in 1896 had produced a 'killed' antityphoid vaccine and tested it during an outbreak of the disease at the lunatic asylum in Maidstone.[75] While the Commission's report was lukewarm about antiplague vaccine, Wright was privately encouraging Haffkine and other laboratory scientists in India. At Netley he was producing a cadre of new recruits into the IMS, who were well versed in, if not full converts to and missionaries for, the latest bacteriological knowledge and techniques.

The value and safety of all vaccines produced in the 1890s was the subject of lengthy disputes, and none was adopted as quickly as the diphtheria antitoxin. Nevertheless, they were used by enthusiasts for medical science, such as George Newman, alongside bacterial diagnosis, antitoxins and antisera, as examples of the practical value of the new laboratory medicine in preventive medicine.[76] Given that bacteriologically minded MOsH were stressing personal infection, the proliferation of vaccines was ideologically welcome as they too symbolised personal protection. There was little or no interest in preventive medicine in immunological theories. Rather, doctors were interested in immunological products and were quite happy to continue to use

73 A. E. Wright and D. Bruce, 'On Haffkine's Method of Vaccination against Asiatic Cholera', *BMJ*, 1893, i: 227. W. J. Simpson, who first reported the trials in Britain in December 1895, offered cautious endorsement, though he noted that as cholera infection did not give subsequent immunity the vaccine was at best only likely to give temporary immunity. Cunningham was also sceptical of the value of a vaccine as if the primary site of infection was the gut, how would changing the blood's chemistry and biology help? *PH*, 1895–96, 8, 92. M. P. Sutphen, 'Not What, But Where: Bubonic Plague and the Reception of Germ Theories in Hong Kong and Calcutta, 1894–97', *JHM*, 1997, 52: 81–113.
74 A. Cunningham, 'Transforming Plague: The Laboratory and the Identity of the Infectious disease', in A. Cunningham and P. Williams, eds., *The Laboratory Revolution in Medicine*, Cambridge, Cambridge University Press, 1993, 209–44. Haffkine used bacteria sent to him by French and German investigators from the British possession of Hong Kong in 1894.
75 D. H. M. Grosöschel and R. B. Hornick, 'Who Introduced Typhoid Vaccination: Almroth Wright or Richard Pfeiffer', *Reviews of Infectious Diseases*, 1981, 3: 1251–4.
76 G. Newman, 'The Fundamental Principles of Vaccination and Antitoxin Inoculation', *Medical Magazine*, 1898, 267–8.

the old vaccination analogy to explain what was going on; it was familiar and perhaps falsely reassuring.

DIPHTHERIA, 1880–1900

While British public health doctors took satisfaction from the absence of cholera epidemics in the country since 1866 and the decline of other zymotic diseases, they were worried about the rising incidence of diphtheria. Established preventive methods were seemingly having little effect, and it was even thought that certain celebrated achievements of the Victorian era might actually be making matters worse. Compulsory school attendance was increasing opportunities for the disease to spread by personal contact, while sewers provided an underground network in which dangerous gases could diffuse and seep into homes. In the early 1890s, the problem in London was attracting public and medical attention with over 1,600 child deaths per year.[77] However, mortality from the disease fell rapidly from the mid-1890s as the result of two applications of bacteriological science: laboratory diagnosis and an antitoxin to cure sufferers.[78] The epidemiological significance of these two innovations is not my concern; what I focus on is their impact on public health medicine and the wider position of bacteriology in Britain.[79]

What is now seen as the definitive work on the isolation of the diphtheria *bacillus* by Klebs and Loeffler in 1883 and 1884, respectively, was not immediately accepted in Britain. Indeed, there was considerable dissent over the status of this particular organism, especially its form and mode of action.[80] Significantly, it was not shown by Cheyne at the Parkes Museum in 1884, nor was it mentioned by Klein in the first edition of his *Micro-organisms and Disease*; however, Loeffler's key paper was included in Cheyne's *Recent Essays* volume in 1886.[81] There were two main problems with the Klebs–Loeffler *bacillus*: it was not present in all cases of the disease; and often when it was present there was no disease.[82] Matters were complicated in 1887 when Loeffler announced the pseudodiphtheria *bacillus*, a different species that had the same physical characteristics as the 'true' Klebs–Loeffler *bacillus* but reduced virulence. The Pasteurian account of these organisms, developed by Roux and Yersin, unsurprisingly argued that they were the same species, with the pseudobacillus an

77 Seaton, 'A Report', 57–4; J. F. J. Sykes, 'The Cause of the Increase in Mortality from Diphtheria in London', *PH*, 1894–95, 7: 331.
78 R. Muir and J. Ritchie, *Manual of Bacteriology*, Edinburgh, Young J. Pentland, 1899, 353.
79 Hardy, *Epidemic Streets*, 80–109.
80 For a contemporary assessment, see: *Lancet*, ii: 1884, 741.
81 W. Watson Cheyne, W. H. Corfield and C. E. Cassell, *Public Health Laboratory Work*, International Health Exhibition, 1884. E. Klein, *Micro-organisms and Disease*, London, John Murray, 1884.
82 W. W. Cheyne, ed., *Recent Essays by Various Authors on Bacteria in Relation to Disease*, London, New Sydenham Society, 1886.

attenuated form.[83] In the 1880s, microscopy and cultures of material taken from
he mouth and throat revealed a rich flora of microorganisms, as they had with
he gut in studies of cholera, so it remained possible that diphtheria was the
result of some complex association of germs. There were two reactions to all of
his amongst MOsH: first, to suggest that bacteriologists' claim to have found
he specific germ of diphtheria was premature, and, second, to take the evidence of variable virulence of bacteria and interpret it in sanitary and epidemiological terms. This was translated into Pettenkofer-type notions that the
morbidific agent' might gain virulence in sewer gas or damp soil.[84] However,
t was not only in the environment that the 'agent' might change; doctors
assumed that in the milieu of the inflammatory products of sore throats benign
organisms might develop diphtheric properties.

Throughout the late 1880s diphtheria was fought as both a 'filth disease'
preventable by sanitary measures and a 'dangerous infective disease' preventable by isolation. Edward Seaton, in his address to the International Congress on Hygiene and Demography in 1891, concentrated on predisposing
sanitary conditions, especially the role of sewer gases, while in the same year
Richard Thorne Thorne's Milroy Lectures focused on personal infection,
especially school attendance and the dangers from the milk supply.[85]
However, in the face of rising incidence there was pressure to find new
approaches or settle which existing measures were most effective. An editorial in the *Times* in October 1893 observed that, 'Unfortunately, it is a disease
which is excessively obscure. Despite laborious investigations, by many skilled
observers, we know little as to its origins, its mode of spread, the precautions
to be taken for checking it, or the best mode of treating it'.[86] The new
approaches suggested by exclusive-minded MOsH required direct intervention in homes and schools.[87] They wanted greater powers to close schools
and exclude children, as well as to influence parenting and domestic conditions, especially house ventilation and the health of pets, whom Thorne in
particular, following Klein, suspected as sources of infection.[88]

In 1893, certain MOsH also began to advocate the use of laboratory
diagnosis of diphtheria based on the presence-absence of the Klebs–Loeffler

3 W. W. Spink, *Infectious Diseases: Prevention and Treatment in the Nineteenth and Twentieth Centuries*, Minneapolis, MH, University of Minnesota Press, 1978, 169–76.
4 *BMJ*, i: 1884: 405, 1293
5 R. Thorne Thorne, *Diphtheria: Its Natural History and Prevention: Being the Milroy Lectures, 1891*, London, Macmillan, 1892.
6 *Times*, 30 October 1893, 7e. In 1890–2, the mean annual death rate in England and Wales was 192 per million living, and in London it was 377.
7 See the discussion at the Annual Meeting of the BMA in the summer of 1893, especially the views of Arthur Newsholme. *BMJ*, 1893, ii: 409–10.
8 In the early 1890s, Klein achieved some notoriety with his idea that domestic cats could harbour and spread diphtheria. He still carried the stigma of his evidence to the Royal Commission on Vivisection in 1875 and was the model for a number of demonic medical men in late Victorian fiction. C. Lansbury, *The Old Brown Dog: Women, Workers and Vivisection in Victorian and Edwardian England*, Madison, WI, University of Wisconsin Press, 1985.

bacillus. Their immediate aim was to save money by reducing hospital admissions and stop conflicts with general practitioners over misdiagnoses.[89] These ideas received a welcome boost in the summer of 1894, when Hermann M. Biggs, who ran the municipal diphtheria testing programme in New York, visited London and extolled the value of his service.[90] The service provided free laboratory tests, including specimen collection and reporting of results, aiming to give better control of admissions to hospitals and more accurate mapping of the disease in the community. The influence of Biggs's visit has tended to be overshadowed by the introduction of the diphtheria antitoxin later in the year. However, laboratory diagnoses were a prior and initially separate initiative. They were pursued by provincial MOsH such as John Robertson in St Helens and D. S. Davies in Bristol, neither of whom rushed to adopt the antitoxin.[91] However, the arrival of the antitoxin did lead the MAB to adopt laboratory diagnoses in October 1894. The Board asked German Sims Woodhead if the London Conjoint Laboratories could provide the service, though the aim was to identify 'true' cases to ration the scarce supplies of antitoxin, not to control admissions or improve surveillance.[92] As with cholera and the comma *bacillus*, the use of laboratory diagnosis did not imply acceptance that the Klebs–Loeffler *bacillus* was the specific cause.[93] The tension between laboratory and clinical diagnoses was recognised, though the advocates of bacteriology sought to avoid conflict.[94] For example, D. S. Davies's letter to general practitioners on the introduction of a diagnostic service in Bristol stated that

It is considered advisable not to examine bacteriologically and report upon diphtheria cultures except for 'notified' cases, as the intention is not to make, but to confirm a diagnosis; for clinical observation is not necessarily contradicted by a negative bacteriological result and precautions are necessary in all suspicious cases.[95]

When Woodhead reported that no bacilli were found in approximately one-quarter of the cases admitted to MAB hospitals, he conceded that many of these were probably due to failed cultivations and hence 'were clinically, and probably truly, diphtheria'.[96] Elsewhere laboratory diagnosis was described as a 'coadjudicator', and because the clinician and bacteriologist were so often in agreement, 'confidence was inspired in both'.[97] However,

89 This work was done by the Conjoint Laboratory for only two years; from January 1897 it was taken over by the hospitals themselves. *ARCP*, 40, 1896–98: 57. Ayers, *England's First*, 196–7.
90 *PH*, 1893–94, 6: 338; 1894–95, 7: 311.
91 *PH*, 1898–99, 11: 602. The first service seems to have been established by D. J. Hamilton in Aberdeen in 1894.
92 *ARCP*, 39, 1894–96: 67   93 *BMJ*, 1894, i: 106, 1391.
94 As late as 1923, a Medical Research Council report stated that 'the diagnosis of the *disease* of diphtheria – is the province of the clinician alone'. F. W. Andrewes et al., eds., *Diphtheria: Its Bacteriology, Pathology and Immunology*, London, MRC, 1923, 235.
95 *PH*, 1895–96, 8: 403   96 G. S. Woodhead, 'Diagnosis of Diphtheria' *PH*, 1896–97, 9: 356.
97 H. Beale Collins (MOH, Kingston, Surrey), *BMJ*, 1894, ii: 1067; *PH*, 1896–97, 9: 67.

others highlighted direct conflicts between bacteriologists and clinicians. For example, James Niven, on the basis of a mere thirty-five percent positives in bacteriological tests of clinically diagnosed patients in Manchester, stated that 'it is abundantly clear that no conclusion can be drawn from previous allocations of the disease'.[98]

These initiatives with laboratory diagnosis were soon overtaken by the demands on laboratories and laboratory workers to produce and test the new antitoxic serum treatment for diphtheria. Antitoxin was first used in Britain in the summer of 1894, though trials had been in progress in Germany and France for many months, and the possibility of an antitoxic treatment had been trailed by chemically minded bacteriologists for many years.[99] The original laboratory studies on which the treatment was based had been made in the late 1880s, and Behring and Kitasato had not been shy in publicising their ideas on the antibacterial properties of the blood and other tissues to medical audiences. Behring's and Kossel's paper on serum treatment was summarised in the medical press in May 1893, though it was presented as yet another remedy from German laboratories, where biological treatments were being added to their chemical range. Exactly a year later a similar report, this time based on the results obtained by Ehrlich, Kossel and Wassermann, was printed in the Epitome of the *BMJ*; interestingly, it was given no more column inches than yet another new treatment based on the local application of antiseptics to the throat. In Britain, public attention was drawn to the treatment by Sir Henry Roscoe in June 1896, who used it to advance the general claims of experimental medicine in Britain and the particular needs of the struggling British Institute for Preventive Medicine (BIPM).

The idea for a BIPM had emerged from the failed attempts to create a Pasteur Institute in Britain in the late 1880s. The huge success of Pasteur's antirabies vaccine after 1884 had produced demands for the treatment to be made available across the world. The result was the creation of Pasteur Institutes in towns and cities where sufficient private, voluntary or public support could be mobilised to support such a venture. The initial aim was that these institutes would supply only the rabies cure, but the proliferation of Pasteurian vaccines and other bacteriological developments meant that they soon diversified to provide a range of services. Two main reasons were given for not establishing a Pasteur Institute in London: first, geography, as proximity to Paris allowed sufferers to enjoy the best treatment available there in a matter of hours; and, second, it was decided to control rabies as an animal contagion, using quarantines to 'stamp out' the disease.[100] There were other

98 *PH*, 1896–97, 9: 66.
99 *PH*, 1889–90, 3: 281. *BMJ*, 1890, ii: 1317, 1395; *Lancet*, 1890, ii: 1279.
00 This section is largely based on H. Chick et al., *War On Disease: A History of the Lister Institute*, London, André Deutsch, 1971, 19–27.

reasons, too: anti-French sentiment and worries about the actions of anti-vivisectionists. By 1890, the London initiative had transmuted into plans to establish the national centre for bacteriological research that the country lacked. An appeal for funds was launched in 1891, aimed mainly to attract large donations from landed and industrial wealth. The response was luke-warm, except from antivivisectionists, who petitioned against the proposal and mobilised public opposition in London. Nonetheless, at the International Congress on Hygiene and Demography in London in the summer of 1891, the foundation of the BIPM was announced, backed by Lister, Roscoe, William Turner, C. S. Roy, William Humphry, Cheyne and Spencer Wells. It took a further two years to collect enough funds to open the Institute in December 1893, albeit as a very modest affair, based in the rooms of the College of State Medicine (CSM), which the BIPM quickly absorbed. There were only four staff: Armand Ruffer (Director), Allan Macfadyen (bacteriologist), Joseph Lunt (chemist) and William Whittingham (laboratory attendant), though other London doctors and researchers used the laboratories part-time as they had the Conjoint laboratories and those in the CSM.

The diphtheria antitoxin changed the fortunes of the BIPM both materially and ideologically. The antitoxin was produced by inoculating horses, who were nonsusceptible to diphtheria, with the Klebs–Loeffler *bacillus*. The blood of the horse produced antitoxins similar to those elaborated by the human immune response. The size of horses meant that large volumes of blood could be harvested, the antitoxin-bearing serum separated from whole blood and concentrated, and then injected to boost the natural antitoxic reactions of human sufferers. The Institute became a major producer of the new remedy, as well as providing other bacteriological services for towns and cities. The work provided a much-needed income stream for the Institute and associated it with a life-saving medical breakthrough that was all the more potent for bringing children back from near certain death.

The treatment was first used by individual doctors who obtained German-produced serum through London pharmaceutical agents.[101] Two provincial doctors, George Eastes (Folkestone) and Urqhart Walker (Worksop), were in the vanguard and quickly published favourable results. The high cost of imported serum meant that the treatment was restricted to enthusiasts and the wealthy, though very quickly other laboratories and private companies began to market sera. Favourable case reports of the treatment continued to be published during 1894, building up the sense of a modern medical miracle. Statistics from its use in Germany and France pointed to reductions in mortality of over fifty percent.[102] These results excited those doctors supporting the development of experimental medicine,

101 *BMJ*, 1894, ii: 125, 180.
102 *BMJ*, 1894, ii: 889. To the middle of October there were thirty-six cases reported in Britain, with a 5.5 percent mortality.

hough there was some caution as memories of Tuberculin were still
vivid.[103] In France and Germany the treatment was boomed in the popular
press and public subscriptions were started to ensure supplies and to provide
he resources to underpin further research.[104] There was nothing like the same
evel of publicity or public interest in Britain, where the press was more
worried about children being treated as guinea pigs and profiteering by
aboratories. However, the proponents of laboratory medicine had high hopes
hat the diphtheria antitoxin would at last signal therapeutic benefits from
he bacteriological revolution. An editorial in the *Lancet* at the start of 1895
uggested that:

ve have in these 'antitoxins' the *specific* remedies which have been desired since medicine
emerged from pure empiricism.... Unless the whole fabric of bacteriology is unsub-
tantial and visionary there is reason to believe that the path has been opened which may
ead to our mastery over ... acute infective disease.[105]

Antivivisectionists and the government were given equal blame for the fact
hat this innovation in chemical pathology had been developed in Germany,
n an area of research where Britain had been the world leader in the late
880s.

The major problem in Britain in the summer and autumn of 1894 was
he shortage of serum, plus the variable quality of what was available and
uncertainty about dosage. The directors of Britain's few medical laboratories
aw the problems with supply as an opportunity that was too good to miss.
They competed to meet demand, converting research and diagnostic labora-
ories into serum-production facilities, buying horses, and researching ways
of determining the strength of sera. The BIPM was the first laboratory to
offer to supply serum, and they were soon joined by the Conjoint Labora-
ory, the Brown Institution, the Royal Veterinary College and commercial
companies such as Burroughs Wellcome.[106] The idea of a public appeal for
unds for the BIPM, along continental lines, was initially resisted by Lister,
who was perhaps chastened by the failure of earlier attempts to raise funds.
However, once the scale of demand became evident, Lister changed his mind
nd appealed for donations in October 1894. Supplies of antitoxic sera
rom domestic sources increased over the winter months of 1894–95, though
hey continued to be outstripped by demand. Imports continued to be
sed, with worries about their cost, purity, strength and efficacy. In the
utumn it was reported in the press that antitoxin was only being used at

03 *Practitioner*, 1895, 54: 47.
04 P. Weindling, 'From Medical Research to Clinical Practice: Serum Therapy for Diphtheria in the
   1890s', in J. V. Pickstone, ed., *Medical Innovations in Historical Perspective*, London, Macmillan, 1992,
   72–83.
05 *Lancet*, i: 1895, 42.
06 E. M. Tansey, 'The Wellcome Physiological Research Laboratories, 1894–1904: The Home Office,
   Pharmaceutical Firms and Animal Experiments, *MH*, 1989, 33: 1–41.

one of the MAB's hospitals and that the Board would not say which one.[107] The official explanation was that this was because of the shortage of serum. However, journalists speculated that doctors' secrecy was because they were undertaking a huge comparative trial with the capital's children as guinea pigs, where three-quarters of the sufferers were denied the new remedy.

The BIPM had promised that its serum would be stronger than that obtainable from abroad, which doctors hoped would resolve one of the major problems of the treatment – dosage. There were in fact several problems. First, there were doubts about the meaning of the 'units' of strength, let alone the relationship between labels and contents. Next, there was the question of what dose to give. British doctors were reluctant to administer the large doses recommended by German and French authorities, and there were complaints that the lower falls in mortality rates seen in Britain were due to this un-willingness to give large doses early in the illness. The problem was partly technical; for example, in 1895 Burroughs Wellcome serum was given in 250-milliliter or half-pint doses in what was almost a minor operation. Shortages had led doctors to spread what serum they had too thinly amongst sufferers. One response, organised by the *Lancet* rather than the government, was the establishment in the spring of 1895 of a Special Commission to investigate the strengths of antitoxic sera.[108] Much was at stake, for doctors were defend-ing what, in the words of Allan Macfadyen, the new director of the BIPM, was 'the greatest modern advance in the treatment of disease'.[109]

The favourable reception of diphtheria antitoxin in Britain during the summer of 1894 was followed by a more critical reaction. The disputes in Germany over the nature and efficacy of sera were given prominence in the medical press.[110] Indeed, the best results from continental Europe had only brought their diphtheria mortality rates down to those already prevailing in Britain. Was this another example of British sanitary empiricism outshining continental laboratory science? In addition, doctors began to report adverse reactions to the injection of serum and of complications during recovery, for example, skin rashes and kidney failure.[111] Antivivisectionists, who had been surprised by this success for laboratory medicine, went back on the offen-sive. They pointed to the extra cruelty now being perpetrated on animals, especially as the horses used to produce the antitoxin were not protected by legislation, as, like the calves producing vaccine lymph, they were being used for production rather than research. However, the testing and calibration of serum was covered by the Act, a situation reflected in the increase in the number of inoculation experiments licensed under Certificate A of the 1875 Cruelty to Animals Act, which went up from 1,507 in 1894 to 5,217 in 1896.

107 *Times*, 18 December 1894.   108 *Lancet*, 1896, ii: 182–95.
109 PH, 1898–99, 11: 127. Interestingly, he went on to argue that bacteriologists were now fighting diseases by 'Nature's methods'.
110 BMJ, 1894, ii: 947.   111 *Practitioner*, 1898, 50: 371.

Those producing sera also had to battle against the taint of 'commercialism'.[112] Michael Foster spoke at the BMA in Toronto in 1897 against 'the selfish withholding of new scientific truths' and how 'his new alchemy which makes gold out of serum is an ignoble business, and degrades those who pursue it below the level of the vulgar quacksalver'. This was fed in large measure by the wider public perception of doctors charging excessively for their services and the sense that science was public knowledge and hence its results should be public property. The press also questioned the ethics of making profits from suffering children and from a natural substance produced by the noble horse. In this context, the BIPM let it be known that its serum production would be nonprofit-making, while production at the Conjoint Laboratories was subsidised by the Goldsmith's Company.

Although the majority of reports of the treatment were favourable, there was vocal dissent from a minority led by Dr. Lennox Browne, Senior Surgeon at the London Ear, Nose and Throat Hospital.[113] The issues he raised are revealing of some of the tensions between bench and bedside, and how both sides were now using bacteriological ideas. Lennox Browne cleverly used the laboratory evidence that forty percent of the cases of diphtheria were misdiagnosed to suggest that success with antitoxin was being claimed for many patients who never had the disease. Moreover, he argued that the increase in admission rates meant that hospital mortality rates were bound to go down as the proportion of very serious cases admitted had fallen. He pointed out that antitoxin was being used in conjunction with existing antiseptic and stimulant treatments, which with good nursing had already given Britain the best recovery rates in Europe.[114] Another line of criticism was to question the action of antitoxin; how could a remedy injected in different parts of the body affect a membrane in the throat? And if its active principle was a chemical agent, why did it take up to two days to work?[115]

In diphtheria antitoxin's first year, the medical press only contained case reports, and these were from all kinds of practitioners in both private and hospital practice. What both supporters and critics were waiting for was statistics from a more controlled environment, say, from the experiences of a

---

12 *BMJ*, 1897, ii: 232. In 1899, in his famous attack on bacteriology, George Wilson cliamed that the subject was 'steeped in commercial interests'. G. Wilson, 'Bacteriology in its Relation to State Medicine, *JSM*, 1899, 7: 495–501.

13 *Times*, 6 December 1894, 14f; 7 December 1894, 14f, and 31 January 1895, 3d.

14 In February 1896, a journalist, D. C. Boulger, who had recently recovered from diphtheria published an article on treatment regimes at MAB hospitals. He said he was given chlorine gargles, hot linseed oil poultices round the throat, together with iron and brandy to strengthen the system. He reported suffering severe side effects from the antitoxin and said that he owed his life to superior nursing and established treatments. D. C. Boulger, 'Antitoxin, From a Patient's Point of View', *Contemporary Review*, 1896, 69: 177–89.

15 *BMJ*, 1895, i: 49. The implication here was that there was an incubation period, which pointed to the active agent in the antitoxin being a living organism or ferment.

large isolation hospital, such as those of the MAB.[116] The delay in producing figures gave ammunition to the opponents of laboratory medicine and led Lister to write to the superintendent of the Homerton Hospital, Edward Goodall, to encourage prompt publication as the matter was of 'vital importance'.[117] The first statistics from Homerton were published in August 1895 and showed a drop in mortality from 33.6 to 22.8 percent. However, the full MAB results, widely seen as the definitive British trial, were not published until April 1896 and then showed what was seen as a very modest fall in mortality, from 29.6 to 22.5 percent. Several explanations were offered for this result: delays in admission leading to a preponderance of advanced cases; the initial shortage of serum leading to rationing; and delays in treatment due to the need for confirmatory bacterial diagnoses before using scarce material. It was not only the recovery-rate statistics that were against diphtheria antitoxin in 1896. Confidence was not helped when the Lancet Special Commission on Serum Strength reported in July 1896 that the quality of two out of the three main brands of British sera was 'most variable'.[118] Clinicians were clear that the treatment made a difference, especially when high doses were given early in the disease, so whatever spin was put on statistics or laboratory testing, their 'experience' ensured that its use continued.[119]

There was a major difference between London and the remainder of the country regarding diphtheria antitoxin. As a Poor Law organisation, the MAB was able to offer treatment to patients, whereas isolation hospitals elsewhere came under sanitary authorities and, in theory at least, could only be used in a preventive capacity. However, legal restrictions did not stop individual MOsH from administering the remedy. One suggested way around the problem was for provincial MOsH to use antitoxin prophylactically, giving it to families, school children and communities where the disease was incipient or rife.[120] Even in limited outbreaks the costs would have been high, and public resistance to medical intervention with the healthy was anticipated. The limited use of the antitoxin by MOsH outside of London meant that production and testing remained concentrated in the capital, and also in the northwest as a result of earlier initiatives. In the late 1890s, even a city as large as Birmingham sent its bacteriological samples to London.[121] Given their

---

116 Lister wrote to E. W. Goodall, Medical Superintendent at the Homerton Hospital questioning the MAB's apparent secrecy. RCP Archives, Mss. 682/4, letter dated 7 February 1895. Lister also sought information on the normal complications of diphtheria, so that these could be distinguished from the effects of antitoxin.

117 RCP Archives, Mss 628/6 Lister to Goodall 2 June 1897.

118 *Lancet*, 1896, ii: 196, 182–95. Lack of confidence in the quality of serum remained a problem and was still felt to be holding back the adoption of the treatment in 1897. RCP Archives, Minutes of Laboratory Committee, 23 July 1897.

119 *Times*, 6 April 1896, letter from 'FRCS' and 9 April 1896, letter from 'MB'. *Lancet*, 1897, i: 1607, and *BMJ*, 1897, i: 794, 1897; ii: 1267.

120 *BMJ*, 1894, ii: 376; *Times*, 23 November 1894, 3c.

121 A Hill, 'Diphtheria in Birmingham', *PH*, 1895–6, 8; 342.

overall responsibilities for prevention, it is no surprise to find that provincial MOsH continued to focus on the merits of school closure and the environmental factors that caused the waxing and waning of local epidemics, rather than novel therapeutics. On this front a number of MOsH continued to worry about the influence of bacteriologists in leading sanitary authorities to neglect 'extralaboratory work'.[122] Such views were not necessarily hostile to bacteriology; for example, Louis Parkes stressed that MOsH had to be interested in the life history of bacteria beyond the body and, drawing on notions of variable virulence, asked, 'Does not the trend in modern investigation give more and more importance to predisposing causes, and detract from the view originally held that the specific microbe was the be-all and end-all of disease?'[123] As I have shown throughout this volume, there was never a time when the 'seed' explained everything and the role of the 'soil' was ignored; however, it was useful to MOsH in the 1890s to once again stress the importance of the contingencies of contagion as a product of medical progress.

While MOsH wanted to maintain a balance of inclusive and exclusive approaches, they were more enthusiastic than ever about the value of bacteriological diagnoses for mapping disease and identifying epidemic foci. By the summer of 1898, seven London vestries, along with departments in Aberdeen, Bristol, Brighton, Croydon, Dundee, Leeds, Liverpool, Manchester, Newcastle, St Helens and Sheffield, had contracted out, or organised for themselves, bacteriological services. Smaller authorities used the BIPM or the Clinical Research Association. Lister opened many of these provincial laboratories, as in Belfast in January 1897 and Liverpool in October 1898, each time taking the opportunity to promote the recent benefits of bacteriology and experimental medicine, and always citing diphtheria antitoxin as its most wonderful benefit.[124] The model for provincial bacteriological services was that established in Manchester by Sheridan Delépine. In the early 1890s, Delépine, who was Professor of Pathology at the Victoria University, had undertaken a series of ad hoc researches for Manchester Corporation on cholera, tuberculosis, disinfectants and the water supply. This work was encouraged by the university and was routinised in 1895 on a payment for service basis. The volume of work grew rapidly as other local authorities in the Northwest, and soon the rest of northern England and much of the north Midlands, made use of the service. By 1900, the laboratory was making over 100 reports per week, despite losing work as larger towns and cities made their own local arrangements.[125] The highest demand was for the culturing of throat swabs for diphtheria, followed by sputum tests for *Tubercle bacilli*. Delépine and the others were responding to

122 *PH*, 1895–96, 8: 320–1.
123 L. Parkes, 'Sewer Ventilation', *PH*, 1997–98, 10: 267.
124 J. Lister, 'On the Value of Pathological Research, *BMJ*, 1897, i: 317–9; 1898, ii: 1189.
125 *Report of the Advisory Committee on the Building and Opening of the New Laboratory at York Place and the Director's Report for the Session 1904–5*, Manchester, 1905, 6.

initiatives that came 'up' from rank-and-file MOsH, not to proposals coming 'down' from government or elite medical scientists. Aware of the interests of the local political constituencies who were being asked to support new services, MOsH promoted public health laboratories on the grounds of economy and public protection, especially by reducing admissions to isolation hospitals and avoiding the unnecessary disinfecting of properties. They also adopted laboratory screening of isolation hospital patients to determine when they were bacteria-free and could be safely allowed back into the community. Laboratories should not only be seen in practical terms; they were also potent cultural symbols for a modern local authority. Thus, when the Camberwell Vestry in London opened its bacteriological laboratory, the event was marked by an evening that included 'music, microscopes, Roentgen rays, the electrophone and Dr Bousfield's lecture . . . illustrated by microphotographs displayed by limelight'.[126]

The spread and utility of bacteriological testing was valuable ammunition for those physicians and surgeons who were pushing for the development of clinical teaching in infectious disease hospitals as well as the formal inclusion of practical bacteriology in the medical curriculum. The latter topic had been debated since the 1880s, and the position in the late 1890s was that bacteriology was taught in most medical schools, but only in extramural classes and postgraduate qualifications, with instruction in bacterial aetiologies spread across the curriculum. The complaint made by reformers was that there was no requirement for practical training in ordinary medical education. What training a student received depended on where they studied and the interests and enthusiasm of individual staff. In 1894, there were bacteriological laboratories in London at Guy's, University College, King's College and St. Bartholomew's, with teaching at Oxford, Cambridge, Manchester, Durham, Edinburgh, Aberdeen and Glasgow.[127] The department at Guy's had opened in 1888–90 to provide instruction and laboratory facilities for staff, not students.[128] The first lecturer, John Washbourn, who had postgraduate experience in Vienna and Königsberg, initially provided a short course of lectures with practical work voluntary. A demonstrator was appointed in 1894 because of the increase in diagnostic work and practical classes were instituted for candidates in the Diploma of Public Health. Finally, in 1896–97, a course in microscopical pathology, including both bacteriology and morbid histology, became compulsory for all students. At St. Bartholomew's a short course was taught from 1889 by C. B. Lockwood and V. D. Harris, despite the presence of Klein on the staff. Alfred Kanthack was appointed to the new lectureship in bacteriology in 1894, continuing the type of teaching he had introduced in Liverpool in 1892. Such examples show that bacteriology was being taught well before attempts were made to formalise its position. Delépine raised the

126 *BMJ*, 1899, i: 105.   127 *Lancet*, 1894, ii: 487.
128 'The Bacteriological Department, Guy's Hospital', *Guy's Hospital Gazette*, 1915, 141–2.

question of making bacteriology a compulsory subject in initial qualifications in his address to the BMA in the summer of 1896. This prompted William Davy to bring the matter before the Royal College of Physicians in October 1896.[129] The question was put to a special meeting and eventually a Special Committee. The problem was not whether to include the subject in the course for Licentiates, but where to include it without further overloading the curriculum. This proved impossible, as, unsurprisingly, no group of specialists offered to reduce their part of the syllabus. This left bacteriologists to make slow inroads in a number of areas, but especially in pathology practicals.

TYPHOID FEVER: LABORATORY DIAGNOSIS AND VACCINES

The position of typhoid germs remained *sub judice* in Britain from 1884 to 1895, despite the acceptance in Germany and elsewhere that the so-called Eberth–Gaffky *bacillus* was the specific cause. This *bacillus* had been identified by Eberth and Klebs in 1880 as showing more or less constant association with clinically diagnosed cases. Its features were confirmed by Koch and Mayer in 1881, though it was not until 1884 that Gaffky, working in Koch's laboratory, managed to isolate the microorganism on solid plate cultures. However, as with the cholera germs, experimenters could find no animal model in which inoculation with pure cultures produced the disease, denying once again the full establishment of Koch's postulates. In the 1880s, neither Klein nor Crookshank was convinced that the specific agent of typhoid fever had been identified, and both thought that it was premature to rule out a role for the many other *bacilli* found in the gut. They assumed that conditions in the gut were ideal for the transmutation of bacteria and the production of variations in virulence. Not only were doctors adapting notions of variable virulence and evolution into their framework for understanding infectious diseases, they also were using such assumptions to construct the required properties of any candidate *bacillus*. Bacteriological physiology was also mobilised to set further standards for the anticipated typhoid bacterium. For example, in 1891 Sanderson argued that it would have to be among 'less specific' bacteria, because it was adapted both to the aerobic conditions of soil and water and the anaerobic conditions of the human gut.[130] A particular problem by this time was the relation between the Eberth–Gaffky *bacillus* and *Bacillus coli communis* (B. coli, now E. coli) – the commonest microbe found in the gut.[131] The evidence for transmutation between the two came from laboratories in Europe and North America, and from the assumed behaviour of the bacterium in the field. In 1892, the

29 *Lancet*, 1896, ii: 349–51, 664, 777, 845.
30 J. B. Sanderson, 'The progress of discovery relating to the origin and nature of infectious diseases', *BMJ*, 1891, ii: 1136.
31 Hamlin, *Science of Impurity*, 280. *Twenty-Second Annual Report*, 345–65.

Dublin-based bacteriologist E. J. McWeeney reflected on the wider meanings of this work as follows:

The subject, which, from the earlier researches of Eberth and Gaffky seemed a comparatively simple example of the causation of a given disease by a given micro-organism, has within the last two years developed into a network of conflicting possibilities and probabilities, as is to be met in the whole range of scientific medicine.[132]

This statement was typical of a common trope in the 1890s of referring back to an invented past when 'germ-equalled-disease'. McWeeney went on to wonder if things had now returned to the views of Murchison and that the *de novo* origin of epidemics would once again be allowed. The issue of the specificity of the Eberth–Gaffky *bacillus* and its relations with *B. coli* was investigated many times by the Medical Department, and this was the context for Klein's conversion to the Eberth–Gaffky *bacillus* in 1894.[133]

Klein's previous views on the bacteriology of typhoid fever had been congruent with the epidemiological views articulated by the leadership of the Medical Department and those of the wider public health community.[134] They all understood typhoid fever to be spread principally by the faecal contamination of water supplies A dwindling minority of doctors thought aerial transmission possible, and the growing minority implicated contaminated food, especially milk supplies. This construction made typhoid fever 'an exemplary disease' once again for public health medicine. It had to be fought equally with inclusive and exclusive measures.[135] The most dangerous sources of the disease were seen to be typhoid sufferers; hence the first line of defence was for clinicians to ensure that infected bowel discharges were disinfected, and where this was likely to be difficult, as with paupers and the poor, to send sufferers to isolation hospitals. The prevalence of the disease and the difficulties in early diagnosis meant that control by personal infection could never be the whole story, as undetected cases would continue to spread the disease through water supplies and other media. Public health officials used this constant threat to bolster their continuing campaigns for the establishment and maintenance of safe water supplies and sewage systems. However, the threat was not just from sufferers and their wastes; many MOsH continued with Pettenkofer-like statements that in appropriate conditions microbes of 'indefinite form' could acquire virulence or change form to become typhoidal. As McWeeney had anticipated, sanitarian-minded doctors now

132 E. J. McWeeney, 'Some Points in the Aetiology of Typhoid Fever', *JSM*, 1893, 1: 65.

133 PH, 1894–5, 7: 144. The report was based on Klein's reports in the 1894 Report of the Medical Department. *Twenty-Third Annual Report*, Appendix B, 457–68. Also see: E. Klein, Recent Researches on the Identification of the Typhoid bacillus and the Cholera Vibrio', *JSM*, 1896, 4: 285–6, 375–7, 469–71. Also see: E. Klein, 'Recent Researches on the Identification of the Typhoid bacillus and the Cholera Vibrio', *JSM*, 1896, 4: 285–6, 375–7, 469–71.

134 A. Hardy, 'On the Cusp: Epidemiology and Bacteriology at the Local Government Board, 1890–1905', *MH*, 1998, 42: 328–46.

135 L. G. Stevenson, 'Exemplary Disease: the Typhoid Pattern', *JHM*, 1982, 37: 159–81.

ised such bacteriological ideas to refashion the *de novo* origin of the disease
nd to support 'inclusive' measures.[136]

This agenda, together with the politics of water supplies and the difficul-
ies of managing the disease at the personal level, led to repeated attempts to
ind typhoid and related bacteria in the water supply. As Hamlin has shown,
he matter became fraught with conflicts, not only over what investigators
vere looking for and how to find it, but what the presence of microbes actu-
lly meant.[137] Water supply companies were seeking indicators of water
]uality and safety, whereas doctors were looking for the sources of specific
nfections, often trying retrospectively to find the origins of local outbreaks.
'articularly problematic for sanitarians was the drift in findings towards the
onclusion that public water supplies were mostly free of pathogenic germs
nd that reservoirs became purer, rather than more germ-ridden, over time.
The weight of expectation behind the search for typhoid fever bacteria in
he environment is shown by the number and scope of government-funded
tudies in the late 1890s. Klein published on the bacteriology of soil, Andrewes
nd Parry and Laws on sewer gas, Cautley on milk, Martin on the disinfec-
ion of soil, Klein on the persistence of germ in dead animals and Klein again
n the bacterial ecology of soils.[138] The accumulated results suggested that
o external media were obvious breeding grounds for typhoid agents or for

36 One of the leading advocates of the bacterial explanation of a de novo outbreak was H. R.
   Kenwood, author of a much-used text on bacterial techniques: *Public Health Laboratory Work*,
   London, H. K. Lewis, 1896. Also see the discussion prompted by Klein's paper at the Congress
   of the Sanitary Institute in 1894: *Lancet*, 1894, ii: 767–8, 1058, 1121, 1184, 1247.
37 Hamlin, *Science of Impurity*, Chs. 8 and 9.
38 E. Klein, 'Report on the Etiology of Typhoid Fever', *Supplement to the Twenty-Second Annual Report*,
   345–66; .idem., 'Further Report on the Etiology of Typhoid Fever', *Supplement to the Twenty-Third
   Annual Report*, 457–68; idem., 'Further Report on the Etiology of Typhoid Fever', 399–407, and
   'Report on the Behaviour of the Bacillus of Enteric Fever and of Bacillus Coli in Sewage', *Supplement to the Twenty-Fourth Annual Report*, 407–11; idem., Report on the Abilities of Certain Microbes
   to Maintain their Existence in Water', Ibid., 411–29; T. Cautley, 'Report on the Micro-organisms
   Found in Common Articles of Food'; Ibid., 473–504; idem., 'An Inquiry into the Influence of
   Certain Non-Pathogenic Micro-organisms Liable Gain Access to Food', *Supplement to the Twenty-
   Fifth Annual Report of the LGB, Containing the Annual Report of the Medical Officer for 1895–96*, BPP,
   1896, [C.8214], xxxvii, 297; S. Martin, 'Report on the Growth of the Typhoid Bacillus in Soil', *Sup-
   plement to the Twenty-Sixth Annual Report of the LGB, Containing the Annual Report of the Medical
   Officer for 1896–97*, BPP, 1897, [C.8584], xxxvii, 231–43; T. Cautley, 'Report on the Behaviour of the
   Typhoid Bacillus in Milk'; Ibid., 243–55; A. C. Houston, 'Report on the Chemical and Bacteriological Examination of Soils', *Supplement to the Twenty-Seventh Annual Report of the LGB, Containing
   the Annual Report of the Medical Officer for 1897–98*, BPP, 8197, [c. 8953], xl, 251–307; S. Martin,
   'Report on the Growth of the Typhoid Bacillus in Soil', Ibid., 308–18; E. Klein, 'The Fate of Path-
   ogenic and Other Infective Microbes in the Dead Animal', *Supplement to the Twenty-Eighth Annual
   Report of the LGB, Containing the Annual Report of the Medical Officer for 1899–99*, BPP, 1899, [C. 9445],
   xxxviii, 344–82; S. Martin, 'Report on the Growth of the Typhoid Bacillus in Soil', Ibid., 382–412;
   A. C. Houston, 'Inoculation of Soil with particular Microbes', Ibid., 413–39; S. Martin, 'Further
   Report on the Growth of the Typhoid Bacillus in Soil', *Supplement to the Twenty-Ninth Annual Report
   of the LGB, Containing the Annual Report of the Medical Officer for 1899–1900*, BPP, 1900, [Cd. 299],
   xxxiv, 525–49; J. P. Laws and F. W. Andrewes, *Report of an Investigation on the Micro-organisms of Sewage*,
   London County Council, 1894.

the transformation of other bacteria into typhoid forms. However, such negative evidence left open the possibility that any medium might be dangerous in exceptional circumstances, especially the still mysterious conditions
that sparked local typhoid epidemics.[139] The concentration on field rather
than clinical bacteriology in the early 1890s was also due to the findings that
the typhoid and related germs were rather unexciting chemically and pathologically. Though motile, the Eberth–Gaffky *bacillus* seemed to remain
localised in the gut and did not produce potent toxins, which meant that
there were no powerful antitoxins for laboratory scientists to play with, as in
diphtheria and tetanus. The apparent weakness of the *bacillus* also fed doubts
about its ability to produce severe systemic symptoms.

After 1896, the situation regarding the Eberth–Gaffky *bacillus* and the laboratory changed rapidly, first with the announcement in the summer of a
diagnostic test based on the agglutination of serum, and then with the first
trials of an antityphoid vaccine. The serum diagnostic test became known as
the Widal Reaction, after the French doctor who first published a specific
protocol in June and July 1896. However, the potential of the reaction was
first noticed in the Vienna laboratory of Max von Gruber in April 1894,
where crucial development work was undertaken by two young British students, Herbert E. Durham and Albert S. F. Grunbaum.[140] Both were protégés
of Sherrington, products of Cambridge, and of Guy's and St. Thomas's
Hospitals, respectively, and holders of Grocer's Company travelling scholar-
ships. Agglutination was the name given to the clumping of specific bacteria seen in suspensions of the microorganisms treated with serum from a
person infected with the same pathogen. It was quickly construed as being
due to the action of immune antibodies that disabled bacteria by making
them stick together. Crucially, it seemed that a natural, bodily immune mechanism had been successfully replicated in the laboratory. The diagnostic value
of the phenomenon came from taking serum from a suspected sufferer and
adding it to a suspension of typhoid bacilli. If clumping occurred, the person
had to have produced specific antibodies and hence must have the disease.
No clumping gave the reverse conclusion. The effect was first noticed with
cholera, then with typhoid fever and *B. coli*, and crucially for clinical purposes was observable with the naked eye. Gruber and Durham had been
looking for a simple test for identifying specific bacteria, but recognised the
diagnostic potential in their first publication on the phenomena in 1895.
Durham returned to England and then followed Sherrington to Liverpool
and eventually a career in tropical medicine, leaving the development of the
diagnostic application to Gruber and Grunbaum. Gruber reported their

139 Hardy, 'On the Cusp', 341–2.
140 H. E. Durham, 'On a Special Action of the Serum of Highly Immunised Animals and its Use in
   Diagnostic and Other Purposes', *PRSL*, 1897, 59: 224–6; A. S. Grunbaum, 'Goulstonian Lectures on
   Theories of Immunity and Their Clinical Application', *BMJ*, 1903, i: 653–5, 715–7, 783–6.

uccess in April 1896, though they waited until September to publish their esults, losing priority and the proprietary claim to Widal.[141]

The test depended on using an emulsion of the bacillus, and it was the pecificity of this test, rather than any microscopic or experimental demon- tration, that cemented the position of the Eberth–Gaffky *bacillus* as the pecific cause.[142] The rapid adoption of the Widal test was facilitated by the nfrastructure of bacterial services being created for diphtheria and tubercu- osis testing. The Widal test was simple though delicate, requiring exact stan- lards and dilutions. It was possible to perform it in test tubes and observe he results with the naked eye; however, the test was developed as an intri- ·ate procedure using microscopy. There were several reasons for this outcome.)octors were reluctant to take large quantities of blood due to worries about eptic infection and patient resistance to blood-taking. Thus, bacteriologists levised methods that only required four drops of blood taken from the ear obe, and the agglutination reactions were carried out on hollowed-out nicroscope slides. Microtesting also required smaller quantities of reagents nd was better suited to the postal collection of samples used by most labo- atories.[143] However, the test only worked seven days after infection, so it was nainly used in doubtful and long-lasting cases. In 1897, most of the new bac- eriological laboratories were offering Widal tests, and in the provinces the lemand was often greater than for diphtheria cultures.[144] Indeed, the testing or typhoid fever, diphtheria and tuberculosis was the mainstay of public tealth laboratory work in its first decade.[145] When diagnostic laboratories vere established in hospitals, they were quickly used for clinical research. With yphoid fever, investigators soon reported that *bacilli* often persisted in the ;all bladder long after the illness and were excreted in the urine. There were lso asymptomatic sufferers – a phenomenon that was constituted as the tealthy 'carrier' in the 1900s.[146]

Antityphoid inoculation was developed by Almroth Wright in the 'athology Department of the Army Medical College at Netley. As noted lready, Wright developed a strong laboratory research orientation in the lepartment and was inspired to pursue antityphoid vaccines by Haffkine. Iowever, rather than using live attenuated bacilli, Wright switched to killed acilli after Richard Pfeiffer, from Koch's Institute for Infectious Diseases in ≀erlin, told him that he had obtained a specific immune response in a man

41 For a while the test was known as the Gruber-Widal test, though Sherrington wrote that it ought to have been the Grunbaum test. See quote in 'Leyton, A. S. (Grunbaum): Obituary Notice', *JPB*, 1920, 29: 109–13, 112. During the First World War, Grunbaum changed his name to Leyton. The story with Grunbaum's name written out is given by T. Horton Smith, *Lancet*, 1900, i: 1051.
42 There are obvious parallels with Fleck's work on syphilis and the Wassermann Reaction. L. Fleck, *Genesis and Development of a Scientific Fact*, Chicago, IL, Chicago University Press, 1935, rep. 1979.
43 Editorial, 'Bacterial Diagnosis of Infectious Disease', *BMJ*, 1898, ii: 1357.
44 In 1897, Delépine's laboratory made 318 diphtheria investigations and 623 for typhoid fever.
45 *PH*, 1898–99, 11: 606.
46 J. W. Leavitt, *Typhoid Mary: Captive to the Public's Health*, Boston, MA, Beacon Press, 1996.

inoculated with a heated (killed) culture of bacilli. Working with David Semple, in July 1896 Wright began inoculating himself and 'volunteers' with different dilutions of heated cultures of Eberth–Gaffky *bacilli*, and used the new agglutination test to measure any enhanced immunity produced.[147] The first trial of antityphoid inoculations was with the staff of the Barming Heath Asylum at Maidstone in Kent in 1897.[148] In the same year the government of India, impressed by the success of anti-cholera vaccine, proposed to the Secretary of State for India that Wright be seconded to the government of India for four months to offer antityphoid inoculations to any officer or soldier in India or embarking for service. The proposal was turned down because medical opinion was split, but the letter from the War Office ended by stating that Lord Landsdowne's objection was more 'to the formal authorisation of inoculation at public expense than to voluntary operations at private cost'. In 1898 Wright was appointed to the India Plague Commission and spent from November 1898 to March 1899 travelling in the country. Whilst in India, he used the loophole in Landsdowne's letter and persuaded the medical officers in various stations that voluntary trials of his vaccine were permissible.[149] Record-keeping was poor or nonexistent, but a clear impression grew up in certain sections of the Indian Medical Service that the vaccine worked. This came more from clinical experience than statistical returns. Soldiers who were vaccinated did not necessarily escape the disease, though the consensus amongst elite doctors was that the vaccine improved mortality and morbidity rates.[150] In the spring of 1899, Robert Harvey, Director General of the IMS, recommended dropping the ban on the vaccine, but the government of India was more fulsome. In a letter to the Secretary of State for India in May 1899, Lord Landsdowne stated that 'we are very strongly of the opinion that a more extended trial should be made . . . and we trust your lordship will permit to approve the inoculation at public expense, of all British officers and soldiers who may voluntarily submit themselves'. Government policy was changed, leading to a further 5,999 men being inoculated in 1900 and 4,883 in 1901.

The policy recommended by the government of India was also adopted for the whole army after the outbreak of the South African War in October 1899. Antityphoid inoculations were available on a voluntary basis to officers and troops. Wright's department supplied the vaccines and advice on when and how to vaccinate. The extent to which the procedure was adopted depended on individual medical officers – there were inoculation rates of over fifty percent in some regiments – but the final average for all regiments

147 Grosöschel and Hornick, 'Who Introduced'.   148 *PH*, 1897–98, 10: 183.
149 A. E. Wright and W. B. Leishman, 'Results Which Have Been Obtained by the Antityphoid Inoculations', *BMJ*, 1900, i: 122–4.
150 The Army Medical Report for 1899 reports that during that year of the 4,502 men vaccinated, only 44 (0.98 percent) suffered from the disease, with nine deaths – case mortality of 20.4 percent. This compared with 25,851 nonvaccinated men amongst whom 657 (2.54 percent) suffered the disease, of whom 146 died – giving a similar case mortality of 22.2 percent.

n the war overall was under five percent.[151] In the early months of 1900 a
number of Parliamentary questions were tabled with the aim of pressurising
he army to make inoculations compulsory, but each was rebutted by the
claim that a trial was still in progress. The practice did not become an issue
until the summer of 1900, when William Burdett Coutts launched his attack
in Parliament on the performance of the army medical service in the war.
His revelations focused on appalling hospital conditions and how these had
been the source of epidemics. A Parliamentary debate followed and then a
Royal Commission was appointed, which eventually reported in February
901.[152] Antityphoid inoculation and the uses of laboratory medicine were
in the public eye again in July 1900 when the BMJ published a letter from
Conan Doyle which stated that the one big mistake in the campaign so far
had been that 'Inoculation against enteric fever was not made compulsory'.[153]
The following week, Wright published an article in the same journal on the
experience of typhoid fever in the beleaguered garrison in Ladysmith, which
he treated as a control population. Using data collected by Royal Army
Medical Corps (RAMC) personnel, he showed that of the 12,214 men in
he town, 1,705 (seventeen percent) had been inoculated.[154] The incidence of
he disease amongst the noninoculated was 1 in 7 and the mortality rate 1
in 32; the comparable figures for the inoculated were 1 in 49 and 1 in 213.
Wright introduced many caveats, but the implication was clear: the siege had
in part been endured due to the ability of laboratory medicine to make the
bodily soil' of troops resistant to disease.[155]

SCARLET FEVER: PERSONAL INFECTION AND ISOLATION

n the 1890s, apart from smallpox, the disease that most symbolised personal
infection was scarlet fever.[156] It was the single largest cause of admission to
isolation hospitals, and in London in 1890 the disease accounted for seventy-
eight percent (6,537 cases) of all fever hospital admissions.[157] By 1900, the
proportion of admissions had fallen to forty-eight percent, though the actual
number of admissions had risen to 10,343. The relative fall was due to the

51 A. E. Wright, 'On the Results Which Have Been Obtained by Anti-Typhoid Inoculation', *Lancet*, 1902, ii: 652–3.
52 *Hansard*, 1900, 85: Col. 89–184, 99.
53 A. Conan Doyle, 'The Epidemic of Enteric Fever at Bloemfontein', *BMJ*, 1900, ii: 49–50.
54 These data were based on self-reporting, and Wright noted that it might be an overestimate as it was likely that many men would have confused typhoid fever and smallpox vaccinations.
55 *BMJ*, 1900, ii: 51, 114, 1369. In November 1900, antityphoid inoculations were strongly endorsed by Howard Tooth, who was Assistant Physician at St. Bartholomew's but was currently serving as Physician to the Portland Hospital. He reported statistics in favour of antityphoid inoculation that were more favourable than those from Ladysmith. H. H. Tooth, 'Enteric Fever in the Army in South Africa, with Remarks on Inoculation', *BMJ*, 1900, ii: 1368–9.
56 J. M. Eyler, 'Scarlet Fever and Confinement: The Edwardian Debate over Isolation Hospitals', *BHM*, 1987, 61: 1–24. This debate had its origins in the 1890s, though it became a major issue after 1900.
57 All figures from Ayers, *England's First*, 119, 286.

increased hospitalisation of diphtheria cases and the provision of more beds. By this time three out of four notified cases of scarlet fever in the capital were being hospitalised, over ninety percent of whom were under fourteen years of age. However, it was a disease without a bacterium, no accurate diagnostic test, no antitoxin and no prospect of a vaccine. In fact, a complex streptococcal aetiology was first settled upon in the 1920s, by which time bacteriologists recognised different strains of *Streptococcus*, many of which could produce quite different conditions. The first volume of Allbutt's *System of Medicine*, published in 1897, classified it as one of several 'Diseases of Uncertain Bacteriology', reflecting the faith that it was simply a matter of time before the specific germ was revealed.[158] Klein's *Streptococcal scarlatinae* identified in the Hendon Disease episode in 1885–86 remained the best candidate, but all attempts to associate it consistently with sufferers, let alone to produce inoculation evidence, had failed.[159]

The higher proportion of all scarlet fever cases hospitalised was a product of the falling incidence of the disease, shorter periods of isolation and an increase in beds. Both the Notification of Diseases Act, 1889, and the Isolation Hospitals Act, 1893, were permissive and, as Pickstone and Wohl have shown, the degree to which they were adopted and how they were used depended on local political, social and medical circumstances.[160] The official basis of hospitalisation remained that it was an alternative to home isolation; however, by the 1890s new rationales were being articulated by the MOsH. Bacteriology was used to create a picture of insidious, yet robust organisms, such that those with the microorganism and the disease needed to be contained and treated by experts in special institutions. In many ways, this was the case that surgeons were making for aseptic surgery. The MOsH reported that there was less public resistance to isolation, which is congruent with other evidence of a shift in public attitudes towards hospitals. With infectious diseases, the success of diphtheria antitoxin, the benefits of intensive nursing and the use of antiseptic rituals were all testimony to the power of modern medicine. The MOsH placed great store in ensuring that isolation hospitals were state-of-the-art designs to ensure safety and reduce public anxiety. They campaigned particularly hard for improvements in nonepidemic years, using the fear factor of the inevitable return of killer contagions to induce local authorities to invest in more wards and tighter local rules. There were dissenters from these views, most notably general practitioners, who claimed that hospitalised patients fared no better, and sometimes worse, than those nursed at home. They doubted that the dangers of personal infection were as extreme as many MOsH argued, and worried about the cost of hospitalisation to rate payers and to themselves in lost business. They asked, if these diseases were

158 T. C. Allbutt, *A System of Medicine*, Vol. 2, London, Macmillan, 1897, 122–78.
159 Ibid., 163.
160 Pickstone, *Medicine*, 161–77; Wohl, *Endangered Lives*, 137–40.

o contagious, why risk cross-infections by aggregating patients together
n large hospitals? The MOsH pointed out that in the larger and more efficient hospitals, with separate blocks for different diseases, the chances of cross-
infection were reduced.[161] Indeed, in the late 1890s many MOsH attempted
o rationalise hospital provision across local authority boundaries to obtain
economies of scale and to avoid the logistic and political difficulties of empty
wards in nonepidemic periods. One tactic that the MOsH used to keep their
hospitals full was to isolate a greater number of infections, progressively
adding cases of measles, whooping cough, enteritis, meningitis and
poliomyelitis to their wards. After 1898, wards were also converted into tuberculosis sanatoria.

The high rates of hospitalisation for all infectious diseases was a significant
accomplishment by the MOsH and shows the extent to which notification,
isolation and disinfection dominated preventive policy. It was a particular
achievement with scarlet fever because the disease was amongst the most difficult to diagnose in its early stages and its severity was quite variable. The
main evidence that isolation made any difference was long-run correlations
between the introduction of isolation and the decline in the mortality rate,
plus anecdotal evidence of the absence of the disease in families whose children went to hospital.[162] In his Milroy Lectures in 1896, Edward Seaton spent
more time saying how hard it was to show the benefits of isolation, because
of the possible changes in the character of the disease and the different policies towards hospitalisation across the country, than setting out the positive
case.[163] The latter depended mostly on clinical rather than statistical data, particularly the fall in case-mortalities in hospital, from ten percent in the 1880s
to five percent in the 1890s.[164]

In March 1896 a new factor entered the story – increased worries about
the dangers of hospitalisation. In a court case in Birmingham, damages were
awarded against the City Council after the death from scarlet fever of the
brother of a child discharged as recovered by the city's Infectious Diseases
Hospital.[165] This was the most dramatic instance yet of a worrying new
feature of scarlet fever isolation, the number of so-called 'return cases', that
is, 'any patient coming to hospital with scarlet fever from the house to
which a patient discharged from hospital had recently returned'.[166] 'Return
cases' need not, of course, have caught the disease from a recovered sufferer,

61 *BMJ*, 1898, ii: 1505.
62 A. Newsholme, 'The Utility of Isolation Hospitals in Diminishing the Spread of Scarlet Fever',
   Journal of Hygiene, 1900, 1: 145–52.
63 E. Seaton, 'The Value of Isolation and Its Difficulties', *Lancet*, 1896, i: 698–70.
64 T. A. Green, 'Some Difficulties Met with in the Isolation of Infectious Diseases, *PH*, 1900–1, 13:
   422–9.
65 *PH*, 1995–96, 8: 244. The MOH was the defendant, and it is no surprise to find that the family's
   General Practitioner gave evidence on their behalf. The council was fined £50, though negligence was not found.
66 E. Millard, 'The Etiology of "Return Cases" of Scarlet Fever', *BMJ*, 1898, ii: 614–8.

especially in an epidemic year, but the likelihood was that they had. The problem was a relatively small one, representing less than five percent of the total admissions nationally. Nonetheless, it became a problem for the MOsH, as the discharge of patients became as controversial as admission. This matter was also an issue with diphtheria, especially as bacteriological examinations of throat swabs often showed the persistence of the Klebs–Loeffler *bacillus*, or the pseudobacillus, long after the symptoms had disappeared. If the function of isolation hospitals had been to cure the sick, this would not have been an issue; but as their role was preventive, the MOsH felt that they had a duty to retain potential disease-carriers. The problem with scarlet fever was that there was no bacteriological test and, in fact, no microorganism from which to infer the degree of infectivity of a patient. The assumption that doctors made was that 'the infective poison . . . is found to reside chiefly in the scales which peel off the skin in the period of convalescence'.[167] This meant that the disease was most contagious in its later stages. This also meant that isolation need not be rushed and could be left until the full development of the fever and rash, but discharge was likely to be delayed; indeed, in 1900 the average length of stay for scarlet fever in MAB hospitals was over three months.

The need to account for return cases exercised many MOsH, and they mostly used bacterial analogues.[168] The usual explanation was that some form of the poison or bacterium had collected in the nose and throat of sufferers and, once they developed a cold, material was released into the atmosphere.[169] Another possibility was that scarlet fever might be like syphilis, with a long incubation period, or was a virus that could persist in a dormant state for many months or even years.[170] In the absence of a specific microscopical entity, doctors' attention fell mainly on desquamation (shedding skin) and the notion that the poison-virus accumulated in scales and other discharges at the end of the disease. Amongst the best evidence for such convictions and of the assumed power of personal infection were the 'Bathing-Out Rules' introduced in Birmingham in the wake of the 1896 verdict.[171] Children were subjected to an antiseptic ritual in a special pavilion, being bathed in strong Izal solutions, washed with carbolic soap, their hair was rubbed with carbolic oil (adults' hair was dipped in formalin), and finally they were dried with a clean bath sheet. The ears and nose were then syringed with 1 in 2,000 formalin and the patient was allowed to dress in clothes brought in for them, before a final examination in the 'finishing room' by the medical officer.

Throughout the 1890s the sense in public health medicine was that an announcement of the specific bacterial organism responsible for scarlet fever was imminent. However, the problems over return cases and the wider

167 G. Thin, 'Contagium of Scarlet Fever', *BMJ*, 1887, ii: 402–8. *Lancet*, 1896, ii: 1066.
168 *Lancet*, 1895, ii: 1295.   169 *PH*, 1899–1900, 12: 726.   170 *Lancet*, 1896, ii: 304.
171 Millard, 'Etiology', 616.

criticisms of isolation finally led the Medical Department to commission specific investigations. Edward Klein started publishing once again on the problem in 1896 and 1897, with Dr. Mervyn Gordon following up in 1898, 1899 and 1900.[172] This research still failed to produce a specific organism, with Gordon finding the *Streptococcus conglomeratus* as often as Klein's *S. scarlatinae.* The question of milk-borne epidemics was debated again, this time initiated by the wider concerns about milk raised by the antituberculosis campaign.

Bacterial germ theories of disease became the *lingua franca* of public health medicine between 1880 and 1900. In the 1880s, support for bacterial models of disease was associated with those MOsH who wanted to prioritise more targeted, person-centred, 'exclusive' methods of disease prevention. However, by the 1890s both sides of the inclusive–exclusive divide used bacterial theories, especially as ideas of changing virulence and bacterial evolution were used to support all programmes. Such was the power of bacterial theory that public health doctors found no problem with working with yet-to-be-discovered bacteria, such as those of smallpox and scarlet fever, or to embark on research programmes with discoveries in mind. Indeed, investigators used epidemiological and clinical properties to predict the nature of specific microorganisms and directed their research accordingly. Between 1880 and 1900 many germs and bacteria became less powerful, as the contingencies of contagion came to the fore once again. The establishment of a bacterial disease in an individual was seen to depend on many things, though amongst the most important were its portal of entry, the number of organisms entering, their virulence and the condition of the human body's immune system. With no disease was the bacterium the whole story. Public health doctors of all persuasions used the seed and soil metaphor to adapt their germ theories of epidemic and endemic diseases to mesh with the clinical and epidemiological experiences of the variability of individual cases, seemingly spontaneous outbreaks and long-term trends in morbidity and mortality.

In the last quarter of the nineteenth century, public health was dominated by the linked policies of notification, isolation and disinfection. However, these policies were radically changed by developing bacterial aetiologies and pathologies, as these came to concentrate on pathogens in, on and immediately around individuals, rather than on the wider environment. The triad were given new rationales and there were important changes in detail, for example, in methods of disinfection and the length of isolation. Notification was more widely accepted by the medical profession and there were major, albeit uneven, investments in isolation hospitals, which became symbols of

172 *Supplement to the Twenty-Sixth Annual Report,* 263–6; *Supplement to the Twenty-Seventh Annual Report,* 326–34; *Supplement to the Twenty-Eighth Annual Report,* 480–97; *Twenty-Ninth Annual Report,* 385–457.

the power of personal infection. Public health medicine was not touched directly by bacteriological laboratory work until the mid-1890s, but from then on there were revolutionary changes with certain diseases – diphtheria, typhoid fever and tuberculosis, respectively, due to antitoxins, vaccines and laboratory diagnoses.[173] Any 'Bacteriological Era' in public health began in 1894, not earlier. Many established practices, such as Jennerian vaccination and disinfection, having been remade as germ practices, were made yet again as exemplary bacteriological practices. There were sanitarian-minded MOsH who worried about the reductionism and curative tendencies in the new public health, though in most cases the new methods were added to the old, rather than replacing them, though the introduction of antisera and vaccines suggested that exclusive measures were becoming very personal, looking to change the properties of the human soil.

173 G. S. Woodhead, 'Harben Lectures on the Bearing of Recent Bacteriological Investigations on Public Health', *JSM*, 1897, 5, 289, 357, 405, 453.

Conclusion

n the closing years of the nineteenth century, doctors produced many reflec-
ions on recent changes in their profession, its work and ideas. In Britain
here was a burst of reflections, prompted by the Jenner Centenary in 1896,
Queen Victoria's Diamond Jubilee in 1897 and the celebrations of the cen-
ennial in 1899 and 1900.[1] The elite surgeons and physicians who spoke at
meetings and wrote in journals agreed that the previous 60 to 100 years had
been momentous changes, but there was no consensus over what the most
mportant transitions had been. The developments mentioned most were
naesthesia, antisepsis and the overall fall in mortality, which they attributed
argely to sanitary reform and preventive medicine. Authors represented these
evelopments first and foremost as humanitarian, in reducing suffering and
aving lives. When it came to medical knowledge, everyone agreed that
medicine had become more 'scientific', in the sense of having become more
recise, exact and empirical. These largely positivist reflections presented the
evelopment of medicine as continuous and cumulative. The theories of cells,
erms and immunity were hardly mentioned; authors seem to have assumed
hat they had become 'fact'. Instead, they concentrated on the new pathol-
gy and bacteriology, maturing disciplines with exact methods and expand-
ng bodies of knowledge. They also stressed the utility of the new disciplines,
n important though often ignored feature of the positivist view of science.
he key change here was how new understandings of aetiologies and the
mechanisms of diseases had enabled doctors to make more precise and effec-
ve preventive, diagnostic and curative interventions.[2] In 1900, bacteriology
lso embraced what later became known as immunology, though at this time

'Jenner Centenary Number', *BMJ*, 1896, i: 1245–1307; 'Special Jubilee Edition', *Practitioner*, 1897,
58: 560–690; 'Queen's Commemoration Number', *BMJ*, 1897, i: 1521–672; F. T. Roberts, 'The
Progress of Medicine in the Nineteenth Century', *Lancet*, 1899, ii: 996–1000; H. G. Howse, 'A
Review of Surgery during the Past 100 Years', *Lancet*, 1899, ii: 1717–24; B. Bramwell, 'Thirty-Five
Years of Medical Progress', *BMJ*, 1899, ii: 898–902.
S. Delépine, 'On the Development of Modern Ideas on Preventive, Protective and Curative
Treatment of Bacterial Diseases, and on the Immunity or Refractoriness to Disease', *Lancet*, 1891,
i: 241–4.

medical interest was on practices and products, such as vaccine development, antitoxin therapy and serum diagnosis. Bacteriology, in all its guises, was still portrayed as a new subject that had yet to fulfil its potential; hence there was a strong sense amongst commentators that medicine was at the start, not the end, of a period of rapid change.

The conclusions that I draw from this volume, about the place of germ science and technology in late Victorian medicine, are in many ways closer to those of doctor-historians at the turn of the twentieth century than to views that have characterised histories of the germ-theory of disease since. My study has not shown an all-conquering germ-theory of disease nor have I identified a 'bacteriological revolution', a 'scientific revolution', a 'laboratory revolution' or a clear switch from physiological to ontological conceptions of diseases. Rather, I have argued that the development and uses of germ theories varied across medicine, with groups constituting germs differently, depending on their interests, resources and work. The spread of germ theories, practices and ideologies showed uneven and combined development, which militates against any talk of revolutions, if we take that term to refer to rapid and radical change. There were pivotal moments: the impetus that the cattle plague gave to contagionism after 1865; Lister making antiseptic surgery an icon of living-germ theory in the late 1860s; Tyndall's pro-germ pronouncements over dust and Klein's typhoid fever germs in the early 1870s; the demise of spontaneous generation in the late 1870s, together with the eclipse of chemical theories and nonbacterial germ theories; the spread of standard bacteriological techniques in the early 1880s; the potential to produce artificial vaccines after 1880; and, last but not least, the arrival of antitoxins and antisera in the mid-1890s. However, over the period 1865 to 1900, the changes in disease theories and medical practices associated with germs and bacteriology were evolutionary, though nonetheless profound for that.

DISEASE THEORIES

Hindsight has led many historians to identify 'germs' exclusively with bacteria and to ignore the many other things that disease-germs were said to be, or might have been. The starting point for this volume was to recapture this indeterminacy and to establish the sense that disease-germs could have been constituted as something other than 'bacteria' or nothing at all. This meant giving appropriate weight to the views of those scientists and medical practitioners who promoted chemical theories and nonbacterial germ theories, as well as to those who denied the very existence of disease-germs. There were two broad phases in the development and spread of germ theories of disease: from 1865 to 1882, the era of 'germs', and from 1882 to 1900 and beyond, the era of 'bacteria'.

After 1865, doctors and scientists 'theorised' about four main questions: Did disease-germs exist? What were they? Where did they come from? How did they act? It was in this context that it is unavoidable not to talk about germ-*theories* of disease, as there were many ideas, principles and findings on each of these questions. Contemporary references to *the* germ-theory, not theories, were made in specific contexts. In surgery, the term was borrowed from Pasteur's 'germ theory of putrefaction', and was only used for a single process – sepsis. Listerian surgeons still assumed that systemic disease was produced by poisonous chemical breakdown products from sepsis. In public health medicine, a minority of doctors and scientists began designating *contagium viva* and zymotic poisons as living, disease-causing germs. In doing so they conflated two meanings of the word germ: that *contagium viva* (or their germs in the sense of seeds or spores) were exciting causes of disease, and that zymotic poisons were living organisms rather than chemicals. Tyndall was the first person to pull all of these strands together publicly into a general theory in 1870, though his single principle brought down on him the wrath of the medical profession for speculative oversimplification and generalisation. At stake here, as well as particular germ theories, was the meaning and political uses of 'theory' in medicine. Germ theorists liked to think that they subscribed to a single principle – a high-level generalisation. To admit that between them they held many principles would have damaged their authority and the credibility of their ideas. On the other side, opponents of 'germ-theory' highlighted the theory as speculation and rationalism, and hoped that references to the number of theories would damage the germ theorists' project. During the 1870s, across medicine and the biological sciences, disease-germs were imagined to be many things and to act in various ways, a situation reflected in Drysdale's review in 1877.[3] However, by this time, germ theorists were already thinking, writing and speaking less about 'germs'. Increasingly they were talking about specific, observable microorganisms, especially bacteria, linking their form and function more explicitly to disease states and using new techniques to observe and experiment with these organisms.

The acceptance and spread of standard bacteriological techniques and exemplary aetiological demonstrations, especially around anthrax and tuberculosis, promised to settle important questions about germ theories of disease. The first and most important issue, which went away rather than being settled, was spontaneous generation. Support for spontaneous generation amongst medical practitioners was strong in Britain, so its demise was critical to altering terms of discussion over the issue of germs and disease, and the *de novo* origin of disease in individuals and populations. At the same time the 'reality' of disease-germs became harder to deny, with the best candidates – bacteria – being constituted by botanists, microscopists and medical investigators as living microorganisms with ancestries, life cycles and

J. J. Drysdale, *The Germ Theories of Infectious Diseases*, London, Baillière, Tindall and Cox, 1878.

specific properties. However, the principle 'that the origin of many diseases lay in the pathogenic actions of certain micro-organisms when introduced into the body' left open questions about the actions of germs and body's reactions.[4] In the early 1880s, only enthusiastic germ theorists felt that the establishment of two or three well-articulated bacterial aetiologies – anthrax, relapsing fever and tuberculosis – was sufficient grounds to build a single bacterial model for all infectious and contagious diseases. Indeed, the very idea of specific bacteria being linked to specific diseases implied that there might be a whole range of aetiological and pathological models. Germ theorists, who increasingly styled themselves as bacteriologists from the mid-1880s, continued to develop new principles and theories, not least as to try to embrace the growing range of possible causal agents, and the variety of actions and reactions that field and laboratory investigations in the new science of bacteriology threw up.

In the eyes of many doctors and scientists, bacteriology seemed to limit what could count as disease-germs. Only bacteria that were susceptible to display by particular techniques (microscopy and plate cultures) with pathogenic actions demonstrable by new standards of proof (Koch's postulates) seemed to be acceptable. However, neither criterion was rigorously applied. The limitations of the new techniques were evident as early as 1883 in the dispute over the cholera vibrio, when Koch's microscopy was seen by many to be unconvincing and when he was unable to satisfy his own postulates. More importantly, despite the failure of bacteriologists to produce the specific bacteria of a large number of infections, this did not stop many diseases from being seen and classified as 'germ' or 'bacterial' conditions. With hindsight, the last quarter of the nineteenth century seems full of discoveries, but over the period as a whole, as many infectious diseases were without specific bacterial causes as had them. The cultural power of the bacterial model within medicine was such that alternative, nonbacterial theories of infections ceased to be articulated. All of these points show the value of thinking about the establishment of bacterial aetiologies as a process rather than a discovery event. These processes involved the construction, adoption, spread and use of ideas and practices, but not in a linear sequence. Ideas and practices were reconstructed at every stage. Adoption was rarely once and for all, as ideas and practices were taken up, dropped and readopted, frequently in modified form, while the spread and use of ideas and practices was uneven and variable across the profession and within its subcultures.

By 1900 it was commonplace for medical scientists to create histories where early versions of the living germ theories of disease had simply equated

---

4 This definition from the *Oxford English Dictionary* is based on the given in H. Power and L. W. Sedgwick, *New Sydenham Society's Lexicon of Medicine and the Sciences*, London, New Sydenham Society, 1881. J. K. Crellin, 'The Dawn of Germ Theory: Particles, Infection and Biology', in F. N. L. Poynter, ed., *Medicine and Science in the 1860s*, London, WIHM, 1966, 57–76.

he germ with the disease. In contrast, the latest bacteriological understand-
ng of disease had moved on from such crude ontological thinking to more
dvanced and complex ideas:

t is now fully acknowledged that it is not enough to have a poison germ on the one
and to acquire the disease on the other. There are intermediate or antecedent circum-
tances of dosage, acquired susceptibility, or that subtle malformation of tissue in certain
rgans which is inherited or renders them weak to certain forms of attack.[5]

The notion that once-upon-a-time the attacking germ was accepted as the
ole explanation of any disease is mistaken. Germ theories of disease, explic-
tly or implicitly, always included ideas about the interactions between germs
nd bodies. Every chapter in this book has shown that the seed and soil
nalogy, or some variant, was routinely used to explain both disease and its
bsence from the first uses of modern germ theories of all types.

The military metaphor of invading enemy germs and bodily defences, used
n the above quotation, only came to the fore in the 1880s; its use was coin-
ident with the elaboration of immunological models of defensive ranks of
ctive phagocytes and the body's arsenal of potent antitoxins and antisera.
Previously, the body's immunity to living germs had been seen to be holis-
ic and passive, for example, to lie in the absence of suitable nutrients for the
erms, to depend on the resilience of tissues, or to be determined by the
oint of entry or where germs settled. In surgery, the notion of 'vital resis-
ance' and the different properties of infective and putrefactive germs was
lways a factor, though in early Listerian practice, if not theory, it tended to
bscure pathological complexities. Also, it was to the advantage of anti-
ermists, like Benjamin Ward Richardson, to caricature Listerism as exclu-
ively germ-oriented. Similarly in public health, the contingencies of germ
ontagion were always evident; the assumption of multifactorial aetiologies
tructured thinking and practice. However, critics again tried to paint germ
heorists as proposing simplistic aetiological models and dangerously 'exclu-
ve' preventive policies. The intellectual and political power of the sanitarian
nindset led germ theorists to construct aetiologies and pathologies that were
ongruent with the contingencies of epidemiological understandings.

In Britain, germ and bacteriological principles and practices were con-
tructed, developed, interpreted and spread by 'theorists' who mostly had
nedical training, who were active in clinical work, or who worked in disease
revention where interests had focused on the external, exciting agents of
isease. I have identified a group of germ theorists in Britain from the early
870s, though whether they constituted an 'army', as suggested in the *Lancet*
n 1877, is a moot point. They faced opponents until the late 1870s, led by
Charlton Bastian and Benjamin Ward Richardson, who lacked the support of
ne scientific elite, but who enjoyed the support, albeit passive rather than

active, of medical practitioners at all levels. The main national figures were Joseph Lister, John Tyndall, Lionel Beale, Edward Klein, William Watson Cheyne and John Burdon Sanderson, though there were also advocates and investigators in local provincial and specialist groups. Before 1880, not all germ theorists believed that disease-germs were independent, specific, living microorganisms. I have included Lionel Beale in my list of leading germ theorists, and at lower levels I would include the followers of Pettenkofer, such as Lewis and Cunningham, the contagionists in veterinary medicine, and those doctors who used the term metaphorically for the sources of fungal and parasitic diseases. The transformation of germ theorists into bacteriologists occurred around 1880, with Cheyne playing a key but short-term role in the spread of Kochian methods and models after 1882. Thereafter, the new discipline was developed by diverse groups, though its technical character and demands put pathologists in the driving seat.

There were three competing schools of British bacteriology in the 1880s, centred around Cheyne at King's College, London; Klein at the Brown, College of State Medicine and St. Bartholomew's; and Woodhead in Edinburgh. Klein's group was the most important, because its influence spread across public health, surgery and medicine, but an essential feature of British medical bacteriology was that it was fragmented, small-scale and subordinate to other medical disciplines. Given the importance of the seed and soil metaphor, it might be argued that British bacteriology was a synthesis of the Koch and Pasteur schools. This case has been made from British immunology, where Almroth Wright's opsonin theory postulated the existence of chemical substances that made infective agents more attractive to phagocytes, as Wright seemed to combine German humoral and French cellular models.[6] However, I have argued that British bacteriology is best understood as an indigenous product. Protobacteriologists and then bacteriologists had weak institutional positions, which meant that the aims and assumptions of their work were heavily influenced by clinical and preventive interests. Their work was disease-centred, but this was structured around different combinations of physiological and ontological conceptions. Hence, the widespread use of the seed and soil metaphor and variants, such as sparks and combustible matter, the occult dry rot fungus, and parasites and hosts. The first generation of British bacteriologists were almost all part-timers whose main careers were in other areas. Indeed, clinical and teaching careers claimed many figures, such as Cheyne, Ogston, Horsley, Greenfield, Roberts and Sanderson, who might have built a well-resourced and dynamic specialism in the mid- to late 1880s. This situation is one factor in explaining why British scientists and doctors were so poor at staking discovery claims and making them stick. This was not simply because their claims were 'wrong' or were later overridden,

6 D. J. Bibel, *Milestones in Immunology: A Historical Explanation*, Madison, WI, 1988, Science Tech, 174–5.

hough Klein's problems with sheep-pox, typhoid fever, scarlet fever, cholera nd other germs did not help. If we regard recognition for discoveries as chievements rather than rewards, then it seems that other researchers, espe-ially those around Koch in Germany, were better at managing the profes-ional politics of science. Thus, the works of Sanderson, Ogston, Wright, Klein, Greenfield, Durham, Martin and others were never converted into chievements. An additional factor was that the practical context of British germ science and bacteriology meant that finding the 'seed' on its own was ever seen to be that important. In this context, it is worth noting that many ontemporary histories of British medicine in the nineteenth century tended o celebrate practical innovations rather than scientific discoveries. The great hifts in understanding – localised pathology, cellular pathology and bacterial etiology – were conceded to France and Germany, but every first-rank dvance in the 'art of medicine' was claimed for Britain.[7] The 'captain of ewels in the carcanet' were vaccination (Edward Jenner), chloroform anaes-hesia (James Simpson), antiseptic surgery (Joseph Lister) and sanitary science John Snow, Edmund Parkes, John Simon). The picture was of Britain as the workshop of the medical world', whose citizens on average enjoyed longer ives and better levels of health, just as they enjoyed the higher standards of ving brought by industrialisation.

Temkin suggested that the most significant consequence of germ theories f disease in medicine was the manner in which they changed the meaning f health and disease:

Diseases could be bound to definitive causes; hence the knowledge of the cause was eeded to elevate a clinical entity or a syndrome to the rank of a disease. Moreover, an nfection had a beginning and it ended after the annihilation of the invading microbe. Between these two points in time the person in question was sick; before and after he vas healthy; consequently health was absence of disease.[8]

The suggestion that nonbacterial diseases came to be defined by the same etiological standards as bacterial diseases has much to recommend it. For xample, cancer became quite germlike, as rogue cells progressively colonised he host body; previously, it was understood as an altered state of bodily struc-ure and function on the way to death. But how widely and rapidly did onto-ogical conceptions spread? I have shown that there were few instances of a raightforward switch from holistic, physiological notions to reductionist ntological constructions, even with highly contagious diseases. With many iseases, different conceptions were used by different groups within medicine

W. Osler, 'Medicine in Greater Britain', BMJ, 1897, ii: 578. An implicit parallel was with Britain as the workshop of the industrial world.
O. Temkin, The Double Face of Janus, Baltimore, MD, Johns Hopkins University Press, 1977, 436.
Cf. A. Cunningham, 'Transforming the Plague: The Laboratory and the Identity of Infectious Disease', in A. Cunningham and P. Williams, eds., The Laboratory Revolution in Medicine, Cambridge, Cambridge University Press, 1992, 209–44.

and outside the profession, as with tuberculosis between clinicians, MOsH, veterinarians, farmers and the public. Also, doctors seem to have found no difficulty working with quite contradictory ideas and ideals, separating theory and practice, tailoring approaches to different problems and individuals, or simply following the maxim that in medicine it is better not to be wrong than to be right. With bacterial diseases, doctors used the seed and soil analogy to combine physiological and ontological conceptions, as in cholera, where the state of the body not only affected receptivity but was also believed to alter the form and activity of the bacillus.

The best example of this synthesis was in the campaign against consumption at the end of the century, orchestrated by the National Association for the Prevention of Consumption (NAPC); note that it was not aimed against Tuberculosis or TB. The NAPC had many linked activities and ideas. At one level it aimed to educate the public in holistic ways to reduce their chances of acquiring an 'openness' to infection, or to compensate for any inherited weaknesses. At the same time, NAPC propaganda sought to teach the public to avoid the *Tubercle bacillus* by specific measures, such as collecting, sterilising or burning sputum; washing food utensils; and avoiding sleeping near sufferers in unventilated rooms. The Association also promoted the sanatorium treatment to produce cures. This was described as a 'specific' remedy, offering rest and overfeeding to strengthen the constitution, in a model hygienic, even aseptic, environment. Attempts at merely attacking the *Tubercle bacillus* with antiseptic sprays, irrigating lungs and surgery were scoffed at. All doctors knew that the bacillus was a necessary but not on its own a sufficient cause of the development of the disease in any individual. By 1900, it was accepted that most people infected with the *Tubercle bacillus* never developed the disease. Indeed, some doctors were saying that the presence of the bacillus in the body improved health, as it stimulated immunity in what seemed like an example of natural vaccination.

The place that specific bacteria were accorded in the causation of infectious and other diseases was a powerful exemplar for ontological conceptions of disease. However, it would be wrong to link the rise of ontological conceptions solely with living-germ theories of disease. Other developments also contributed, for example, localised pathology, the expansion of surgery, the development of preventive medicine in public health and the acceptance of the specificity of more and more diseases. The great attraction of ontological ideas for all doctors was that they offered more and better defined opportunities to intervene in the mechanisms of disease: to destroy or remove causal entities (e.g. surgical removal, antisepsis, anti-inflammatory methods), or to prevent causal entities from reaching the body (isolation and disinfection), and to boost the ability of the body to resist or counter the effects of causal entities (e.g. regimens and tonics, to vaccines and antitoxins), or all of these.

The importance of the metaphor of seed and soil raises the question of the ction of germs-bacteria in different groups of people. Doctors discussed this nostly in terms of the strengths and weaknesses of individuals with a common, •asic physiology – what was called the 'personal factor' in disease in the 1900s.[9] There was surprisingly little consideration of the action of germs on the soils of lifferent social classes, races or sexes. In preventive medicine, the working class vas seen to be the most vulnerable to epidemics, both from their higher rates •f infection due to their living in overcrowded and filthy conditions, and their cquired weaknesses from those same conditions. The relative decline in the nfluence of epidemiology signalled declining interest in social factors, as lisease was constituted in relations between bacteria and individual bodies, vhere personal behaviour, not social structures and social relations, determined he balance of disease and health. At the end of the 1870s, as germs became bac- eria, they were transformed from environmental contaminants of a germless •ody to much more intimate dangers. In surgery, they were present on the skin nd on instruments; in public health they spread on the breath and where •odies were close together; and in medicine they lurked in the mouth, gut, ings and eventually in healthy tissue.

There was a general rule in geographical pathology, where people suffered ∍ss from local, native diseases and most from newly imported ones.[10] Thus, ∛engalis were believed to be less susceptible to cholera than Europeans, nd Europeans less vulnerable to smallpox than 'virgin soil' populations in ∍mote regions. Between 1865 and 1900, the explanation of such phenome- on switched from acquired characteristics, such as habituation to poisons, to iherited evolutionary adaptations of pathogen–host relationships. There is iore work to be done on these topics in Britain and its Empire, especially ✓ith changing ideas on acclimatisation. Their neglect at present is probably ue to the absence of large-scale migrations into Britain in the period, and ie way in which the history of health in colonial populations has followed ie ontological path and emphasised parasites and vectors.[11] However, it is irprising that historians of eugenics have not had more to say on the rela- ons between disease-germs and germ plasm.[12]

Germ theories of disease and health were not particularly gendered. On ie whole, germs were considered to be asexual, first when thought to derive

⁾ S. MacKenzie, 'The Powers of Natural Resistance, or the Personal Factor in Disease of Microbe Origin', *TMSL*, 1902, 25: 302–18.

⁾ A. Hirsch, *Handbook of Geography and Historical Pathology* (Trans. by C. Creighton), London, New Sydenham Society, 1883.

ₓ On the influence of migration of American medical ideas, see: A. M. Kraut, *Silent Travelers: Germs, Genes, and the 'Immigrant Menace'*, New York, Basic Books, 1994. On tropical medicine and parasitology, see: M. Worboys, 'Germs, Malaria and the Invention of Mansonian Tropical Medicine: From "Diseases in the Tropics" to "Tropical Disease"', in D. Arnold, ed., *Warm Climates and Western Medicine: The Emergence of Tropical Medicine, 1500–1900*, Amsterdam, Rodopi, 1996, 181–208.

₂ B. Harris and W. Ernst, eds., *Race, Science and Medicine*, London, Routledge, 1999.

from ordinary cells and later when they were thought to be seeds, spores or fission-fungi whose reproduction was by simple division. Botanists had ascribed bacteria to the *Schistomycetes*, a group defined by their asexual, largely splitting mode of reproduction. There are a few examples where germs were construed as eggs, and a single reference to germs having 'spermatic virtue', because of their abilities to enter bodies and initiate cellular changes. If anything, germ and bacterial theories tended to unsex diseases, which shows once again the slow movement from physiological to ontological conceptions. For example, Childbed fever, a condition specific to parturating women, became just another type of septic infection due to streptococcal infection. Bacteriologists eventually reshaped syphilis and gonorrhoea to be thoroughly contagious and to have similar pathologies in both sexes. Previously, they had been seen to exhibit differences between men and women, with both conditions more likely to arise spontaneously in the interiority of the female reproductive organs. At the level of health care, responses to bacterial models of disease, especially their reductionist tendencies, have been seen as potentially gendered, with women doctors more inclined to develop holistic, hygienist views than their male counterparts.[13] In British surgery there was a tacit division of labour between male surgeons' local management of the wound and female nurses' role in maintaining a hygienic environment and sustaining the holistic care that strengthened the human soil.[14] In public health, the role of women sanitary inspectors was successively inclusive and exclusive; initially they were agents of sanitary cleansing, though later they pursued the reform of more personal behaviour in domestic and occupational settings.[15] In this role they became missionaries in the antigerm crusade, extolling the powers of carbolic soap, Izal disinfectant and Condy's fluid, plus the virtues for families of notification and isolation of sick children, and improved motherhood.[16]

MEDICAL PRACTICE

Germ science and technology was promoted by its enthusiasts as potentially revolutionary. Germ theorists offered completely safe surgery, the abolition of zymotic diseases and the extinction of tuberculosis, while later bacteriologists held out the prospect of preventive vaccines for every infectious disease,

13 Regina Morantz, 'Mary Putnam Jacobi and Elisabeth Blackwell and Germ Theory', *American Studies*, 1986.
14 C. E. Rosenberg, 'Florence Nightingale on Contagion: The Hospital as a Moral Universe', in C. E. Rosenberg, ed., *Healing and History: Essays for George Rosen*, New York, Science History Publications, 1979, 116–36.
15 C. Davies, 'The Health Visitor as Mother's Friend: A Woman's Place in Public Health, 1900–1914', *SHM*, 1988, 1: 39–60.
16 N. Tomes, *The Gospel of Germs: Men, Women, and the Microbe in American Life*, Cambridge, MA, Harvard University Press, 1998.

cures' from antibacterial and antitoxic therapy and specific constitutional
regimes. In 1900, doctors and scientists who wanted to accentuate the positive could find examples of success, or a promising start on all fronts.
However, sceptics could point to the failure of Tuberculin, the absence of
proven vaccines for any major infectious disease, the new evidence on the
limitations of antisepsis, the limited extension of antitoxin therapy beyond
diphtheria, and that the great antituberculosis crusade relied on established
hygienic measures.[17] Historians have also tended to argue that the immediate practical benefits from adopting germ theories and developing bacteriology were limited, suggesting that effects on long-run mortality trends did not
come until the twentieth century, with antibiotics and mass vaccinations.[18]
This was essentially Thomas McKeown's argument in denying any major role
for curative or preventive medicine in population growth in Britain.[19] His
assessment of preventive medicine has been challenged by Szreter and Hardy,
who argue that changes in policies and practices in the second half of
the nineteenth century impacted significantly on mortality.[20] I have made
no claims about the 'outcomes' of any of the new preventive and curative
measures that were given a germ or bacteriological pedigree between 1865
and 1900. However, I have shown that germ science and bacteriology was
used to guide, legitimate and give meaning to practices old and new at every
level, from specific local antigerm measures, as in antiseptic surgery, to general
health programmes that aimed to strengthen populations, as in the antituberculosis campaign at the end of the 1890s. It is impossible to assess the
influence of specific measures on therapeutic outcomes, due to the number
of variables involved, as shown only too well in the debates over antiseptic
surgery, but the evidence presented in this volume shows that germ theories
and bacteriology gave doctors powerful resources to explore new ways to
prevent, diagnose and treat diseases.

Before 1900, germ theorists and bacteriologists were understood to have
offered the most to disease prevention. This was principally because they
had shifted the medical gaze from the internal order and functioning of the
body, where opportunities for intervention were limited, to its external
relations and to 'things' entering the body, where it was supposedly easier for
doctors to act. Moreover, the external environment was constituted in
new ways. Instead of quite general conditions influencing the whole body,
remotely and indirectly by the *configuration* of material and social conditions,

17 Cf. J. H. Warner, *The Therapeutic Perspective: Medical Practice, Knowledge and Identity in America, 1820–1885*, Princeton, NJ, Princeton University Press, 1986, 258–83.
18 A. Digby, *Making a Medical Living: Doctors and Patients in the English Market for Medicine, 1720–1911*, Cambridge, Cambridge University Press, 1994, 97, 311.
19 T. McKeown, *The Rise of Modern Population*, London, Edward Arnold, 1976.
20 S. Szreter, 'The Importance of Social Intervention in Britain's Mortality Decline, c. 1850–1914: A Reinterpretation of the Role of Public Health', *SHM*, 1988, 1: 1–38; A. Hardy, *The Epidemic Streets: Infectious Disease and the Rise of Preventive Medicine, 1856–1900*, Oxford, Clarendon Press, 1993.

germ theorists proposed that medical interest should focus on specific *contaminants*, their movements and their specific effects. There were continuities, with the *predisposition* of individuals and communities a factor in both configurational and contaminationist accounts of the causes of disease. Yet, over the period 1865 to 1900, a new balance of forces was drawn up where *contamination* became more important than *configuration*, and more diseases were constituted as due to, or likely to be due to, specific *contaminants*.[21] It is interesting that in both surgery and public health from the late 1860s, germ theorists were almost always linked with proposals to introduce narrow, exclusive policies. This was not a necessary connection. The best way to prevent the transmission of germs, as Simon argued with cholera, might well have been general sanitary improvements, sorting out problems at the source and dealing with many diseases with a single measure. The linkage of living-germ theories and bacteriology with exclusivity was in part dictated by opponents, who sought to link the new ideas to risky policies. On issues of public safety, especially with lay audiences, the programme of inclusive measures was easier to defend, though it remained hard to implement for economic and political reasons. Germ theorists and bacteriologists denied that they wanted to be wholly exclusive. Their policy principles were to try to be more cost-effective, by targeting specific points of passage of disease-agents, and to be more efficient, by avoiding unnecessary measures and concentrating on relatively circumscribed technical problems, avoiding local politics.

The new germ and bacterial therapies developed after 1870 aimed both at the exciting and predisposing causes of disease – attacking seeds and improving the soil. While many of these therapies may not have cured patients, judged by the standards established by antibiotics in this century, there is no doubt that after 1865 the 'experience' of many doctors was that they 'worked'. Everything here depends on what is understood by the term 'worked'. The most important criterion in the late-Victorian period was 'clinical experience'. This might appear to be a vague notion by modern standards, but late-Victorian doctors were confident that their work was rooted in the best practices that had been learned formally and informally, and had been reinforced or adapted in use. There were competing ideas of best practice held by groups, as well as for individual variation within any consensus. Anyone doubting the power of this approach need only remember that the double-blind clinical trial was invented in the mid-twentieth century, and so-called evidence-based medicine came into vogue in the closing decades of the twentieth century. A second sense in which germ therapies 'worked' was in enabling germ theorists and bacteriologists to contrast their improved powers

21 I am using here Rosenberg's triad of concepts for understanding changing constructions of epidemics: *configuration, predisposition* and *contamination*. This framework can be very usefully applied to all diseases, not just epidemics. C. E. Rosenberg, 'Explaining Epidemics', in C. E. Rosenberg, *Explaining Epidemics and Other Essays*, Cambridge, Cambridge University Press, 1992, 287.

f intervention with the therapeutic scepticism and fatalism of the older gen-
ration of doctors, trained in mid-Victorian times. So, the use and spread of
he following practices amongst late-Victorian doctors is testimony to the
ower and influence of new germ-based theories. Surgeons used more anti-
eptics and for more conditions, and undertook more minor operations to
emove infected tissue. MOsH promoted the building of isolation hospitals;
dvised patients and the public to avoid specific sources of infection; and used
ntisera, antitoxins and vaccines. Doctors generally revised their constitutional
egimes and used them with more optimism, used antiinflammatory reme-
ies to counter the presumed effects of germs, and paid more attention to
he patient, and possible germs within and without their body. What I am
eferring to here are changes in the 'management' of patients, not anachro-
istic assessments of the successes of clinical outcomes.[22]

Much has been written recently about the extent to which germ theories
nd bacteriology 'worked' in facilitating changes in the identity of the medical
rofession. Germ theorists and bacteriologists saw themselves in the vanguard
f the reform of medicine along scientific lines, in every area from educa-
ion to research. Hence, the common observation that germ theories of
isease and bacteriology were used to symbolise and legitimatise medicine as
modern, science-based, socially useful profession. There is much to be said
or this view, but it needs to be qualified by a recognition of the continu-
ng professional and public ambivalence towards vaccination, vivisection, and
he reductionist and materialist associations of positivist science. However, the
890s saw medical science tarred with new problems, notably, the failures of
mmune products and the stigma of commercialism given to them by lay
ritics and some university scientists worried about the sullying of pure
cience. Nonetheless, both the science and technologies of bacteriology had
elped to move the cost-benefit analysis of science to medicine towards
enefits, both within the profession and in its external relations.[23]

The eventual establishment of germ science in the technical discipline of
acteriology has led historians to focus on the development of laboratory
ractices such as microscopy, culture techniques, the use of animals as ex-
erimental models and the production of vaccines and antisera, not to forget
bandoned techniques such as light beams and serial dilutions. All of these
nnovations were crucial in the conversion of living-germ theories of disease
ito bacteriological science. However, this should not obscure the equally
nportant development of germ ideas and practices in the fields of clinical
nd preventive medicine. Indeed, the links between laboratory and field were
wo-way and reciprocal. Many established field practices were given new

2 W. F. Bynum, *Science and the Practice of Medicine in the Nineteenth Century*, Cambridge, Cambridge
   University Press. 1994, 226.
3 R. H. Shryock, *The Development of Modern Medicine: An Interpretation of the Social and Scientific
   Factors Involved*, Madison, WI, University of Wisconsin Press, 1936, Ch. 16.

meanings: during the cattle plague epizootic, quarantines were turned into measures that prevented the importation of disease-germs; antisepsis was remade as a struggle against living, powerful and panspermic disease-germs; and 'true' vaccination had been thought of as germ-practice long before Pasteur appropriated the term after 1880. The ease with which the meaning of this term changed shows the pervasiveness of germ theories before 1880.

The growing importance of the link between field and laboratory was clear in the reception of laboratory work on anthrax from the 1860s. Thus, Koch's work is best seen as part of an ongoing series of investigations that had created an audience of investigators interested in attending to his 'theatre of proof'. Koch widened his audience by correlating the life cycle of the bacillus with epidemiological and clinical experience and interests. On the other hand, his subsequent work on traumatic infections did not find the same audience, especially in Britain and even amongst Listerians. The new investigations, based on inoculation experiments and microscopy, were seen by clinicians to lack relevance to human disease for many reasons. As in studies of tuberculosis, inoculations were seen to produce an 'artificial' disease, there were doubts about whether what happened in small animals was relevant to humans, and the relations between types of septic disease were uncertain. British germ theorists were also unreceptive. They did not trust microscopy to the same degree as Koch; they had difficulties repeating inoculation experiments; and, most important of all, Cheyne, a home grown investigator working in Lister's department, had shown that micrococci were nonpathogenic. The key moments in the development of laboratory practices in Britain came at the International Medical Congress in London in the summer of 1881, when Koch showed his advanced microscopy and solid plate culture techniques for seeing and manipulating 'bacteria', and then just over six months later, when he showed the value of these methods with *Tubercle bacilli*. While many germ theorists rejoiced that germ 'theory' had became germ 'fact', the meaning of the new facts remained to be settled and the reliability of the techniques had to be validated. The application of Koch's theoretical and technical innovations were soon shown to have general and specific limitations: many 'bacteria' were still too small or elusive to be seen by microscopy; matter that supposedly contained bacteria would often not culture; similarly cultured 'bacteria' would not always reproduce specific diseases in animal models; and there remained the overarching question of what, if anything, the behaviour of bacteria in ever more elaborate and 'artificial' laboratory experiments told one about their actions in the real world of human (and animal) interactions.

The first deployment of the bacteriological techniques was to try and construct more aetiological demonstrations following the exemplars of anthrax and tuberculosis; hence the scramble to Egypt and India to secure cholera 'bacteria'. Another major research programme was how best to kill different germs. This led to classic studies of the value of chemicals and heat, as well

s to different ways of disinfecting the body, from local applications of
mproved antiseptics, through to attempts at systemic antibiosis with 'bacte-
iotherapy' – the injection into the body of nonpathogenic bacteria that were
he enemies or competitors of pathogenic organisms. However, the most
mportant research for medicine was on the production of altered 'bacteria'
s vaccines and the use of pathogenic organisms to produce antitoxins, anti-
era and other materials as therapeutic agents. This work was crucial politi-
ally as well as practically, as it brought laboratory products into the fields of
reventive and clinical work. British medicine was denied the boon of the
abies vaccine, which French medical scientists gained so much from, by the
overnment's decision to stamp out rabies by veterinary administrative mea-
ures, though, given my earlier points, it is unlikely that this would have
rompted the Pasteurisation of Britain. The impact of bacteriological work
cross a number of areas of medical practice provided the stimulus of the
nstitutionalisation of medical investigations as laboratory research, rather
han clinical, epidemiological or therapeutic research. In Britain, laboratory
esearch had developed in a piecemeal way relying on voluntary, private and
overnment support. There was no coordinated attempt to develop central,
tate-funded research until 1911. Before then, and, indeed, from before 1865,
overnment support of research developed in an ad hoc fashion to support
epartmental work. Thus, in 1900, medical laboratory work was being funded
y local authorities, the War Office, the India Office, the Colonial Office, the
eterinary Department and the Medical Department of the Local Govern-
ent Board, with all vivisection work monitored by the Home Office.

Diagnostics, the great achievement and icon of Victorian medicine, gained
ast and last from germ science and technology, and then only in limited
reas; indeed, the establishment of service laboratories for public health and
ospital work is largely a twentieth-century story. In the early 1880s the
xpectation amongst germ theorists seems to have been that bacteriological
echniques would become as commonplace as auscultation and thermome-
ry. Bacteriology was initially taught and written about as a do-it-yourself
cience. The system of specialised service laboratories, and a division of labour
etween bench and bedside, only emerged from the late 1890s. It is inter-
sting to reflect how inevitable this change was. Certainly, bacteria were
ound to be more varied and difficult to work with than first thought likely,
hough it is also the case that, in the hands of pathologists and laboratory
cientists, techniques were made complex and costly.[24] Indeed, the full inves-
gation of Koch's postulates required the mastery of three different techni-
al systems: microscopy, culturing and inoculations of experimental animals.
acterial diagnoses also used all three systems plus, from the late 1890s, serum
iagnosis, which was changed into a specialised laboratory test. The routine

O. Amsterdamska, 'Medical and Biological Constraints: Early Research on Variation in Bacteriology', *Social Studies of Science*, 1987, 17: 657–87.

use of bacteriological methods only began in the late 1890s, aided by the facilities created to support preventive medicine, rather than surgery and clinical medicine. Even then, the demand for tests was mostly met by part-time staff in university departments, as in Manchester, or was absorbed by independent research institutions, as in London with the Conjoint Laboratories and the British Institute of Preventive Medicine. Hospital bacteriologists who tended to be young and junior, usually worked part-time. Their main employment and future prospects were as clinicians; full-time laboratory careers were but the dream of a few enthusiasts. The cost, delays and difficulties in obtaining bacteriological tests before 1900, not to mention the higher status of the clinicians compared to laboratory workers, meant that any conflicts were between unequal parties. Usually, laboratory diagnoses were ancillary and secondary to those made at the bedside; the only times they were decisive were when signs and symptoms were difficult to read, or in a protracted illness, when clinicians had already conceded authority to laboratory workers.

By 1900, bacteriology represented above all the conversion of medicine and surgery to specific aetiological and pathological understandings of disease. This change was not wholly the product of bacteriology; developments in physiology, therapeutics and other medical specialisms had also moved medicine in the same direction. The new models of disease were not constructed entirely in mechanistic, reductionist terms, nor were ontological conceptions of disease dominant. Doctors did think more in terms of causes, and tried to relate causes to effects, but there were differences by area of work, age, training, interests and, no doubt, personal inclination. In no case did doctors construct causes or effects as simple and direct. The most decisive change was not the establishment of specific aetiological and pathological models, though certain exemplars structured expectations; rather, it was the spread of the assumption that the mechanisms of disease ought to be knowable and demonstrable, and that such understandings were the road to more effective preventive and curative interventions. This was a vision that both followed and fed the changing identity of the medical profession as an improving, expert body whose science-based work served individuals and society. The hope of bacteriologists, which had spread to most of the profession, was that doctors would not only be able to prevent and cure diseases more effectively, but that they would be able to intervene directly and indirectly to maintain and improve individual 'health' – issues that became much more important in early twentieth-century medicine and welfare.

SELECT BIBLIOGRAPHY

ABBREVIATIONS OF PUBLISHED WORKS

BHM	Bulletin for the History of Medicine
BJHS	British Journal of the History of Science
BMJ	British Medical Journal
BM-CR	Bristol Medico-Chirurgical Review
BMR	Birmingham Medical Review
BPP	British Parliamentary Papers
CR	Contemporary Review
DJMS	Dublin Journal of Medical Science
DNB	Dictionary of National Biography
DQJMS	Dublin Quarterly Journal of Medical Science
EMJ	Edinburgh Medical Journal
GMJ	Glasgow Medical Journal
IMC	International Medical Congress
IMS	Indian Medical Service
CPT	Journal of Comparative Pathology and Therapeutics
HM	Journal of History of Medicine and Allied Sciences
PB	Journal of Pathology and Bacteriology
RAS	Journal of the Royal Agricultural Society
RMS	Journal of the Royal Medical Society
SM	Journal of State Medicine
MR	London Medical Review
IH	Medical History
MMJ	Monthly Microscopical Journal
MTG	Medical Times and Gazette
H	Public Health
MSL	Proceedings of the Medical Society of London
RSL	Proceedings of the Royal Society of London
TRSL	Philosophical Trans. of the Royal Society of London
QJMS	Quarterly Journal of Medical Science
MJ	Quarterly Medical Journal
HM	Social History of Medicine
Rec	Sanitary Record

SRev	Sanitary Review
TESL	Trans. of the Epidemiological Society of London
TMSL	Trans. of the Medical Society of London
TPSL	Trans. of the Pathological Society of London
TRSE	Trans. of the Royal Society of Edinburgh
TSI	Trans. of the Sanitary Institute
TSMOH	Trans. of the Society of Medical Officers of Health
VH	Veterinary History
VJ	Veterinary Journal
VR	Veterinary Review

PARLIAMENTARY PAPERS

1865. *First Report of the Commission Appointed to Inquire into the Origin and Nature of the Cattle Plague*, [3591], xxii, 1.

1866. *Second Report of the Commission Appointed to Inquire into the Origin and Nature of the Cattle Plague*, [3600], xxii, 227.

1866. *Third Report of the Commission appointed to inquire into the origin and nature of the cattle plague*, [3653], lix, 321.

1867. *Ninth Annual Report of the Medical Officer of the Privy Council for 1866*, [3949], xxxvii, 1.

1867–68. *Report of the Cholera Epidemic in England, 1866: Supplement to the Twenty Ninth Annual Report of the Registrar-General of Births, Deaths and Marriages in England*, [4072], xxxvii, xi.

1867–8. *Report on Cattle Plague in Great Britain during the years 1865, 1866 and 1867*, [4060], xviii, 220.

1867–8. *Tenth Report of the Medical Officer of the Privy Council for 1867*, [4004], xxxvi, 413.

1868. *Eleventh Report of the Medical Officer of the Privy Council for 1868*, [4127], xxxii, 1.

1870. *Twelfth Annual Report of the Medical Officer of the Privy Council for 1869*, [C.208], xxxviii, 591.

1871. *Thirteenth Annual Report of the Medical Officer of the Privy Council for 1870*, [C.349] xxxi, 48.

1874. *Report of the Medical Officer of Privy Council and Local Government Board, New Series, No. 2: Supplementary Report on Inquiries in 1874*, [C.1066] xxxi, 33.

1874. *Report of the Medical Officer of the Privy Council and LGB, New Series, No. 3, Report on Scientific Investigations, 1874*, [C.1068], xxxi, 5.

1875. *Report of the Medical Officer of the Privy Council and LGB, New Series, No 6: Report on Scientific Investigations*, [C.1371], xl, 5.

1876. *Report of the Medical Officer of the Privy Council and LGB, New Series, No 8: Report on Scientific Investigations*, [C.1608], xxxviii, 455.

1876. *Report of the Royal Commission on the Practice of Subjecting Live Animals to Experiments for Scientific Purposes*, [C.1397], xli, 1.

1878. *Supplement to the Sixth Annual Report of the LGB, Containing the Report of the Medical Officer of Health for 1876*, [C.1608], xxxvii, Pt. ii, 455.

1878. *Supplement to the Seventh Annual Report of the LGB, Containing the Report of the Medical Officer for 1877*, [C.2130–1] xxxvii, Pt. ii, 403.

1879. *Supplement to the Eighth Annual Report of the LGB, Containing the Report of the Medical Officer for 1878*, [C.2452], xxix, 1.

882. Report of the Royal Commission on Smallpox and Fever Hospitals, [C.3314], xxxix, 1.

884–85. Supplement to the Fourteenth Annual Report of the LGB, Continuing the Report of the Medical Officer for 1884, [C.4516], xxxiii, 227.

886. Annual Report of the Agricultural Department on Contagious Diseases Inspection and the Transit of Animals for 1885, xix, [C.4703], 6.

887. Supplement to the Sixteenth Annual Report of the LGB, Containing the Report of the Medical Officer for 1886, [C.5171], xxxvi, 619.

888. Annual Report of the Agricultural Department of the Privy Council on Contagious Diseases, etc. for 1887, [C.5340], xxxiii, 7.

888. Report of the Departmental Committee appointed to inquire into Pleuropneumonia and Tuberculosis in the United Kingdom, [C.5461], xxxii, 267.

888. Report on Eruptive Diseases of the Teats and Udder in Cows in Relation to Scarlet Fever in Man, [C.5481], xxxii, 1.

889. Annual Report of the Agricultural Department of the Privy Council on Contagious Diseases, etc. for 1888, [C.5679], xxvii, 3.

894. Supplement to the Twenty-Second Annual Report of the LGB, Containing the Report of the Medical Officer for 1892–93, [C.7412], xxxix, 261.

894. Supplement to the Twenty-Third Annual Report of the LGB, Containing the Report of the Medical Officer for 1893–94, [C.7538], xl, 363.

895. Royal Commission Appointed to Enquire into the Effects of Food from Tuberculous Animals on Human Health, [C.7992],xlvi, 11.

895. Supplement to the Twenty-Fourth Annual Report of the LGB, Containing the Report of the Medical Officer for 1894–95, [C.7906], li 391.

896. Supplement to the Twenty-Fifth Annual Report of the LGB, Containing the Report of the Medical Officer for 1895–96, [C.8214], xxxvii, 297.

897. Supplement to the Twenty-Sixth Annual Report of the LGB, Containing the Report of the Medical Officer for 1896–97, [C.8584], xxxvii, 1.

897. Supplement to the Twenty-Seventh Annual Report of the LGB, Containing the Report of the Medical Officer for 1897–98, [C.8953], xl, 1.

899. Supplement to the Twenty-Eighth Annual Report of the LGB, Containing the Report of the Medical Officer for 1899–99, [C.9445], xxxviii, 1.

900. Supplement to the Twenty-Ninth Annual Report of the LGB, Containing the Report of the Medical Officer for 1899–1900, [Cd.299], xxxiv, 1.

WORKS PUBLISHED BEFORE 1900

Aitken, W. 1888. 'On the Progress of Scientific Pathology', BMJ, ii: 348–59.

Ballard, E. 1868. On Vaccination: Its Value and Alleged Dangers, London, Longmans, Green.

Bastian, H. C. 1869. 'The Origin of Life', BMJ, i: 312–3, 569–70; ii: 157–8, 214–15, 270–2, 473–4, 665–6.

Bastian, H. C. 1871. 'Epidemic and Specific Contagious Diseases: Considerations as to Their Nature and Mode of Origin', BMJ, ii: 400–9.

Bastian, H. C. 1871. The Modes of the Origin of Lowest Organisms, London, Macmillan.

Bastian, H. C. 1872. The Beginnings of Life, London, Macmillan.

Bastian, H. C. 1873. 'Dr Sanderson's Experiments and Archeobiosis', Nature, 1873, 8: 485.

Bastian, H. C. 1873. 'On the Temperature at which Bacteria, Vibriones and their Supposed

Germs are Killed when Immersed in Fluids or Exposed to Heat in a Moist State', *PRSL*, 21: 220–32.

Bastian, H. C. 1874. *Evolution and the Origin of Life*, London, Macmillan.

Bastian, H. C. 1876. 'The Germ Theory', *Lancet*, i: 294–5.

Bastian, H. C. 1876. 'Remarks on a New Attempt to Establish the Truth of the Germ-Theory', *BMJ*, i: 157–9.

Bastian, H. C. 1878. 'Spontaneous Generation: A Reply', *Nineteenth Century*, 3: 261–77.

Beale, L. S. 1854. *The Microscope, and its Application to Clinical Medicine*, London, S. Higley.

Beale, L. S. 1861. *How to Work with the Microscope*, London, Churchill.

Beale, L. S. 1866. 'Observations on the "Granular Matter" and "Complex Albuminoid Matter" ', *MTG*, ii: 658–9.

Beale, L. S. 1870. *Disease Germs: Their Real Nature*, London, Churchill.

Beale, L. S. 1870. *Disease Germs: Their Supposed Nature*, London. Churchill.

Beale, L. S. 1872. *Bioplasm: An Introduction to the Study of Physiology and Medicine*, London, Churchill.

Beale, L. S. 1872. *Disease Germs, Their Nature and Origin*, London, Churchill.

Beale, L. S. 1872. 'The Nature and Origin of Contagious Disease Germs', *BMR*, 1: 31–4.

Beale, L. S. 1876. 'A Germ Theory: Remarks on Some of Dr Tyndall's Recent Observations', BMJ, i: 223–4

Beatson, G. T. 1879. 'Some Remarks on the Exciting Causes of Expense in the Antiseptic Treatment of Surgical Cases', *GMJ*, 11: 440–51.

Bennet, J. Henry 1867. 'The Treatment of Pulmonary Consumption', *BMJ*, ii: 137.

Bennett, J. Hughes 1867. 'The Atmospheric Germ Theory', *EMJ*, 13: 810–34.

Bennett, J. Hughes 1971. 'Phthisis pulmonalis', Reynolds, *System of Medicine*, 3: 554–67.

Blyth, A. Winter 1890. *A Manual of Public Health*, London, Macmillan.

Boulger, D. C. 1896. 'Antitoxin, From a Patient's Point of View', *Contemporary Review*, 69: 177–89.

Bowlby, A. A. 1887. *Surgical Pathology and Morbid Anatomy*, London, Churchill.

Bradley, S. M. 1879. 'The Prevention of Blood Poisoning', *BMJ*, ii: 446.

Braidwood, P. M. and Vacher, F. 1875. 'First Contribution to the Life History of Contagion', *BMJ*, ii(Suppl.): 18–22.

Braidwood, P. M. and Vacher, F. 1882. 'Third Contribution to the Life History of Contagion', *BMJ*, i: 41–3, 77–9, 107–13, 143–6, 181–4, 219–22, 257–68.

Bramwell, B. 1899. 'Thirty-Five Years of Medical Progress', *BMJ*, ii: 898–902.

Brunton, T. L. 1875. 'Another Aspect of the Tyndall Typhoid Controversy', *Practitioner*, 24: 62–67.

Brunton, T. L. 1875. 'Dr Klein and the Pathology of Small-pox and Typhoid Fever', *Practitioner*, 24: 4–10.

Buist, J. B. 1887. *Vaccinia and Variola: A Study of Their Life History*, London, Churchill.

Callender, W. 1873. 'Isolation and the Treatment of Wounds' *BMJ*, ii: 256–7.

Calwell, W. 1898. 'The Hygienic Treatment of Consumption Independently of Sanatoria', *BMJ*, ii: 947.

Cameron, C. 1881. 'Micro-organisms and Disease', *BMJ*, ii: 583–7, 585.

Carpenter, A. 1876. *On the Right of the State to Obtain Early Information of the Appearance of Epidemic and Infectious Disease*, London, P. S. King.

Carpenter, A. 1879. 'On the First Principles of Sanitary Work', *BMJ*, ii: 643–8.

Carpenter, A. 1879. 'The Dual Requirements which Are Necessary for the Production of

Enteric Fever, and a Consideration of the Fallacies which Are Based upon a Narrow View of the Germ Theory', *BMJ*, i: 336–7.

Cautley, T. 1895. 'Report on the Micro-organisms Found in Common Articles of Food', *Supplement to the Twenty-Fourth Annual Report*, 473–504.

Cautley, T. 1896. 'An Inquiry into the Influence of Certain Non-Pathogenic Micro-organisms Liable Gain Access to Food', *Supplement to the Twenty-Fifth Annual Report*, 297.

Cautley, T. 1897. 'Report on the Behaviour of the Typhoid Bacillus in Milk', *Supplement to the Twenty-Sixth Annual Report*, 243–55.

Cayley, W. 1880. 'Croonian Lectures on Some Points on the Pathology and Treatment of Typhoid Fever', *BMJ*, i: 391–3.

Cheyne, W. W. 1879. 'On the Relation of Organisms to Antiseptic Dressings', *TPSL*, 30: 557–82.

Cheyne, W. W. 1882. *Antiseptic Surgery: Its Principles, Practice, History and Results*, London, Smith, Elder.

Cheyne, W. W. 1883. 'Report to the AAMR on the Relation of Micro-Organisms to Tuberculosis', *Practitioner*, 30: 240–320.

Cheyne, W. W. 1885. *The Antiseptic Treatment of Wounds*, London, Smith, Elder.

Cheyne, W. W. 1886. *Recent Essays by Various Authors on Bacteria in Relation to Disease*, London, New Sydenham Society.

Cheyne, W. W. 1889. *Suppuration and Septic Diseases*, Edinburgh, Young J. Pentland.

Cheyne, W. W. 1891. 'The Value of Tuberculin in the Treatment of Surgical Tuberculosis', *BMJ*, i: 951, 1043, 1070, 1097.

Cheyne, W. W. 1894. *The Treatment of Wounds, Ulcers and Abscesses*, Edinburgh, Young J. Pentland.

Cheyne, W. W. 1925. *Lister and His Achievement*, London, Longmans Green, 1925.

Cheyne, W. W. et al. 1884. *Public Health Laboratory Work*, London, Williams Clowes and Sons.

Chiene, J. and Ewart, J. C. 1878. 'Do Bacteria or Their Living Germs Exist in the Organs of Healthy Animals?', *Journal of Anatomy and Physiology*, 12: 498–53.

Coats, J. F. 1881. *Discussion on the Pathology of Phthisis Pulmonalis*, Glasgow, A. MacDougall.

Coats, J. F. 1883. *A Manual of Pathology*, London, Longmans Green.

Coats, J. F. 1891. 'The Spontaneous Healing of Tuberculosis', *BMJ*, ii: 933–8.

Cobbett, L. 1898. 'Anti-streptococcal Sera', *Lancet*, i: 986–92.

Cohn, F. 1872. 'Bacteria and their Relations to Putrefaction and Contagion', *QJMS*, 12: 208.

Copeman, S. M. 1891–2. 'Bacteriology of Vaccine Lymph', *TESL*, 11: 70–80.

Copeman, S. M. 1898. 'The Milroy Lectures on the Natural History of Vaccinia', *BMJ*, i: 1185–9, 1245–50; 1312–18.

Copeman, S. M. and Blaxall, F. R. 1898. *Report on the Influence of Glycerine in Inhibiting Growth of Micro-organisms in Vaccine Lymph*, London, Eyre and Spottiswoode.

Corfield, W. H. 1874. 'On the Alleged Spontaneous Development of the Poison of Enteric Fever', *PH*, 2: 155–8.

Crace Calvert, F. 1873. *On Protoplasmic Life and the Action of Heat and Antiseptics Upon It*, Manchester, W. H. Clegg.

Creighton, C. 1876. 'Note On Certain Unusual Coagulation Appearances Found in Mucus and other Albuminoid Fluids', *PSRL*, 24: 140–4.

Crookshank, E. M. 1886. *Manual of Bacteriology*, London, H. K. Lewis.

Crookshank, E. M. 1887. *Photomicrography of Bacteria*, London, H. K. Lewis.

Crookshank, E. M. 1888. 'The History and Present Position of the Germ Theory of Disease', *PH*, 1: 16–19, 53–6.

Crookshank, E. M. 1889. *The History and Pathology of Vaccination*, Vol. I, London, H. K. Lewis.

Crookshank, E. M. 1896. *A Textbook of Bacteriology: Including Etiology and Prevention of Infective Diseases and a Short Account of Yeasts, Moulds, Haematozoa and Psorosperms*, London, H. K. Lewis.

Crowfoot, W. M. 1882. 'The Germ-Theory of Disease', *BMJ*, ii: 554.

Cullimore, H. 1880. *Consumption as a Contagious Disease* (trans. of Professor Cohnheim's pamphlet 'Die Tuberklose vom Standpunkte der Infections-Lehre'), London, Baillière, Tindall and Cox.

Dallinger, W. H. and Drysdale, J. J. 1873. 'Further Researches into the Life History of Monads', *MMJ*, 10: 245–9; 11: 7–10, 69–72; 97–113; 12: 261–9; 13: 185–97.

Dallinger, W. H. and Drysdale, J. J. 1873. 'Researches on the Life History of Cercomonad: A Lesson in Biogenesis', *MMJ*, 10: 53–8.

de Chaumont, F. 1881. 'Pettenkofer's Views on the Parasitic Theory of the Causation of Cholera', *SRec*, 2: 247.

Delépine, S. 1891. 'On the Development of Modern Ideas on Preventive, Protective and Curative Treatment of Bacterial Diseases, and on the Immunity or Refractoriness to Disease', *Lancet*, i: 241–4.

Delépine, S. 1898–9. 'The Prevention of Tuberculosis', *PH*, 99, 11: 469–78.

Dickinson, W. H. 1891. 'On the Uses of Prospects of Pathology', *BMJ*, ii: 247–50.

Dobell, H. 1861. *Lecture on the Germs and Vestiges of Disease and on the Prevention of the Invasion and Fatality of Disease by Periodic Examination*, London, Churchill.

Dreschfeld, J. 1883. 'Micro-organisms in Their Relation to Disease', *BMJ*, ii: 1055–8.

Drysdale, C. R. 1872. *Syphilis and its Nature with a Chapter on Gonorrhoea*, London, Baillière, Tindall and Cox.

Drysdale, J. J. 1878. *The Germ Theories of Infectious Diseases*, London, Baillière, Tindall and Cox.

Duncan, J. 1883. 'Germs and the Spray', *EMJ*, 28: 778.

Durham, H. E. 1897. 'On a Special Action of the Serum of Highly Immunised Animals and its Use in Diagnostic and Other Purposes', *PRSL*, 59: 224–6.

Elliott, G. F. 1870. 'The Germ Theory', *BMJ*, i: 488–9.

Erichsen, J. E. 1869. *The Science and Art of Surgery*, Fifth Ed., London, J. Walton. Further edns. published by Longmans, Green: 1872, 1877, 1884, 1888, 1895.

Erichsen, J. E. 1874. *Hospitalism and the Causes of Death after Operations and Surgical Injuries*, London, Longmans, Green.

Ewart, J. C. 1878. 'The Life History of Bacterium termo and Micrococcus, with Further Observations on Bacillus', *PSRL*, 26: 474–85.

Ewart, J. C. 1878. 'The Life History of the Bacillus Anthracis', *QJMS*, 18: 161.

Farr, J. 1864 'Miss Nightingale's "Notes on Hospitals" ', *MTG*, i: 186–8; 491–2.

Fleming, G. 1871. *Animal Plagues: their History, Nature and Prevention*, London, Chapman and Hall.

Fleming, G. 1875. *A Manual of Veterinary Sanitary Science and Police*, London, Chapman and Hall.

Fleming, G. 1877. 'The Part Played by Minute Organisms in Disease', *VJ*, 4: 118–20.

Fleming, G. 1878. 'The Transmissibility of Tuberculosis', *BFM-CR*, 54: 461–86.

Fleming, G. 1882. 'Vivisection and the Diseases of Animals', *Nineteenth Century*, 11: 468–78.

Fleming, G. 1886. *Pasteur and His Work: From an Agricultural and Veterinary Point of View*, London, William Clowes.

Flügge, C. 1890. *Micro-organisms: with special reference to the etiology of infective disease*, (Trans. second edition of *Fermente und Mikroparasiten* by W. W. Cheyne), London, New Sydenham Society.

Fowler, J. K. 1888. *The Localisation of Phthisis, in Relation to Diagnosis and Prognosis*, London.

Fowler, J. K. 1892. *Arrested Pulmonary Tuberculosis*, London, Churchill.

Fox, C. B. 1876. 'Is Enteric Fever Ever Spontaneously Generated', *BMJ*, i: 374–7.

Fox, J. M. 1874. 'Typhoid Fever and Sanitary Administration', *PH*, 2: 7–9; 20–3.

Fox, W. 1868. *On the Artificial Production of Tubercle in the Lower Animals*, London, Macmillan.

Fox. W. 1873. 'Anatomical Relations of Pulmonary Phthisis to Tubercle of the Lung', *TPSL*, 24: 284–8 *et seq.*

Gamgee, S. 1878–9. 'On Wound Treatment', *Lancet*, ii: 869–71; i 342–8, 456–8.

Gamgee, S. 1883. *On the Treatment of Wounds and Fractures*, London, Churchill.

Gibbes, H. 1881–3. 'Bacteria and Micrococci: Bacilli in Tuberculosis', *PMSL*, 6: 314–20.

Gibbes, H. 1883. *Practical Histology and Pathology*, London, H. K. Lewis.

Gowan, P. 1878. *Consumption: Its Nature, Symptoms, Causes, Prevention, Curability and Treatment*, London, Churchill.

Green, T. H. 1871. *An Introduction to Pathology and Morbid Anatomy*, London, Henry Renshaw.

Green, T. H. 1878. *The Pathology of Pulmonary Consumption: Three Lectures*, London, Henry Renshaw.

Green, T. H. 1882. 'Lectures on Phthisis', *Lancet*, i: 813–5; 1065–7.

Green, T. H. 1883. 'A Lecture on the Tubercle-Bacillus and Phthisis', *BMJ*, i: 194.

Greenfield, W. S. 1881. 'Pathology, Past and Present', *Lancet*, ii, 738–41; 781–6.

Greenfield, W. S. 1881. 'Report on an Experimental Investigation of Anthrax and Allied Diseases, made at the Brown Institution', *JRAS*, 42: 30–44.

Grunbaum, A. S. 1903. 'Goulstonian Lectures on Theories of Immunity and Their Clinical Application', *BMJ*, i: 653–5, 715–7; 783–6.

Gull, W. 1884. 'An Address on the Collective Investigation of Disease', *BMJ*, 1884, ii: 305–8.

Hamilton, D. J. 1883. *On the Pathology of Bronchitis, Catarrhal Pneumonia, Tubercle and Allied Lesions of the Human Lung*, London, Macmillan.

Hankin, E. H. 1890. 'A Bacteria-Killing Globulin', *PRSL*, 48: 93–107.

Harley, G. 1881. 'Some New Facts Conected (sic) with the Action of Germs in the Production of Human Diseases', *MTG*, ii: 570–3, 596–8, 651–3, 705–7; iii: 732–4.

Harris, T. 1889. 'The Curability of Phthisis', *BMJ*, ii: 1385–8.

Hassall, A. H. 1885. *The Inhalation Treatment of Diseases of the Organs of Respiration, including Consumption*, London, Longmans Green.

Heath, C. 1886. *Dictionary of Surgery*, Vol. 1, London, Smith, Elder.

Heron, G. A. 1883. 'Some of the More Recent Facts and Observations Concerning the Bacillus of Tubercle', *BMJ*, i: 805–7.

Heron, G. A. 1885–6. 'The Cholera Bacillus of Koch', *TSMOH*, 17–32.

Hirsch, A. 1883. *Handbook of Geography and Historical Pathology*, (Trans. by C. Creighton), London, New Sydenham Society.

Hogg, J. 1870. 'The Organic Germ Theory of Disease', *MTG*, i: 659–61; 685–7.

Holmes, T. 1874. 'Pyaemia in Hospital and Private Practice', *BMJ*, i: 269–70; ii: 142–5.

Holmes, T. 1888. *A Treatise on Surgery: Its Principles and Practice*, (revised by T. Pickering Pick), London, Smith Elder.

Holmes, T. ed. 1870–1. *System of Surgery*, 5 vols., London, Longmans, Green.

Horsley, V. 1889. 'On Rabies: Its Treatment by M. Pasteur, and on the Means of Detecting Suspected Cases', *BMJ*, i: 342.

Horsley, V. and Mott, F. W. 1880–2. 'On the Existence of Bacteria or their Antecedents in Healthy Tissues', *Journal of Physiology*, 3: 188, 296.

Houston, A. C. 1897. 'Report on the Chemical and Bacteriological Examination of Soils', *Supplement to the Twenty-Seventh Annual Report*, 251–307.

Houston, A. C. 1899. 'Inoculation of Soil with Particular Microbes', *Supplement to the Twenty-Eighth Annual Report*, 413–39.

Howse, H. G. 1899. 'A Review of Surgery during the Past 100 Years', *Lancet*, ii: 1717–24.

Humphry, F. A. 1886. 'The Medical Aspect of Surgery', *BMJ*, ii: 307.

Hutchinson, J. 1874. 'The Hospital Plagues', *BMJ*, i: 161–3.

Jaccoud, S. 1885. *The Curability and Treatment of Pulmonary Phthisis*, London, Kegan Paul, Trench.

Jervoise, J. Clarke 1882. *Infection, with Remarks by Miss Nightingale*, London, Vacher and Sons.

Keetley, C. 1881. *Index of Surgery*, London, Smith, Elder.

Kenwood, H. R. 1893. *Public Health Laboratory Work*, London, H. K. Lewis.

Kern, L. 1872. *Deutsche Bakteriologie im Spiegel englischer medizinischer Zeitschriften, 1875–1885*, Zurich, Juris Druck and Verlag.

Klein, E. 1874. 'Research on Smallpox of Sheep', *PRSL*, 22: 338–41.

Klein, E. 1876. 'Note on the Mycelium Described in My Paper on Smallpox of Sheep', *PRSL*, 25: 259–60.

Klein, E. 1878. 'Enteric or Typhoid Fever of the Pig', *Supplement to the Sixth Annual Report*, 455.

Klein, E. 1878. 'Infectious Pneumo-Enteritis in the Pig', *Supplement to the Seventh Annual Report*, 169–280.

Klein, E. 1878. 'Experimental Contribution to the Etiology of Infectious Diseases, with Special Reference to *Contagium vivum*', *QJMS*, 18: 170–6.

Klein, E. 1881. 'Aetiology of Miliary Tuberculosis', *Practitioner*, 27: 83.

Klein, E. 1884. *Micro-organisms and Disease*, London, Macmillan. Further edns: 1885, 1886, 1896.

Klein, E. 1884. 'Micro-organisms and Disease', *Practitioner*, 32: 170–86, 241–64, 321–52, 401–26; 33: 21–40, 81–112, 161–80; 241–57.

Klein, E. 1884. 'The Bacteria of Swine Plague', *Journal of Physiology*, 5: 1–13.

Klein, E. 1885. 'The Relation of Bacteria to Asiatic Cholera', *PRSL*, 1885: 154–7.

Klein, E. 1885. 'The Etiology of Asiatic Cholera', *BMJ*, i: 650–2.

Klein, E. 1887. 'The Etiology of Scarlet Fever', *Supplement to the Sixteenth Annual Report*, Appendix B, 367–414.

Klein, E. 1889. *The Bacteria in Asiatic Cholera*, London, Macmillan.

Klein, E. 1894. 'Further Report on the Etiology of Typhoid Fever', Supplement to the *Twenty-Third Annual Report*, 457–68.

Klein, E. 1894. 'On the Etiology of Vaccinia and Variola', *Supplement to the Twenty-Second Annual Report*, 693–7.

Klein, E. 1894. 'Report on Psorosperms in their Relation to the Etiology of Cancer', Supplement to the Twenty-Third Annual Report, 479–93.

Klein, E. 1894. 'Report on the Etiology of Typhoid Fever', Twenty-Second Annual Report, 345–66.

Klein, E. 1895. 'Further Observations on the Microbes of Vaccinia and Variola', Supplement to the Twenty-Fourth Annual Report, 267–86.

Klein, E. 1895. 'Further Report on the Etiology of Typhoid Fever', Supplement to the Twenty-Fourth Report, 399–407.

Klein, E. 1895. 'Report on the Abilities of Certain Microbes to Maintain their Existence in Water', Supplement to the Twenty-Fourth Annual Report, 411–29.

Klein, E. 1895. 'Report on the Behaviour of the Bacillus of Enteric Fever and of Bacillus Coli in Sewage', Supplement to the Twenty-Fourth Annual Report, 407–11.

Klein, E. 1896. 'Recent Researches on the Identification of the Typhoid Bacillus and the Cholera Vibrio', JSM, 4: 285–6, 375–7, 469–71.

Klein, E. 1899. 'The Fate of Pathogenic and Other Infective Microbes in the Dead Animal', Supplement to the Twenty-Eighth Annual Report, 344–82.

Koch, R. 1880. Investigations into the Etiology of Traumatic Infective Diseases, (transl. by W. W. Cheyne), London: New Sydenham Society.

Koprowski H. and Oldstone, M. B. A., eds. 1996. Microbe Hunters: Then and Now, New York, Medi-Ed Press.

Lewis, T. R. and Cunningham, D. D. 1872. A Report of Microscopical and Physiological Researches into the Nature of the Agent or Agents of Cholera, Calcutta, Office of the Superintendent of Government Printing.

Lewis, T. R. 1879. The Microscopic Organisms Found in the Blood of Man and Animals and Their Relation to Disease, Calcutta, Office of the Superintendent of Government Printing.

Lister, J. 1858. 'On the Early Stages of Inflammation', PTRSL, 2: 645–702.

Lister, J. 1867. 'On a New Method of Treating Compound Fractures, Abscess, etc.', Lancet, i: 336–9, 357–9, 387–9, 507–9, ii: 95–6.

Lister, J. 1867. 'On the Antiseptic Principle in the Practice of Surgery', Lancet, ii: 353–7, 668–9.

Lister, J. 1868. 'An Address on the Antiseptic System of Treatment in Surgery', BMJ, ii: 53–6, 101–2, 461–3, 515–7.

Lister, J. 1870. 'On the Effects of the Antiseptic System of Treatment upon the Salubrity of a Surgical Hospital', Lancet, i: 4–6, 40–42.

Lister, J. 1870. 'Further Evidence Regarding the Effects of the Antiseptic Treatment on the Salubrity of a Surgical Hospital', Lancet, ii: 287–9.

Lister, J. 1871. 'On Some Cases Illustrating the Results of Excision of the Wrist for Caries', EMJ, 17: 144–50.

Lister, J. 1871. 'The Address in Surgery [Antiseptic treatment of Wounds]' BMJ, ii: 225–33.

Lister, J. 1873. 'A Further Contribution to the Natural History of Bacteria and the Germ Theory of Fermentative Changes', QJMS, 13: 380–408.

Lister, J. 1873. 'On a Case of Rupture of the Axillary Artery', EMJ, 18: 829–31.

Lister, J. 1873. 'On the Germ Theory of Putrefaction and Other Fermentative Changes', Nature, 8: 212–4, 232–3.

Lister, J. 1874. 'A Case of Rodent Ulcer', EMJ, 20: 268–70.

Lister, J. 1874. 'Cases Illustrating Antiseptic Management', EMJ, 20: 556–7.

Lister, J. 1874. 'Cases of Omental hernia', EMJ, 20: 69–73.

Lister, J. 1875. 'A Contribution to the Germ Theory of Putrefaction and Other

Fermentative Changes, and the Natural History of Torulae and Bacteria', *TRSE*, 27: 313–44.

Lister, J. 1875. 'Demonstrations of Antiseptic Surgery', *EMJ*, 21: 195–6, 481–7.

Lister, J. 1875. 'On Recent Improvements in the Details of Antiseptic Surgery', *Lancet*, i: 365–7, 401–2, 434–6, 468–70, 603–5, 717–9, 787–9.

Lister, J. 1877. 'On Lactic Fermentation and its Bearing on Pathology', *TPSL*, 29: 425–67.

Lister, J. 1878. 'On the Nature of Fermentation', *QJMS*, 18: 177–94.

Lister, J. 1881. 'An Address on the Treatment of Wounds', Lancet, ii: 863–6, 901–3.

Lister, J. 1881. 'On the Relation of Micro-Organisms to Disease', *QJMS*, 21: 330–42.

Lister, J. 1881. 'On the Relation of Micro-Organisms to Inflammation', *Lancet*, ii: 695–8.

Lister, J. 1885. 'Corrosive Sublimate as a Surgical Dressing', *TMSL*, 8: 2–19.

Lister, J. 1890. 'An Address on the Present Position of Antiseptic Surgery', *BMJ*, ii: 377–9.

Lister, J. 1890. 'On a New Antiseptic Dressing', *TMSL*, 13: 32–50.

Lister, J. 1893. 'The Essentials of Antiseptic Surgery', *BMJ*, ii: 1014.

Lister, J. 1893. 'An Address on the Antiseptic Management of Wounds', *BMJ*, i: 161–2, 277–8, 337–9.

Lister, J. 1894. 'On the Simplification of the Antiseptic Treatment', *GMJ*, 41: 434–9.

Lister, J. 1897. 'On the Value of Pathological Research', *BMJ*, i: 317–9.

Lockwood, C. B. 1890. 'Preliminary report on aseptic and septic surgical cases', *BMJ*, ii: 943–7.

Lockwood, C. B. 1892. 'Further Report on Aseptic and Septic Surgical Cases, with Special Reference to Infection from the Skin', *BMJ*, i: 1127–37.

Lockwood, C. B. 1894. 'Report on Aseptic and Septic Surgical Cases', with Special Reference to the Disinfection of the Skin, Sponges and Towels', *BMJ*, i: 175–83.

Lockwood, C. B. 1895–6. 'A Brief Note on Aseptic Surgery; Advocating the More Frequent Use of Scientific Tests', *QMJ*, 4: 118.

Lockwood, C. B. 1896. *Aseptic Surgery*, Edinburgh, Young, J. Pentland.

Low, R. B. 1880. 'The Origin of Enteric Fever in Isolated Rural Districts', *BMJ*, i: 733–6.

Lowe, J. 1883. 'The Germ Theory of Disease', *BMJ*, ii: 53–5.

Lund, E. 1872. *Antisepticity in surgery*, Manchester, J. E. Cornish.

MacCormac, W. 1880. *Antiseptic Surgery*, London, Smith Elder.

MacCormac, W. 1888. 'Old and New Surgery', *BMJ*, ii: 865.

MacKenzie, S. 1902. 'The Powers of Natural Resistance, or the Personal Factor in Disease of Microbe Origin', *TMSL*, 25: 302–18.

Maclagan, T. J. 1876. *The Germ-Theory Applied to the Explanation of the Phenomena of Disease*, London, Macmillan.

Maclagan, T. J. 1884. 'On Methods of Therapeutic Research', *BMJ*, ii: 260–1.

Martin, S. 1890. 'The Chemical Products of the Growth of Bacillus Anthracis and their Physiological Action', *PRSL*, 48: 78–80.

Martin, S. 1892. 'Phagoctosis and Immunity', *BMJ*, i: 496.

Martin, S. 1892. 'Chemical Pathology of Diphtheria Compared with Anthrax, Infective Endocarditis and Tetanus', *BMJ*, i: 641, 696, 755.

Martin, S. 1897. 'Report on the Growth of the Typhoid Bacillus in Soil', *Supplement to the Twenty-Sixth Annual Report*, 231–43.

Martin, S. 1898. 'Croonian Lectures on the Chemical Products of Pathogenic Bacteria', *BMJ*, i: 1569–72, 1644–6; ii: 11–15, 73–6.

Martin, S. 1898. 'Report on the Growth of the Typhoid Bacillus in Soil', *Supplement to the Twenty-Seventh Annual Report*, 308–18.

Martin, S. 1899. 'Report on the Growth of the Typhoid Bacillus in Soil', *Supplement to the Twenty-Eighth Annual Report*, 382–412.

Martin, S. 1900. 'Further Report on the Growth of the Typhoid Bacillus in Soil', *Supplement to the Twenty-Ninth Annual Report*, 525–49.

McDonald, J. 1878. *A Few Remarks on the Germ Theory and its Relation to the Germ Theory of Disease*, MD Thesis, University of Glasgow.

McVail, J. V. 1880. 'Ten Years' Surgery in the Kilmarnock Infirmary' *Lancet*, ii: 340–4.

McWeeney, E. J. 1893. 'Some Points in the Aetiology of Typhoid Fever', *JSM*, 1: 65.

M'Fadyean, J. and Woodhead, G. S. 1891. 'On the Communicability of Tuberculosis from Animals to Man', *BMJ*, ii: 412–3, 635–6.

Millard, E. 1898. 'The Etiology of "Return Cases" of Scarlet Fever', *BMJ*, ii: 614–18.

Morris, J. G. 1867. *Germinal Matter and the Contact Theory: An Essay on Morbid Poisons, their Nature, Sources, Effects, Migrations, and the Means of Limiting their Noxious Agency*, London, Churchill.

Moxon, W. and Goodhart, J. F. 1875. 'Observations on the Presence of Bacteria in the Blood and Infective Products of Septic Fever and the "Cultivation" of Septicaemia', *Guy's Hospital Reports*, 20: 229–60.

Muir, R. and Ritchie, J. 1899. *Manual of Bacteriology*, Edinburgh, Young, J. Pentland.

Murchison, C. 1862. *Continued Fevers of Great Britain*, London, Parker, Son and Bourne.

Newman, G. 1898. 'The Fundamental Principles of Vaccination and Antitoxin Inoculation', *Medical Magazine*, 267–8.

Newman, G. 1899. *Bacteria in Relation to the Economy of Nature, Industrial Processes and the Public Health*, London, John Murray.

Newsholme, A. 1892. *Hygiene: A Manual of Personal and Public Health*, London, George Gill.

Newsholme, A. 1900. 'The Utility of Isolation Hospitals in Diminishing the Spread of Scarlet Fever', *Journal of Hygiene*, 1: 145–52.

Niven, J. 1897. 'On the Notification of Tuberculosis', *Medical Chronicle*, 7: 1–15.

Notter, J. Lane 1877. 'The Chemical Theory of Contagion, Compared with the Corpuscular Theory', *BMJ*, ii: 301.

Notter, J. Lane and Firth, R. H. 1896. *The Theory and Practice of Hygiene*, London, Churchill.

Notter, J. Lane, ed. 1891. *Parkes Manual of Practical Hygiene*, 8th edition, London, Churchill.

Ogston, A. 1879. 'Bacteria and Disease', *BMJ*, i: 592.

Ogston, A. 1880. 'Über Abscesse', *Arch. f. Klin. Chir.* 225: 588–600.

Ogston, A. 1881. 'Micro-organisms in Surgical Diseases', *BMJ*, i: 369–75.

Ogston, A. 1882–3. 'Micrococcus Poisoning', *Journal of Anatomy and Physiology*, 16: 526–67; 17: 24–58.

Parkes, E. A. 1864. *A Manual of Practical Hygiene*, London, Churchill; Third edition, 1869; Fowlt edition, 1873.

Parkes, L. 1889. *Hygiene and Public Health*, London, H. K. Lewis.

Pasteur, L. 1882. 'Sur le rouget, ou mal rouge de porcs', *Comptes Rendus*, 95: 1120–3.

Pollock, J. E. 1865. *The Elements of Prognosis in Consumption*, London, Longmans, Green.

Pollock, J. E. 1883. 'Croonian Lectures: Modern Theories and Treatment of Phthisis', *MTG*, i: 261–2, 320–2, 378–80, 431–3, 577–9, 605–7.

Power, H. 1886. 'Bacteriology in its Relations to Surgery', *Lancet*, ii: 1111–6.

Quain, R. ed. 1882. *A Dictionary of Medicine, Vol. 1*, London, Longmans Green.

Ransome, A. 1882. *Consumption: Its Causes and Its Prevention*, Manchester and Salford Sanitary Association.

Ransome, A. 1890. *The Causes and Prevention of Consumption*, London, Smith, Elder.

Ransome, A. 1892. *A Campaign Against Phthisis*, Manchester, John Heywood.

Ransome, A. 1895. 'The Consumption Scare', *Medical Chronicle*, 2: 241–9.

Rawlinson, R. 1880. 'Old Lessons in Sanitary Science Revived, and New Lessons Considered', *TSI*, 2: 127–30.

Report 1874. 'Debate on Pyaemia' 1874 *BMJ*, i: 146, 234–40, 306–11, 324–5, 380–6.

Report 1875. 'Debate on the Germ Theory of Disease', *TPSL*, 26: 255–345.

Reynolds, J. 1871. *A System of Medicine*, 3 Vols., London, Macmillan.

Richardson, B. W. 1867. 'Styptic Colloid', *MTG*, i: 383–5, 409–10.

Richardson, B. W. 1867. *The Poisons of the Spreading Diseases*, London, Churchill.

Richardson, B. W. 1870. 'The Medical Aspect of the Germ-Theory', *MTG*, ii: 510–12, 539–41.

Richardson, B. W. 1877. 'The Glandular Origin of Contagious Diseases', *MTG*, ii: 235–6.

Roberts, F. T. 1873. *A Handbook of the Theory and Practice of Medicine*, London, H. K. Lewis.

Roberts, F. T. 1899. 'The Progress of Medicine in the Nineteenth Century', *Lancet*, ii: 996–1000.

Roberts, W. 1877. *On Spontaneous Generation and the Doctrine of Contagium Vivum*, Manchester, Cornish.

Roberts, W. 1877. 'The Doctrine of Contagium vivum and its Applications to Medicine', *BMJ*, ii: 168–73.

Rose, W. and Carless, W. 1898. *A Manual of Surgery*, London, Baillière, Tindall and Cox.

Ross, J. 1872. *The Graft Theory of Disease*, London, Churchill.

Roy, C. S. 1887. 'Preliminary Report on the Pathology of Asiatic Cholera (as Observed in Spain in 1885)', *PRSL*, 41: 173–81

Sanderson, J. B. 1867. 'Report on the Inoculability and Development of Tubercle', *Tenth Report*, 91–125.

Sanderson, J. B. 1868. 'Further Report on the Inoculability and Development of Tubercle', *Eleventh Report*, 91–125.

Sanderson, J. B. 1870. 'The Intimate Pathology of Contagion', *Twelfth Report*, 58–9, 229–56.

Sanderson, J. B. 1871. 'Further Report on the Intimate Pathology of Contagion', *Thirteenth Report*, 48.

Sanderson, J. B. 1871. 'The Origin of Bacteria', *QJMS*, 11: 323.

Sanderson, J. B. 1872. 'Preparation Showing the Results of Certain Experimental Inquiries Relating to the Nature of the Infective Agent in Pyaemia', *TPSL*, 23: 303–8.

Sanderson, J. B. 1875. 'The Occurrence of Organic Forms in Connection with Contagious and Infective Diseases', *BMJ*, i: 69–71, 199–200, 403–5, 435–7.

Sanderson, J. B. 1877. 'Contagium Vivum', *PH*, 7: 59–63.

Sanderson, J. B. 1877–8. 'The Infective Processes of Disease', *BMJ*, ii: 879–81, 913–5; i: 1–2, 45–7, 119–20, 179–83.

Sanderson, J. B. 1878. 'Remarks on the Attributes of the Germinal Particles of Bacteria, in Reply to Professor Tyndall', *PRSL*, 26: 416–26.

Sanderson, J. B. 1880. 'Report on experiments on anthrax conducted at the Brown Institution, February 18 to June 30, 1878', *JRAS*, 41: 267.

anderson, J. B. 1882. 'Lumleian Lectures on Inflammation', *Lancet*, i: 553–6.

anderson, J. B. 1883. 'Inflammation', in Holmes, T. and Hulke, J. W. eds., *System of Surgery*, Third edition, London, Longmans, Green, 1–98.

anderson, J. B. 1891. 'The Progress of Discovery Relating to the Origin and Nature of Infectious Diseases', *BMJ*, ii: 983–7, 1033–7, 1083–7, 1135–59.

ansom, A. E. 1870. 'On Putrefaction, Fermentation and Infection', *Lancet*, ii: 671.

ansom, A. E. 1871. *The Antiseptic System: A Treatise on Carbolic Acid and its Compounds*, London, Gillman.

aundby, R. 1882. 'Recent Researches on Tubercle and their Bearings on the Treatment of Consumption', *Practitioner*, 29: 178–83.

avory, W. 1879. 'Address in Surgery', *BMJ*, ii: 210–7.

eaton, E. 1868. *A Handbook of Vaccination*, London, Macmillan.

eaton, E. 1894. 'A Report on the Present State of Knowledge Respecting the Etiology and Prevention of Diphtheria', *BMJ*, ii: 573–77.

eaton, E. 1896. 'The Value of Isolation and Its Difficulties', *Lancet*, i: 698–70.

edgwick, L. W. 1869. 'A Report on the Parasitic Theory of Disease', *Transactions of the St Andrew's Graduates Association*, 116–48.

helley, C. E., ed., 1892. *Transactions of the Seventh International Congress of Hygione and Demography*, 13 vols. London, Eyre and Spottiswoode.

hepherd, A. B. 1877. *Goulstonian Lectures on the Natural History of Pulmonary Consumption*, London, Smith Elder.

hingleton Smith, R. 1883. 'The Proofs of the Existence of Phthisical Contagion', *BM-CJ*, 1: 1–41.

hrimpton, C. 1866. *Cholera: Its Seat, Nature, and Treatment*, London, Churchill.

imon, J. 1867. 'Postscript, with Particular Reference to the Cholera-Conference Recently Held at Weimar', *Ninth Report*, 29–34.

imon, J. 1867. 'Proceedings Against Cholera under the Disease Prevention Acts and Otherwise', *Ninth Report*, 1.

imon, J. 1870. 'Inflammation', in Holmes, T., ed. *System of Surgery*, London, Longmans, Green, 1–113.

imon, J. 1874. 'Filth Diseases and Their Prevention', *Report of the Medical Officer, New Series, No. 2*, 33.

imon, J. 1882. 'Contagion' in Quain, R., ed. *A Dictionary of Medicine, Vol. 1*, London, Longmans, Green, p. 294.

imon, J. 1890. *English Sanitary Institutions*, London, Cassell and Co.

impson, J. Y. 1868. 'A Proposal to Stamp Out Smallpox', *MTG*, i: 5–6, 32–3, 264, 537.

impson, J. Y. 1869. *Hospitalism: its Effects on the Results of Surgical Operations*, Edinburgh, Reprinted from Edinburgh Medical Journal.

kerritt, E. Markham 1883. 'Clinical Evidence Against The Contagiousness of Phthisis', *BM-CJ* 1: 48–70.

mart, A. 1884. 'A Chronological History of the Discovery of Germs', *BMJ*, ii: 565.

mith, S. C. 1882. 'Modern Study of Micro-Organisms and its Influence of Medical Thought', *Lancet* i: 309.

pear, J. 1875. 'The "Woolsorters' Disease" or Anthrax Fever', *TESL*, 4: 277–300.

quire, J. E. 1893. *The Hygienic Prevention of Consumption*, London, C. Griffin.

Squire, J. E. 1896. 'The Influence of Bacillary Theory of Tuberculosis on the Treatment of Phthisis', *BMJ*, i: 208.

Squire, W. 1873. 'On the Development and Propagation of Epidemic Diseases', *PH*, 1: 161.

Steel, J. H. 1879. 'Principal Facts Hitherto Ascertained Concerning Bacteria', *VJ*, 9: 156, 238.

Stevens, J. L. 1883. 'The Tubercle Bacillus and its Relations to Phthisis Pulmonalis', *GMJ*, 19: 348–54.

Stevenson, T. and Murphy, S. F. 1892–4. *A Treatise on Hygiene and Public Health*, Vols. 1 and 2, London, Churchill.

Stokes, W. 1888. 'The Altered Relations of Surgery to Medicine', *BMJ*, i: 1197–1202.

Swanson, J. 1890. *Consumption: A Curable Disease*, Glasgow, W. & R. Holmes.

Sykes, J. F. J. 1894–5. 'The Cause of the Increase in Mortality from Diphtheria in London', *PH*, 7: 331.

Syson, E. J. 1877. 'The Antiseptic Treatment of Zymotic Diseases', *PH*, 8: 301–3.

Thin, G. 1887. 'Contagium of Scarlet Fever', *BMJ*, ii: 402–8.

Thomson, W. 1879. 'Blood Poisoning and Antiseptics', *BMJ*, ii: 446–8.

Thomson, W. 1879. 'Typhoid Fever: Contagious, Infectious and Communicable', *BMJ*, i: 343–5.

Thorne, R. Thorne 1892. *Diphtheria: Its Natural History and Prevention: Being the Milroy Lectures, 1891*, London, Macmillan.

Thorne, R. Thorne 1899. *The Administrative Control of Tuberculosis*, London, Baillière, Tindall and Cox.

Treves, F. 1895–6. *A System of Surgery*, London, Cassell and Co.

Turner, G. 1887. 'Report on the Experience of Diphtheria, Especially its Relations to Lower Animals', *Sixteenth Annual Report*, 619.

Tyndall, J. 1870. 'On Dust and Haze', *MTG*, i: 130–1.

Tyndall, J. 1870. 'On Dust and Disease' *Proc. of the Royal Institution of Great Britain*, 6: 1–14.

Tyndall, J. 1876. 'Fermentation and its Bearing on the Phenomenon of Disease', *Fortnightly Review*, 20: 567.

Tyndall, J. 1877. 'Further Research on the Deportment and Vital Resistance of Putrefactive and Infective Organisms', *PRSL*, 26: 228–38.

Tyndall, J. 1878. 'Notes on Dr Burdon Sanderson's Views on Ferments and Germs', *PRSL*, 26: 353–6.

Tyndall, J. 1878. 'Spontaneous Generation', *Nineteenth Century*, 3: 22–47.

Tyndall, J. 1878. 'Spontaneous Generation: The Last Word', *Nineteenth Century*, 3: 497–508.

Tyndall, J. 1881. *Essays on the Floating Matter of the Air in Relation to Putrefaction and Infection*, London, Macmillan.

Tyndall, J. 'The Germ Theory', *Lancet*, i: 262–3.

von Niemeyer, F. 1870. *Clinical Lectures on Pulmonary Consumption*, London, New Sydenham Society.

Walley, T. 1887–8. 'Animal Tuberculosis in Relation to Man', *EMJ*, 33: 984–97, 1078–89.

Walsham, W. J. 1889. *Surgery: Its Theory and Practice*, second edition, London, Churchill.

Watson, E. 1869. 'On the Theory of Suppuration, and the Use of Carbolic Acid Dressings', *GMJ*, 2: 133–4.

Watson, T. 1877. 'The Abolition of Zymotic Diseases', *Nineteenth Century*, 1: 380–96.

Watson, T. 1879. *The Abolition of Zymotic Diseases*, London, Kegan Paul.

Weber, H. 1885. 'The Hygienic and Climatic Treatment of Chronic Pulmonary Phthisis', *BMJ*, i: 517, 641, 688, 725, 744.

Wells, T. S. 1864. 'Some causes of excessive surgical mortality after surgical operations', *BMJ*, ii: 384.

Wells, T. S. 1875. 'On the Relation of Puerperal Fever to the Infective Diseases and Pyaemia', *Trans. of the Obstetrical Society*, 17: 90–130.

Wells, T. S. 1884. *The Revival of Ovariotomy and its Influence on Modern Surgery*, London, Churchill.

West, S. 1883. 'The Bacilli of Tubercle Found in the Contents of Cavities and not in Lung Tissue', *TPSL*, 34: 16–28.

White, S. 1899–1900. 'Aseptic Surgery', *QMJ*, 8: 14–25.

Whitelegge, B. Arthur. 1890. *Hygiene and Public Health*, London, Cassell.

Williams, C. J. B. and Williams, C. T. 1887. *Pulmonary Consumption: Its Etiology and Treatment, with an Analysis of 1,000 Cases to Exemplify its Duration and Modes of Arrest*, London, Longmans, Green.

Williams, C. T. 1883. 'The Contagion of Phthisis', *BMJ*, ii: 618–21.

Wilson, G. 1873. *A Handbook of Hygiene and Sanitary Science*, London, Churchill; eigth edition, 1898.

Wilson, G. 1899. 'Bacteriology in its Relation to State Medicine', *JSM*, 7: 495–501.

Wood, J. 1885. 'The Bradshawe Lecture on Antiseptics in Surgery', *BMJ*, 1885, ii: 1095–7, 1147–9.

Woodhead, G. S. 1892. 'Address in Bacteriology', *Lancet*, i: 238.

Woodhead, G. S. 1897. 'Harben Lectures on the Bearing of Recent Bacteriological Investigations on Public Health', *JSM*, 5, 289, 357, 405–53.

Woodhead, G. S. and Hare, A. W. 1885. *Pathological Mycology*, Edinburgh, Young J. Pentland.

Woodhead, G. S. and M'Fadyean, J. 1886. 'Notes on the Microparasites of Domestic Animals', *Veterinarian*, 59: 591.

Woodhead, G. S. and M'Fadyean, J. 1887. 'Tubercle in the Dairy', *BMJ*, ii: 673.

Wooldridge, L. C. 1893. *On the Chemistry of the Blood and Other Scientific Papers*, (arranged by Victor Horsley and Ernest Starling), London, Kegan, Paul, Trench, Truebner.

Wright, A. E. 1902. 'On the Results Which Have Been Obtained by Anti-Typhoid Inoculation', *Lancet*, ii: 652–3.

Wright, A. E. and Bruce, D. 1893. 'On Haffkine's Method of Vaccination against Asiatic Cholera', *BMJ*, i: 227.

Wright, A. E. and Leishman, W. B. 1900. 'Results Which Have Been Obtained by the Antityphoid Inoculations', *BMJ*, i: 122–4.

Yeo, J. B. 1882. *The Contagiousness of Pulmonary Consumption and its Antiseptic Treatment*, London, Churchill.

Yeo, J. B. 1884. 'Clinical Lectures on the Treatment of Disease', *MTG*, ii: 772.

WORKS PUBLISHED SINCE 1900

Ackerknecht, E. 1948. 'Anticontagionism between 1821 and 1867', *BHM*, 22: 562–93.

Adam, A. 1988. *Spontaneous Generation in the 1870s: Victorian Scientific Naturalism and its Relationship to Medicine*, PhD thesis, C.N.A.A.

Amsterdamska, O. 1987. 'Medical and Biological Constraints: Early Research on Variation in Bacteriology', *Social Studies of Science*, 17: 657–87.

Aronowitz, R. A. 1998. *Making Sense of Illness: Science, Society and Illness*, Cambridge, Cambridge University Press.

Ayers, G. M. 1971. *England's First State Hospitals and the Metropolitan Asylums Board, 1867–1930*, London, WIHM.

Baldry, P. E. 1965. *The Battle Against Bacteria*, Cambridge, Cambridge University Press.

Baron, A. L. 1958. *Man Against Germs*, London, Robert Hale.

Bashford, A. 1998. *Purity and Pollution: Gender, Embodiment and Victorian Medicine*, London, Macmillan.

Bibel, D. J., ed. 1988. *Milestones in Immunology: A Historical Exploration*, Madison, WI, Science Tech.

Bishop, W. J. 1959. *A History of Surgical Dressings*, Chesterfield, Robinson and Sons.

Brand, J. L. 1965. *Doctors and the State: The British Medical Profession and Government Action in Public Health, 1870–1912*, Baltimore, MD, Johns Hopkins University Press.

Brandt, A. M. 1985. *No Magic Bullet: A Social History of Venereal Disease in the United States since 1880*, New York, Oxford University Press.

Brieger, G. H. 1966. 'American Surgery and the Germ Theory of Disease', *BHM*, 40: 135–45.

Brock, T. D. 1988. *Robert Koch: A Life in Medicine and Bacteriology*, Madison, WI, Science Tech.

Brock, W. H. et al., eds. 1981. *John Tyndall: Essays on a Natural Philosopher*, Dublin, Royal Dublin Society.

Brock, W. H. 1998. *Justus von Liebig: The Chemical Gatekeeper*, Cambridge, Cambridge University Press.

Bruce, J. M. 1910. 'The Dominance of Etiology in Modern Medicine', *BMJ*, ii: 246–7.

Bryder, L. 1988. *Below the Magic Mountain: A Social History of Tuberculosis in Twentieth Century Britain*, Oxford, Oxford University Press.

Bulloch, W. 1938. *The History of Bacteriology*, London, Oxford University Press.

Bynum, W. F. 1983. 'Darwin and the Doctors: Evolution, Diathesis and Germs in Nineteenth Century Britain', *Gesnerus*, 40: 43–53.

Bynum, W. F. 1990. ' "C'est un malade": Animal models and concepts of human disease', *JHM*, 45: 397–413.

Bynum, W. F. 1994. *Science and the Practice of Medicine in the Nineteenth Century*, Cambridge, Cambridge University Press.

Bynum, W. F. and Porter, R. 1993. *Companion Encyclopaedia of the History of Medicine*, London, Routledge.

Carter, K. Codell 1985. 'Koch's Postulates in relation to the work of Jacob Henle and Edwin Klebs', *MH*, 29: 353–74.

Carter, K. Codell 1991. 'The Development of Pasteur's Concept of Disease Causation and the Emergence of Specific Causes in Nineteenth Century Medicine', *BHM*, 65: 528–48.

Cartwright, F. F. 1963. *Joseph Lister, the Man who made Surgery Safe*, London, Weidenfeld and Nicolson.

Cartwright, F. F. 1967. *The Development of Modern Surgery*, London, Arthur Barker.

Chick, H. et al. 1971. *War On Disease: A History of the Lister Institute*, London, André Deutsch.

Churchill, E. D. 1965. 'The Pandemic of Wound Infection in Hospitals', *JHM*, 1965, 19: 390–414.

Clarke, A. E. and Fujimura, J. H., eds. 1992. *The Right Tools for the Job: At Work in Twentieth Century Life Sciences*, Princeton, NJ, Princeton University Press.

Coleman, W. 1987. 'Koch's Comma Bacillus: The First Year', *BHM*, 61: 315–42.

Collard, P. 1976. *The Development of Microbiology*, Cambridge, Cambridge University Press.

Crellin, J. K. 1965. *Spontaneous Generation and the Germ Theory (1860–1880): The Controversy in Britain and the Work of F. Crace Calvert*, MSc dissertation, University of London.

Crellin, J. K. 1965. 'The Disinfectant Studies of Frederick Crace Calvert', *Die Vortrage der Hauptversammlung der Internationalen Gesellschaft fuer Gemeinchte der Pharmacie*, Stuttgart, 61–7.

Crellin, J. K. 1966. 'The Dawn of Germ Theory: Particles, Infection and Biology', Poynter, *Medicine and Science*, 57–76.

Cunningham, A. and Williams, P., eds. 1992. *The Laboratory Revolution in Medicine*, Cambridge, Cambridge University Press.

D'Arcy Thompson, R. 1974. *The Remarkable Gamgees: a Story of Achievement*, Edinburgh, Ramsey Head.

de Kruif, P. 1926. *The Microbe Hunters*, London, Jonathan Cape.

Debré, P. 1998. *Louis Pasteur*, Baltimore, MD, Johns Hopkins University Press.

Digby, A. 1994. *Making a Medical Living: Doctors and Patients in the English Market for Medicine, 1720–1911*, Cambridge, Cambridge University Press.

Dowling, H. W. 1977. *Fighting Infection: Conquests of the Twentieth Century*, Cambridge, MA, Harvard University Press.

Dubos, R. 1960. *Pasteur and Modern Science*, New York, Anchor Books.

Dubos, R. and J. 1952. *The White Plague: Tuberculosis, Man and Society*, Boston, MA, Little Brown and Co.

Dukes, C. 1924. *Lord Lister, 1827–1912*, London, Leonard Parsons.

Eyler, J. M. 1979. *Victorian Social Medicine: The Ideas and Methods of William Farr*, Baltimore, MD, Johns Hopkins University Press.

Eyler, J. M. 1980. 'The Conversion of Angus Smith: The Changing Role of Chemistry and Biology in Sanitary Science, 1850–1880', *BHM*, 54: 216–34.

Eyler, J. M. 1987. 'Scarlet Fever and Confinement: The Edwardian Debate over Isolation Hospitals', *BHM*, 61: 1–24.

Eyler, J. M. 1997. *Sir Arthur Newsholme and State Medicine, 1885–1935*, Cambridge, Cambridge University Press.

Farley, J. 1977. *The Spontaneous Generation Controversy from Descartes to Oparin*, Baltimore, MD, Johns Hopkins University Press.

Farley, J. 1992. 'Parasites and the Germ Theory of Disease', in C. E. Rosenberg, J. Golden, eds., *Framing Disease; Studies in Cultural History*, New Brunswick, NJ, Rutger University Press, 33–49.

Fee, E. and Acheson, R., eds. 1991. *A History of Education in Public Health: Health that Mocks the Doctors' Rules*, Oxford. Oxford Medical Publication.

Feldberg, G. 1996. *Disease and Social Class: Tuberculosis and the Shaping of North American Society*, New Brunswick, NJ, Rutgers University Press.

Fisher, J. R. 1979. 'Professor Gamgee and the Farmers', *Veterinary History*, 1 (2): 50.

310   *Select Bibliography*

Fisher, J. R. 1993. 'British Physicians, Medical Science, and the Cattle Plague, 1865–88', *BHM*, 67: 651–69.

Fisher, R. B. 1977. *Joseph Lister, 1827–1912*, New York: Stein and Day.

Fleck, L. 1935. *Genesis and Development of a Scientific Fact*, Chicago, Chicago University Pressrep. 1979.

Foster, W. D. 1961. *A Short History of Clinical Pathology*, Edinburgh, E. & S. Livingstone.

Foster, W. D. 1970. *A History of Medical Bacteriology and Immunology*, London, Heinemann.

Fox, N. J. 1988. 'Scientific Theory Choice and Social Structure: The Case of Joseph Lister's Antisepsis, Humoral Theory and Asepsis', *History of Science*, 1988, 26: 367–97.

Fraser, S. M. F. 1980. 'Leicester and Smallpox: The Leicester Method', *MH*, 24: 315–32.

Frazer, W. M. 1950. *A History of English Public Health, 1834–39*, London, Baillière, Tindall and Cox.

French, R. D. 1975. *Antivivisection and Medical Science in Victorian England*, Princeton, NJ, Princeton University Press.

Geison, G. L. 1974. 'Louis Pasteur', in C. C. Gillespie, ed. *The Dictionary of Scientific Biography*, New York, Charles Scribner, 350–416.

Geison, G. L. 1978. *Michael Foster and the Cambridge School of Physiology*, Princeton, NJ, Princeton University Press.

Geison, G. L. 1995. *The Private Science of Louis Pasteur*, Princeton, NJ, Princeton University Press.

Gillispie, C. C., ed. 1974. *Dictionary of Scientific Biography*, New York, Charles Scribner's Sons.

Godlee, R. J. 1924. *Lord Lister*, Oxford: Clarendon Press.

Golinski, J. 1998. *Making Natural Knowledge: Constructivism and the History of Science*, Cambridge, Cambridge University Press.

Gossel, P. 1992. 'A Need for Standard Methods: The Case of American Bacteriology', in A. E. Clarke and J. H. Fujimura, ed., *The Right Tools for the Job: At Work in Twentieth Century Life Sciences*, Princeton, NJ, Princeton University Press, 287–309.

Granshaw, L. 1992. '"Upon this principle I have based a practice": The Development of Antisepsis in Britain, 1867–90', in J. V. Pickstone, ed., *Medical Innovation in Historical Perspective*, London, Macmillan, 17–46.

Grosöschel, D. H. M. and Hornick, R. B. 1981. 'Who Introduced Typhoid Vaccination: Almroth Wright or Richard Pfeiffer', *Reviews of Infectious Diseases*, 3: 1251–4.

Hamilton, D. J. 1982. 'The Nineteenth Century Surgical Revolution – Antisepsis or Better Nutrition?', *BHM*, 56: 30–40.

Hamlin, C. 1985. 'Providence and Putrefaction: Victorian Sanitarians and the Natural Theology of Health and Disease', *Victorian Studies*, 28: 381–411.

Hamlin, C. 1988. 'Muddling in Bumbledon: Local Governments and Large Sanitary Improvements: The Cases of Four British Towns, 1855–1885', *Victorian Studies*, 32: 55–83.

Hamlin, C. 1988. 'Politics and Germ Theories in Victorian Britain: The Metropolitan Water Commissions of 1867–9 and 1892–3', in R. MacLeod, ed., *Expertise and Government: Specialists, Administrators and Professionals, 1860–1919*, Cambridge, Cambridge University Press, 111–23.

Hamlin, C. 1990. *A Science of Impurity: Water Analysis in Nineteenth Century England*, Bristol, Adam Hilger.

Hamlin, C. 1992. 'Predisposing Causes and Public Health in Early Nineteenth Century Medical Thought', *SHM*, 5: 43–70.

Hamlin, C. 1998. *Public Health and Social Justice in the Age of Chadwick: Britain, 1800–54*, Cambridge, Cambridge University Press.

Hardy, A. 1983. 'Smallpox in London: Factors in the Decline of the Disease in the Nineteenth Century', *MH*, 27: 111–38.

Hardy, A. 1993. 'Cholera, Quarantine and the English Preventive System, 1850–1895', *MH*, 37: 252–69.

Hardy, A. 1993. *Epidemic Streets: Infectious Disease and the Rise of Preventive Medicine, 1856–1900*, Oxford, Clarendon Press.

Hardy, A. 1998. 'On the Cusp: Epidemiology and Bacteriology at the Local Government Board, 1890–1905', *MH*, 42: 328–46.

Harrison, M. 1994. *Public Health in British India: Anglo-Indian Preventive Medicine, 1859–1914*, Cambridge, Cambridge University Press.

Howard-Jones, N. 1975. *The Scientific Background to the International Sanitary Conferences, 1851–1938*, Geneva, WHO.

Hughes, S. 1977. *The Virus: A History of a Concept*, New York: Science History.

Isaacs, J. D. 1998. 'D. D. Cunningham and the Aetiology of Cholera in British India, 1869–1897', *MH*, 42: 279–305.

Kewesbury, E. C. O. 1936. *The Life and Work of C. B. Lockwood, 1856–1914*, London, H. K. Lewis.

Jewson, N. D. 1978. 'The Disappearance of the Sickman from Medical Cosmology, 1770–1870', *Sociology*, 10: 225–44.

Kawaita, Y. et al., eds. 1990. *History of Therapy: Proceedings of the Tenth International Symposium of Comparative Medicine: East and West*, Tokyo, Ishiyaku EuroAmerica Inc.

Kraut, A. M. 1994. *Silent Travelers: Germs, Genes, and the 'Immigrant Menace'*, New York, Basic Books.

Lambert, R. 1963. *Sir John Simon 1816–1904 and English Social Administration*, London, MacGibbon and Kee.

Lansbury, C. 1985. *The Old Brown Dog: Women, Workers and Vivisection in Edwardian England*, Madison, WI, University of Wisconsin Press.

Latour, B. 1988. *The Pasteurization of France*, Cambridge, MA, Harvard University Press.

Lawrence, C. 1980. 'Sanitary reformers and the medical profession in Victorian England', Ogawa, T., ed., *Public Health: Proceedings of the Fifth International Symposium on Comparative History of Medicine: East and West*, Tokyo, Saikon, 145–68.

Lawrence, C. 1985. ' "Incommunicable Knowledge": Science, Technology and the Clinical "Art" in Britain, 1850–1910', *Journal of Contemporary History*, 20: 503–20.

Lawrence, C. 1992. 'Democratic, Divine and Heroic: The History and Historiography of Surgery', in Lawrence, *Medical Theory*, 1–47.

Lawrence, C. and Dixey, R. 1992. 'Practising on Principle: Joseph Lister and the germ theories of disease', in C. Lawrence, ed., *Medical Theory: Surgical Practice*, London, Routledge, 153–215.

Lawrence, C., ed. 1992. *Medical Theory, Surgical Practice*, London, Routledge.

Lawrence, C. 1994. *Medicine and the Making of Modern Britain, 1700–1920*, London, Macmillan.

Leavitt, J. W. 1996. *Typhoid Mary: Captive to the Public's Health*, Boston, Beacon Press.

Lechevalier, H. A. and Solotorovsky, M. 1965. *Three Centuries of Microbiology*, New York, McGraw Hill.

Loudon, I. S. L. 1995. *Childbed Fever: A Documentary History*, London, Garland.

Luckin, W. 1977. 'The Final Catastrophe: Cholera in London, 1866', *MH*, 21: 32–42.

MacLeod, R. 1967. 'Law, Medicine and Public Opinion: The Resistance to Compulsory Health Legislation, 1870–1907: Part II', *Public Opinion*, 189–207.

MacLeod, R. 1967. 'The Frustrations of State Medicine, 1880–1899', *MH*, 11: 15–40.

MacNalty, A. S. 1950. *A Biography of Sir Benjamin Ward Richardson*, London, Harvey and Blythe.

Maulitz, R. 1978. 'Rudolf Virchow, Julius Cohnheim and the Programme of Pathology', *BHM*, 52: 162–82.

Maulitz, R. 1979. '"Physician versus Bacteriologist": The Ideology of Science in Clinical Medicine', in M. J. Vogel and C. E. Rosenberg, eds., *The Therapeutic Revolution: Essays in the Social History of American Medicine*, Philadelphia, University of Pennsylvania Press, 99–108.

Maulitz, R. C. 1987. *Morbid Appearances: The Anatomy of Pathology in the Early Nineteenth Century*, Cambridge, Cambridge University Press.

Mazumdar, P. H. 1972. 'Immunity in 1890', *JHM*, 27: 312–24.

McGrew, R. E. 1985. *Encyclopaedia of Medical History*, London, Macmillan.

McKeown, T. 1976. *The Rise of Modern Population*, London, Edward Arnold.

McTavish, J. R. 1987. 'Antipyretic treatment and typhoid fever', *JHM*, 42: 486–500.

Mendelsohn, J. A. 1996. *Cultures of Bacteriology: Foundation and Transformation of a Science in France and Germany, 1870–1914*, Unpublished PhD thesis, Princeton University.

Ministry of Agriculture Fisheries and Food. 1965. *Animal Health: A Centenary, 1865–1965*, London, HMSO.

Morantz, R. 1982. 'Feminism, Professionalism and Germs: The Thought of Mary Putnam Jacobi and Elisabeth Blackwell', *American Studies*, 34: 459–78.

Parish, H. J. 1965. *A History of Immunization*, Edinburgh, E. & S. Livingstone.

Parish, H. J. 1965. *Victory with Vaccines*, Edinburgh, E. & S. Livingstone.

Parsons, G. P. 1978. 'The British Medical Profession and Contagion Theory: Puerperal Fever as a Case-Study', *MH*, 22: 138–50.

Pattison, I. 1981. *John McFadyean: A Great British Veterinarian*, London, J. A. Allan.

Pattison, I. 1983. *The British Veterinary Profession, 1791–1948*, London, J. A. Allen.

Pelling, M. 1978. *Cholera, Fever and English Medicine, 1825–65*, Oxford, Oxford University Press.

Pelling, M. 1993. 'Contagion/Germ Theory/Specificity', in W. F. Bynum and R. Porter, eds., *Companion Encyclopaedia of the History of Medicine*, London. Routledge, 309–34.

Pennington, H. 1994. 'Osteotomy as an Indicator of Antiseptic Surgical Practice', *MH*, 38: 178–88.

Pennington, H. 1995. 'Listerism, its Decline and Persistence: The Introduction of Aseptic Surgical Techniques in Three British Teaching Hospitals', *MH*, 39: 39–47.

Peterson, J. M. 1978. *The Medical Profession in Mid-Victorian London*, Berkeley, University of California Press.

Pickstone, J. V. 1985. *Medicine in an Industrial Society: A History of Hospital Development in Manchester and its Region, 1752–1946*, Manchester, Manchester University Press, 191–3.

Pickstone, J. V. 1993. 'Ways of Knowing: Towards a Historical Sociology of Science', *BJHS*, 26: 433–58.

Pickstone, J. V., ed. 1992. *Medical Innovation in Historical Perspective*, London, Macmillan.

Porter, D. 1991. ' "Enemies of the Race": Biologism, Environmentalism and Public health in Edwardian Britain', *Victorian Studies*, 34: 160–78.

Porter, D. 1991. 'Stratification and its Discontents: Professionalisation and Conflict in the British Public Health service, 1848–1944', in Fee and Acheson, *A History of Education in Public Health: Health that Mocks the Doctors' Rubs*, Oxford, Oxford Medical Publication, 83–113.

Porter, D. 1994. *The History of Public Health and the Modern State*, Amsterdam, Rodopi.

Porter, D. and Porter, R. 1988. 'The Politics of Prevention: Anti-vaccinationist and Public Health in Nineteenth Century England', *MH*, 32: 231–52.

Porter, D. 1999. *Health, Civilisation and the State: A History of Public Health from Ancient to Modern Times*, London, Routledge.

Poynter, F. N. L., ed. 1968. *Medicine and Science in the 1860s*, London, Wellcome Institute for the History of Medicine.

Rang, M. 1954. *The Life and Work of Henry Charlton Bastian, 1835–1915*, London, UCH Medical School Library.

Reid, R. 1974. *Microbes and Men*, London, BBC.

Reiser, S. J. 1978. *Medicine and the Reign of Technology*, Cambridge, Cambridge University Press.

Richmond, P. A. 1954. 'Some Variant Theories in Opposition to the Germ Theory of Disease', *JHM*, 9: 290–303.

Richmond, P. A. 1980. 'The Germ Theory of Disease', in A. M. Lilienthal, ed., *Times, Places and Persons: Aspects of the History of Epidemiology*, Baltimore, MD, Johns Hopkins University Press, 84–93.

Rogers, N. 1992. *Dirt and Disease: Polio Before FDR*, New Brunswick, NJ, Rutgers University Press.

Romano, T. M. 1993. *Making Medicine Scientific: John Burdon Sanderson and the Culture of Victorian Science*, Unpublished PhD Thesis, Yale University.

Romano, T. M. 1997. 'The Cattle Plague of 1865 and the Reception of "Germ Theory" in Mid-Victorian Britain', *JHM*, 52: 51–80.

Rosen, G. 1958. *A History of Public Health*, Baltimore, MD, Johns Hopkins University Press, 1993 edn.

Rosenberg, C. E. 1962. *The Cholera Years: The United States in 1832, 1849 and 1866*, Chicago, Chicago University Press.

Rosenberg, C. E. 1979. 'Florence Nightingale on Contagion: The Hospital as Moral Universe', in C. E. Rosenberg, ed., *Healing and History: Essay for George Rosen*, New York, SHP, 116–36.

Rosenberg, C. E. 1987. *The Care of Strangers*, Baltimore, MD, Johns Hopkins University Press.

Rosenberg, C. E. 1992. *Explaining Epidemics and Other Studies in the History of Medicine*, Cambridge, Cambridge University Press.

Rosenberg, C. E. and Golden, J. 1992. *Framing Disease: Studies in Cultural History*, New Brunswick, NJ, Rutgers University Press.

Rosenberg, C. E., ed. 1979. *Healing and History: Essays for George Rosen*, New York, SHP.

Rosenkrantz, B. G. 1986. 'Koch's Bacillus: Was there a technological fix?', in Ullman-Margalit, E., ed., *The Prism of Science*, Dordrecht, Reidel, 147–60.

Salomen-Bayet, C. and Lécuyer, B. 1986. *Pasteur et la Revolution pastorienne*, Paris, Payot.

Schaffer, S. 1991. 'The Eighteenth Brumaire of Bruno Latour', *Studies in the History and Philosophy of Science*, 22: 174–92.

Shortt, S. E. D. 1983. 'Physicians, Science and Status: Issues in the Professionalisation of Anglo-American Medicine in the Nineteenth Century', *MH*, 27: 51–68.

Shryock, R. H. 1972. 'Germ Theories in Medicine Prior to 1870: Further Comments on Continuity in Science', *Clio Medica*, 7: 81–109.

Shryock, R. H. 1936. *The Development of Modern Medicine: An Interpretation of the Social and Scientific Factors Involved*, Madison, WI, University of Wisconsin Press.

Sigsworth, M. and Worboys, M. 1994. 'The Public's View of Public Health in Mid-Victorian Britain', *Urban History*, 21: 237–50.

Silverstein, A. M. 1989. *A History of Immunology*, San Diego, CA, Academic Press.

Smith, F. B. 1988. *The Retreat of Tuberculosis*, London, Croom Helm.

Stevenson, L. G. 1955. 'Science Down the Drain: On the Hostility of Certain Sanitarians to Animal Experimentation, Bacteriology and Immunology', *BHM*, 29: 1–26.

Stevenson, L. G. 1980. 'Antibacterial and Antibiotic Concepts in Early Bacteriological Studies and in Ehrlich's Chemotherapy', in J. Pascandola, ed., *A History of Antibiotics*, Madison, WI, University of Wisconsin Press, pp. 43–50.

Stevenson, L. G. 1982. 'Exemplary Disease: The Typhoid Pattern', *JHM*, 37: 159–81.

Spink, W. W. 1978. *Infectious Diseases: Prevention and Treatment in the Nineteenth and Twentieth Centuries*, Minneapolis, MN, University of Minnesota Press.

Strick, J. E. 1997. *The British Spontaneous Generation Debates of 1860–1880: Medicine, Evolution and Laboratory Science in the Victorian Context*, Unpublished PhD thesis, Princeton University.

Sturdy, S. 1991. 'The Germs of a New Enlightenment', *Studies in the History and Philosophy of Science*, 22, 163–73.

Sutphen, M. P. 1997. 'Not What, But Where: Bubonic Plague and the Reception of Germ Theories in Hong Kong and Calcutta, 1894–97', *JHM*, 52: 81–113.

Szreter, S. 1988. 'The Importance of Social Intervention in Britain's Mortality Decline, c. 1850–1914: A Reinterpretation of the Role of Public Health', *SHM*, 1: 1–38.

Tansey, E. M. 1989. 'The Wellcome Physiological Research Laboratories, 1894–1904: The Home Office, Pharmaceutical Firms and Animal Experiments', *MH*, 33: 1–41.

Temkin, O. 1977. 'Health and Disease', in O. Temkin, *The Double Face of Janus and Other Essays in the History of Medicine*, Baltimore, MD, Johns Hopkins University Press, 436–8.

Tigertt, W. D. 1980. 'Anthrax: William Smith Greenfield, MD, FRCP, Professor Superintendent, The Brown Animal Sanatory Institute', *Journal of Hygiene*, 85: 415.

Tomes, N. 1997. 'American Attitudes Tward the Germ Theory of Disease: Phyllis Allen Richmond Revisited', *JHM*, 52: 17–50.

Tomes, N. 1998. *The Gospel of Germs: Men, Women and the Microbe in American Life*, Cambridge, MA, Harvard University Press.

Tomes, N. and Warner, J. H. 1997. 'Introduction to Special Issue on Rethinking the Reception of Germ Theory of Disease: Comparative Perspective', *JHM*, 52: 1–18.

Vernon, K. 1990. 'Pus, Sewage, Beer and Milk: Microbiology in Britain, 1870–1940', *History of Science*, 28: 289–325.

Vogel, M. J. and Rosenberg, C. E., eds. 1979. *The Therapeutic Revolution: Essays in the Social History of American Medicine*, Philadelphia, PA, University of Pennsylvania Press.

Warner, J. H. 1980. 'Physiological Theory and Therapeutic Explanation in the 1860s: The British Debate on the Medical Uses of Alcohol', *BHM*, 54: 253–57.

Warner, J. H. 1983. 'Science in Medicine', *Osiris*, 1: 37–85.

Warner, J. H. 1986. *The Therapeutic Perspective: Medical Practice, Knowledge and Identity in America, 1820–1885*, Princeton, NJ, Princeton University Press, pp. 258–83.

Warner, J. H. 1990. 'From Specificity to Universalism in Medical Therapeutics: Transformation in the Nineteenth Century United States', in Y. Kawaita et al., eds., *History of Therapy: Proceedings of the Tenth International Symposium of Comparative Medicine: East and West*, Tokyo, Ishiyaku EuroAmerica Inc., 193–223.

Warner, J. H. 1991. 'Ideals of Science and Their Discontents in Late Nineteenth Century American Medicine', *Isis*, 82: 454–78.

Waterson, A. P. and Wilkinson, L. 1978. *An Introduction to the History of Virology*, Cambridge, Cambridge University Press.

Watkins, D. E. 1984. *The English Revolution in Social Medicine, 1889–1911*, Unpublished PhD thesis, University of London.

Wilkinson, L. 1992. *Animals and Disease: An Introduction to the History of Comparative Medicine*, Cambridge, Cambridge University Press.

Wilkinson, L. 1993. 'Zoonoses and the Development of Concepts of Contagion and Infection', in A. R. Mitchell, ed., *History of the Healing Professions: Parallels between Veterinary and Human Medicine*, Wallingford, CAB International, 73–90.

Wilson, G. 1979. 'The Brown Animal Sanatory Institute', *Journal of Hygiene*, 83: 155–76, 337–52, 501–21.

Wilson, L. G. 1986. 'The Historical Riddle of Milk-borne Scarlet Fever', *BHM*, 60: 321–42.

Wilson, L. G. 1987. 'The Early Recognition of Streptococci as Causes of Disease', *MH*, 31: 403–13.

Winslow, C. E. A. 1943. *Conquest of Epidemic Disease: A Chapter in the History of Ideas*, Madison, WI, University of Wisconsin Press, rep. 1980.

Wohl, A. S. 1983. *Endangered Lives: Public Health in Victorian Britain*, London, J. M. Dent and Sons.

Worboys, M. 1992. 'The Sanatorium Treatment for Consumption in Britain, 1890–1914', in J. V. Pickstone, ed., *Medical Innovation in Historical Perspective*, London, Macmillan, 47–71.

Worboys, M. 1994. 'From Miasmas to Germs: Malaria, 1850–1879', *Parassitologia*, 36: 61–8.

Worboys, M. 1996. 'Germs, Malaria and the Invention of Mansonian Tropical Medicine: From "Diseases in the Tropics" to "Tropical Disease"', in D. Arnold, ed., *Warm Climates and Western Medicine: The Emergence of Tropical Medicine, 1500–1900*, Amsterdam, Rodopi, pp. 181–208.

Wrench, G. T. 1924. *Lord Lister: His Life and Work*, London, T. Fisher Unwin.

Youngson, A. 1979. *The Scientific Revolution in Victorian Medicine*, London, Croom Helm.

INDEX

Wooldridge, Leonard, 220
Woolsorters' disease, 140
wound management, 74–7, 84, 155–8, 162, 165,
      185–7
   cleanliness, 100, 105–7, 181, 183–4, 186,
      191–2
   dressings. *See* antiseptic surgery
   healing by first intention, 33, 76, 167
   open treatment, 80, 83, 105, 155, 166
   styptic colloid, 85
   See also Listerism
Wright, Almroth, 14, 216, 253, 271, 282–3
   anti-typhoid inoculation, 253, 269
   India Plague Commission, 270–1

Yersin, Alexander, 254

zoonoses, 58, 69
zymes, 34, 37, 114
zymosis, 34, 125
   and fermentation, 34–5, 38, 120–1, 124–5,
      244
   chemical theories of, 128
zymotic diseases, 18, 22, 35, 41, 89, 108–9,
      112, 119, 124–5, 128–31, 148, 154, 177,
      198–9, 203, 234, 236–6, 244, 254,
      291
zymotic theory of disease, 15, 34–42, 52, 54, 78,
      93, 98, 102–4, 114–5, 284

Other titles in the series (*continued from the front of the book*)